MRI in Prostate Cancer

MRI in Prostate Cancer

Guest Editors
Milica Medved
Aritrick Chatterjee

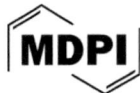 Basel • Beijing • Wuhan • Barcelona • Belgrade • Novi Sad • Cluj • Manchester

Guest Editors

Milica Medved
Department of Radiology
The University of Chicago
Chicago, IL
USA

Aritrick Chatterjee
Department of Radiology
The University of Chicago
Chicago, IL
USA

Editorial Office
MDPI AG
Grosspeteranlage 5
4052 Basel, Switzerland

This is a reprint of the Special Issue, published open access by the journal *Cancers* (ISSN 2072-6694), freely accessible at: https://www.mdpi.com/journal/cancers/special_issues/7PN1RPX5GT.

For citation purposes, cite each article independently as indicated on the article page online and as indicated below:

Lastname, A.A.; Lastname, B.B. Article Title. *Journal Name* **Year**, *Volume Number*, Page Range.

ISBN 978-3-7258-4425-8 (Hbk)
ISBN 978-3-7258-4426-5 (PDF)
https://doi.org/10.3390/books978-3-7258-4426-5

Cover image courtesy of Milica Medved

© 2025 by the authors. Articles in this book are Open Access and distributed under the Creative Commons Attribution (CC BY) license. The book as a whole is distributed by MDPI under the terms and conditions of the Creative Commons Attribution-NonCommercial-NoDerivs (CC BY-NC-ND) license (https://creativecommons.org/licenses/by-nc-nd/4.0/).

Contents

About the Editors vii

Preface ix

Radka Stoyanova, Olmo Zavala-Romero, Deukwoo Kwon, Adrian L. Breto, Isaac R. Xu, Ahmad Algohary, et al.
Clinical-Genomic Risk Group Classification of Suspicious Lesions on Prostate Multiparametric-MRI
Reprinted from: *Cancers* **2023**, *15*, 5240, https://doi.org/10.3390/cancers15215240 1

Juan Morote, Nahuel Paesano, Natàlia Picola, Berta Miró, José M. Abascal, Pol Servian, et al.
Comparing Two Targeted Biopsy Schemes for Detecting Clinically Significant Prostate Cancer in Magnetic Resonance Index Lesions: Two- to Four-Core versus Saturated Transperineal Targeted Biopsy
Reprinted from: *Cancers* **2024**, *16*, 2306, https://doi.org/10.3390/cancers16132306 17

Aritrick Chatterjee, Xiaobing Fan, Jessica Slear, Gregory Asare, Ambereen N. Yousuf, Milica Medved, et al.
Quantitative Multi-Parametric MRI of the Prostate Reveals Racial Differences
Reprinted from: *Cancers* **2024**, *16*, 3499, https://doi.org/10.3390/cancers16203499 27

Kai Zhao, Kaifeng Pang, Alex LingYu Hung, Haoxin Zheng, Ran Yan and Kyunghyun Sung
A Deep Learning-Based Framework for Highly Accelerated Prostate MR Dispersion Imaging
Reprinted from: *Cancers* **2024**, *16*, 2983, https://doi.org/10.3390/cancers16172983 40

Auke Jager, Jorg R. Oddens, Arnoud W. Postema, Razvan L. Miclea, Ivo G. Schoots, Peet G. T. A. Nooijen, et al.
Is There an Added Value of Quantitative DCE-MRI by Magnetic Resonance Dispersion Imaging for Prostate Cancer Diagnosis?
Reprinted from: *Cancers* **2024**, *16*, 2431, https://doi.org/10.3390/cancers16132431 60

Seung Ho Kim, Joo Yeon Kim and Moon Jung Hwang
Magnetic Resonance Elastography for the Detection and Classification of Prostate Cancer
Reprinted from: *Cancers* **2024**, *16*, 3494, https://doi.org/10.3390/cancers16203494 72

Aritrick Chatterjee, Alexander Gallan, Xiaobing Fan, Milica Medved, Pranadeep Akurati, Roger M. Bourne, et al.
Prostate Cancers Invisible on Multiparametric MRI: Pathologic Features in Correlation with Whole-Mount Prostatectomy
Reprinted from: *Cancers* **2023**, *15*, 5825, https://doi.org/10.3390/cancers15245825 83

Andreu Antolin, Nuria Roson, Richard Mast, Javier Arce, Ramon Almodovar, Roger Cortada, et al.
The Role of Radiomics in the Prediction of Clinically Significant Prostate Cancer in the PI-RADS v2 and v2.1 Era: A Systematic Review
Reprinted from: *Cancers* **2024**, *16*, 2951, https://doi.org/10.3390/cancers16172951 99

Dianning He, Haoming Zhuang, Ying Ma, Bixuan Xia, Aritrick Chatterjee, Xiaobing Fan, et al.
A Multiparametric MRI and Baseline-Clinical-Feature-Based Dense Multimodal Fusion Artificial Intelligence (MFAI) Model to Predict Castration-Resistant Prostate Cancer Progression
Reprinted from: *Cancers* **2025**, *17*, 1556, https://doi.org/10.3390/cancers17091556 119

Giulia Nicoletti, Simone Mazzetti, Giovanni Maimone, Valentina Cignini, Renato Cuocolo, Riccardo Faletti, et al.
Development and Validation of an Explainable Radiomics Model to Predict High-Aggressive Prostate Cancer: A Multicenter Radiomics Study Based on Biparametric MRI
Reprinted from: *Cancers* **2024**, *16*, 203, https://doi.org/10.3390/cancers16010203 . . . . **136**

Xiaofeng Qiao, Xiling Gu, Yunfan Liu, Xin Shu, Guangyong Ai, Shuang Qian, et al.
MRI Radiomics-Based Machine Learning Models for Ki67 Expression and Gleason Grade Group Prediction in Prostate Cancer
Reprinted from: *Cancers* **2023**, *15*, 4536, https://doi.org/10.3390/cancers15184536 . . . . **149**

Jade Wang, Elisabeth O'Dwyer, Juana Martinez Zuloaga, Kritika Subramanian, Jim C. Hu, Yuliya S. Jhanwar, et al.
Reasons for Discordance between ^{68}Ga-PSMA-PET and Magnetic Resonance Imaging in Men with Metastatic Prostate Cancer
Reprinted from: *Cancers* **2024**, *16*, 2056, https://doi.org/10.3390/cancers16112056 . . . . **164**

About the Editors

Milica Medved

Milica Medved, PhD DABMP, is a Research Associate Professor at the University of Chicago's Department of Radiology, where she also serves as a Technical Director at the MRI Research Center. She is a Certified Medical Physicist with 26 years of experience in clinical MRI research, primarily in breast and prostate cancer imaging. She has particular expertise in quantitative MRI methods, with a long and successful track record of applying the principles of MRI physics to breast and prostate cancer screening, as well as to other applications such as treatment monitoring. She has extensive experience with dynamic contrast-enhanced MRI, as well as with diffusion imaging- and spectroscopic imaging-based non-contrast MRI methods.

Aritrick Chatterjee

Aritrick Chatterjee is a Research Associate Professor at the Department of Radiology, University of Chicago. His research focuses on the improved diagnosis of prostate cancer using MRI, including the development of new MRI acquisition, analysis and interpretation methods to provide reliable information such as cancer localization, volume, and aggressiveness for deciding optimal treatment options and validating these methods with radiologic–pathologic correlation. He has expertise in developing microstructural imaging techniques and creating MR Virtual Pathology by estimating tissue composition non-invasively using Hybrid Multidimensional MRI and developing risk analysis tools that can effectively detect prostate cancer. His work also focuses on predicting and monitoring response to therapy, quantitative analysis of diffusion imaging, dynamic contrast-enhanced MRI, and artificial intelligence. He has received several grants, including from the NIH, the RSNA and industry.

Preface

This Special Issue focuses on the use of MRI in diagnosing and managing prostate cancer. Prostate cancer is one of the most common types of cancer in men, and it is estimated that one in nine men will be diagnosed with it in their lifetime, representing a major public health concern. While technical developments are ongoing, magnetic resonance imaging (MRI) has increasingly been used to diagnose and monitor prostate cancer. This Special Issue also covers a range of topics, such as the use of MRI for prostate cancer screening, technical developments in MRI sequences and post-processing methods, the relationship of MRI metrics with prostate cancer biology, and the role of radiomics in diagnosing prostate cancer. This Special Issue provides an invaluable resource for researchers, clinicians, and patients interested in the use of MRI in diagnosing and managing prostate cancer.

Milica Medved and Aritrick Chatterjee
Guest Editors

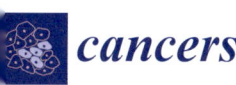

Article

Clinical-Genomic Risk Group Classification of Suspicious Lesions on Prostate Multiparametric-MRI

Radka Stoyanova [1,2,*], Olmo Zavala-Romero [1,†], Deukwoo Kwon [2,3], Adrian L. Breto [1], Isaac R. Xu [1], Ahmad Algohary [1], Mohammad Alhusseini [1], Sandra M. Gaston [1,2], Patricia Castillo [4], Oleksandr N. Kryvenko [1,2,5,6], Elai Davicioni [7], Bruno Nahar [2,6], Benjamin Spieler [1,2], Matthew C. Abramowitz [1,2], Alan Dal Pra [1,2], Dipen J. Parekh [2,6], Sanoj Punnen [2,6] and Alan Pollack [1,2]

1. Department of Radiation Oncology, University of Miami Miller School of Medicine, Miami, FL 33136, USA
2. Sylvester Comprehensive Cancer Center, University of Miami, Miami, FL 33136, USA
3. Department of Public Health Sciences, University of Miami Miller School of Medicine, Miami, FL 33136, USA
4. Department of Radiology, University of Miami Miller School of Medicine, Miami, FL 33136, USA
5. Department of Pathology and Laboratory Medicine, University of Miami Miller School of Medicine, Miami, FL 33136, USA
6. Desai Sethi Urology Institute, University of Miami Miller School of Medicine, Miami, FL 33136, USA
7. Research and Development, Veracyte Inc., San Francisco, CA 94080, USA
* Correspondence: rstoyanova@med.miami.edu
† Current address: Department of Scientific Computing, Florida State University, Tallahassee, FL 32306, USA.

Simple Summary: In this study, we built clinical- and radiomics-based models to predict lesions/patients at low risk based on a combined clinical-genomic classification system. Eighty-three multi-parametric MRI exams from 78 men were analyzed. Several models for lesion classification were built using a minimal clinical variables subset and radiomic features from the lesion and normal tissues. The models were also evaluated for patient classification. In all cases, the radiomic features improved the performance. To the best of our knowledge, this is the first study to demonstrate that machine learning radiomics-based models can predict patients' risk using combined clinical-genomic classification.

Abstract: The utilization of multi-parametric MRI (mpMRI) in clinical decisions regarding prostate cancer patients' management has recently increased. After biopsy, clinicians can assess risk using National Comprehensive Cancer Network (NCCN) risk stratification schema and commercially available genomic classifiers, such as Decipher. We built radiomics-based models to predict lesions/patients at low risk prior to biopsy based on an established three-tier clinical-genomic classification system. Radiomic features were extracted from regions of positive biopsies and Normally Appearing Tissues (NAT) on T2-weighted and Diffusion-weighted Imaging. Using only clinical information available prior to biopsy, five models for predicting low-risk lesions/patients were evaluated, based on: 1: Clinical variables; 2: Lesion-based radiomic features; 3: Lesion and NAT radiomics; 4: Clinical and lesion-based radiomics; and 5: Clinical, lesion and NAT radiomic features. Eighty-three mpMRI exams from 78 men were analyzed. Models 1 and 2 performed similarly (Area under the receiver operating characteristic curve were 0.835 and 0.838, respectively), but radiomics significantly improved the lesion-based performance of the model in a subset analysis of patients with a negative Digital Rectal Exam (DRE). Adding normal tissue radiomics significantly improved the performance in all cases. Similar patterns were observed on patient-level models. To the best of our knowledge, this is the first study to demonstrate that machine learning radiomics-based models can predict patients' risk using combined clinical-genomic classification.

Keywords: prostate cancer; multiparametric MRI; radiomics; Decipher; clinical-genomic risk classification

1. Introduction

Prostate cancer is the most common cancer in American men. In 2022, more than a quarter of a million men was diagnosed with the disease [1]. Clinical decisions related to the choice of treatment, including active surveillance (AS), are multifactorial and complex. Prostate cancer risk assessment governs these decisions across a spectrum of local-regional diseases, from whether to biopsy to whether to intensify treatment using multimodality therapy. RNA transcript marker-based signatures have rapidly been incorporated into such determinations, along with Gleason Score (GS), now termed Grade Group (GG) [2]. While GG remains the standard of care, there has been a paradigm shift to incorporate transcriptomic signatures into clinical decision making. In particular, patients with GG1-3 cancer may be recommended to have either intensified or de-intensified treatment based on a genomic risk score [3,4].

Prostate needle biopsy carried out under multi-parametric MRI (mpMRI) guidance has gained acceptance as a key component of patient management. From the biopsy tissue, both histopathological and genomic biomarkers are used in clinical management. After prostate biopsy, clinicians have various tools for risk assessment, including the National Comprehensive Cancer Network (NCCN) [5] risk stratification schema. The primary goal of the NCCN risk assessment is to predict biochemical recurrence (BCR) rather than survival outcomes such as distant metastasis (DM). To improve the prediction of adverse events, the NCCN classifications were integrated into a three-tier classification system with a commercially available genomic classifier, Decipher (Veracyte Inc., San Francisco, CA, USA) [6], which was optimized to predict the risk of DM [7]. The resultant clinical-genomic classification system, referred to as the Spratt criteria, stratifies patients into low-, intermediate- and high-risk groups [7].

Active surveillance (AS) has emerged as a safe alternative to immediate treatment in low-risk patients [8–10]. AS has been incorporated into many prostate cancer management guidelines, which reduces the burden of overtreatment. While initially reserved for men with low-risk cancer (GS6 or GG1), there has been an increase in the inclusion of men with low-volume favorable intermediate-risk prostate cancer [11]. However, there is still a concern about missing the window for cure in men with greater than GG2 disease, as emerging data with long follow-up show an increased risk of metastasis [12]. Prostate cancer multifocality and heterogeneity [13] are the Achilles heel of prostate cancer risk stratification, and standard ultrasound template biopsies have proven to have poor Negative Predictive Value (NPV) for the detection of clinically significant prostate cancer [14]. We hypothesize that with improved techniques for tumor identification, targeting for biopsies, and classification using quantitative imaging, good candidates for AS would be reliably identified, including some with GG2 disease. We also hypothesize that patients in the low-risk group by the Spratt criteria will constitute patients who are good candidates for active surveillance. The low-risk classification is defined as either (i) low-risk based on NCCN and low- or intermediate-risk based on Decipher; or (ii) low-or-intermediate NCCN risk group and low Decipher group (Supplementary Figure S1).

The use of mpMRI for the detection and classification of prostate cancer is rapidly evolving due to its growing availability and the efforts in the radiology community to standardize the reporting of suspicious prostate lesions (Prostate Imaging Reporting and Data System (PI-RADS) [15] (current version PI-RADSv.2.1) [16]. Computer-aided diagnosis (CAD) techniques for quantitative mpMRI analysis have also been developed for prostate cancer detection and diagnosis [17–22]. The CAD efforts can be divided into two categories based on the main objectives for the analysis: (i) detection/segmentation of the suspicious lesion; and/or (ii) assessment of the aggressiveness of prostate cancer. The Habitat Risk Score (HRS) approach was developed to automatically identify suspicious lesions on mpMRI of the prostate and score the pixels within these regions by aggressiveness [23]. Advanced quantitative mpMRI features, also referred to as radiomic features, are extracted from the lesion volumes, and these variables are then used to build descriptive and predictive models [23].

In this manuscript, we combine clinical and radiomic features to develop a model to classify lesions and, consequently, patients prior to biopsy as low risk according to the Spratt criteria [7]. We utilize HRS to automatically segment on mpMRI the areas of the prostate biopsy and, using our radiomics pipeline [24], extract quantitative imaging features from the segmented region on multiple mpMRI sequences. Patients are classified as low risk if all mpMRI lesions are classified as low risk. To recreate a realistic scenario, only clinical features available a priori to biopsy are considered. The importance of the approach is that this model will allow non-invasive assessment prior to biopsy for patients who are good candidates for AS and may help delay biopsy or de-escalate surveillance biopsies.

2. Materials and Methods

2.1. Study Population

The study cohort comprised patients participating in two institutionally approved and registered trials: a single-arm active surveillance (AS) trial "MRI-Guided Biopsy Selection of Prostate Cancer Patients for Active Surveillance versus Treatment: The Miami MAST Trial"(ClinicalTrials.gov: NCT02242773) and a phase II randomized clinical trial "MRI-Guided Prostate Boosts Via Initial Lattice Stereotactic vs. Daily Moderately Hypofractionated Radiotherapy (BLaStM)" (ClinicalTrials.gov: NCT02307058). Both trials were approved by the Institutional Review Board at the University of Miami and all patients signed appropriate informed consent for treatment and the analysis of MRI and biopsy tissue for research purposes. Patients in both trials underwent mpMRI followed by MRI-ultrasound (MRI-US) fusion biopsies. Patients also agreed to have their tissue sent to Veracyte Inc. (San Francisco, CA, USA), and their data are included in this research. During the initial phase of the trials between 2014 and 2017, all cancer-positive biopsy cores with larger than 1 mm of cancer were sent to Veracyte for gene expression analysis. In addition, if available, positive cores from the patient's diagnostic biopsy (prior to enrollment in the MAST/BLaStM clinical trials) were also sent.

2.2. Multiparametric-MRI of the Prostate

MRI sequences and sequence parameters were consistent with the recommendations for PI-RADSv2 [16]. The exams consisted of axial T2-weighted (T2W) MRI of the male pelvis, Diffusion-Weighted Imaging (DWI) with the generation of Apparent Diffusion Coefficient (ADC) maps and Dynamic Contrast-Enhanced (DCE)-MRI. mpMRI data was acquired using 3T Discovery MR750 (GE, Waukesha, WI, USA), 3T MR Magnetom Trio, Skyra and 1.5T Symphony (Siemens, Erlangen, Germany) magnets. Acquisition parameters of the individual sequences of mpMRI are given in Supplementary Table S1.

2.3. Workflow for Co-Registration of Genomic and Radiomic Data

The image segmentation and the co-registration of the biopsy/gene expression and radiomics of the lesion are illustrated in Figure 1. Prostate and suspicious-for-cancer regions were outlined in Dynacad 5.1 (InVivo, Gainsville, FL, USA) by radiologists with more than ten years of experience in genitourinary (GU) malignancies using PI-RADSv2. The findings were also confirmed by heatmaps generated by HRS, described in detail in Stoyanova et al. [23]. Briefly, HRS is an approach that automatically assigns a score from 1 to 10 to each pixel in the prostate in an increasing fashion related to tumor aggressiveness. HRS combines quantitative characteristics from the diffusion and perfusion sequences of mpMRI and is displayed as a heat map overlaid on the T2-weighted images. HRS was developed in reference to prostatectomy GS and, in particular, HRS6, i.e., the volume comprised by pixels with HRS = 6, which were concordant with the tumor volumes from radical prostatectomy [23].

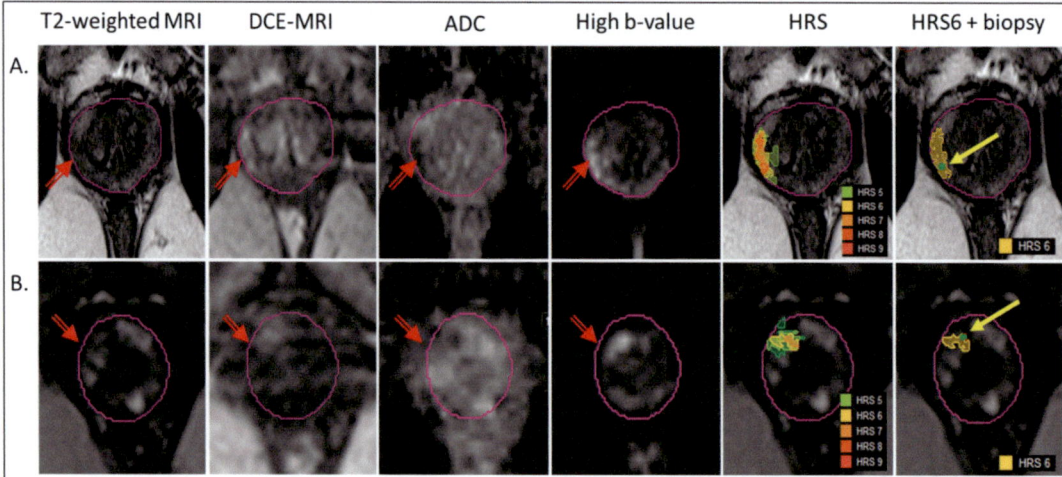

Figure 1. Co-registration of biopsy and segmentation of volumes for radiomics analysis. The radiogenomic pipeline is illustrated in the mpMRI from two patients (**A**,**B**). The lesion is marked with a red arrow on T2-weighted MRI, early enhancing Dynamic Contrast Enhancing (DCE)-MRI, Apparent Diffusion Coefficient (ADC) and High b-value (BVAL) image from the Diffusion-Weighted Imaging (DWI) sequence. Habitat Risk score (HRS) heat maps for HRS $\geq$ 5, associated with the lesion are overlaid on T2-weighted MRI. The last image illustrates the HRS6 volume in yellow, overlapping with the needle track (green dot, yellow arrow).

MRI-US biopsies were carried out in UroNav (InVivo, Gainsville, FL, USA). Tissue from the identified targets was obtained for pathology and gene expression analysis. For patients in BLaStM, only suspicious areas seen on mpMRI were sampled. For patients in MAST, standard template biopsies were also collected.

The biopsy needle track coordinates (beginning and end) were recorded and transferred in MIM 7.2.3 (MIM Software, Cleveland, OH, USA). The tumor Regions of Interest (ROIs) were assigned as the volumes of HRS = 6 coinciding with the individual needle tracks (Figure 1). In cases where the needle tracks were not recorded, the recorded location of the biopsy was used as a guide for selecting the biopsy ROIs. Two regions, representative of the normally appearing tissue peripheral zone PZ (NAPZ) and transition zone TZ (NATZ), were manually selected.

2.4. Normalization of T2W and BVAL Intensities

For normalization of the T2-weighted MRI intensities, a multireference normalization approach was utilized [25]. Using the "Region Growing Utility" in MIM, three reference contours were selected in the gluteus maximus (GM), femoral head, and bladder. The average intensity values from these contours were assigned a fixed reference value. For each patient, a spline function between the average and reference values was fitted. GM was the only anatomical structure that was consistently identified on high b-value images (BVAL) for all patients. BVAL images were normalized by GM.

2.5. Radiomic Analysis

Radiomic features were extracted as described in Kwon et al. [24] using a Java-based plugin in MIM. ROIs intensities (first-order radiomic features) on the three image modalities T2W, ADC and BVAL were characterized using nine histogram descriptors: 10%, 25%, 50%, 75%, 90%, mean, standard deviation, kurtosis, and skewness. Five texture (second-order radiomics) features: energy, entropy, correlation, homogeneity, and contrast, were extracted from T2W, ADC and BVAL using Haralick texture descriptors [26]. The features were calculated using the grey level co-occurrence matrices (GLCM) for each voxel underlying the contoured regions in the image. Voxel-wise texture measures were computed in 3D by sliding a window of size $5 \times 5 \times 5$ across the image region enclosing the tumor volume. Image intensities were rescaled within a 0–255 range within the $5 \times 5 \times 5$ window. The rationale for this local normalization, rather than global volume normalization, is that the objective was to obtain texture estimates in the normal-appearing tissues in addition to the tumor volumes. The GLCM was then computed in 3D using 128 bins in a $5 \times 5 \times 5$ patch centered at each voxel [27]. The texture values for the whole tumor were then summarized using the voxel-wise textures. The nine histogram descriptors described above were calculated for each texture feature. The texture features were computed using C++ and the publicly available Insight ToolKit (ITK 5.2.1) software libraries for imaging (Kitware, Carrboro, NC, USA).

In summary, 162 quantitative imaging variables (Table 1) were analyzed: 3 modalities (T2W, ADC and BVAL) × 6 features (first-order: intensity (int) and second-order: energy (ene), entropy (ent), contrast(con), correlation (cor), and homogeneity (hom)) × 9 descriptors (10%, 25%, 50%, 75%, 90%, mean, standard deviation (SD), kurtosis (Kurt), and skewness (Skew)). In addition, 162 variables were extracted for NAPZ and NATZ, bringing the total analyzed radiomic features to 486. Here, and in the rest of the text, the imaging variables' names are constructed by concatenating the abbreviations of the pertinent ROI (tumor, NATZ or NAPZ), image sequence, radiomics feature, and histogram descriptor (Table 1). For instance, L_ADC_int_50 refers to the 50% of the ADC intensity in the lesion (biopsy ROI).

Table 1. Radiomic variables and the abbreviations used in radiomic variables name-convention *.

ROI	Image Sequence	Radiomics Feature	Histogram Descriptor
Lesion (L)	T2-weighted (t2)	Intensity (int)	10%
Normal Appearing Peripheral Zone (NAPZ)	ADC (adc)	Contrast (con)	25%
Normal Appearing Transition Zone (NATZ)	High b-value (b)	Correlation (cor)	50%
		Energy (ene)	75%
		Entropy (ent)	90%
		Homogeneity (hom)	mean
			standard deviation (SD)
			kurtosis (Kurt)
			skewness (Skew)

Abbreviations: ROI = Region of Interest; ADC = Apparent Diffusion Coefficient. * Variable names are the concatenation of ROI, image sequence, radiomics feature and histogram descriptor for that feature. For example, the lesions' ROI 90% energy texture on ADC will be L_adc_ene_90. Alternatively, NATZ_t2_cor_50 refers to the 50% of the correlation texture variable in NATZ on T2W MRI.

2.6. Genomic Analysis

Tissue microdissection, RNA extraction, and amplification and microarray hybridization were performed in a Clinical Laboratory Improvement Amendments (CLIA)-certified laboratory facility, as described previously in [28]. Amplified products were fragmented and labeled using the Encore Biotin Module (NuGen, San Carlos, CA, USA) and hybridized to Human Exon 1.0 ST GeneChips (Affymetrix, Santa Clara, CA, USA). The Decipher Score is a 22-gene fixed signature or algorithm that ranges from 0.0 to 1.0, with higher scores related to an increased risk of prostate cancer metastasis. The test uses 0.45 and 0.6 as cutoff points to differentiate between low- versus intermediate- and intermediate- versus high-risk, respectively [29].

2.7. Calculation of Spratt Score

The Spratt clinical-genomic risk score is calculated by assigning a numeric value of 0, 1, 2 and 3 to the low, favorable intermediate, unfavorable intermediate, and high/very high NCCN risk groups, respectively [7], and a numeric value of 0, 1, or 2 to the low, intermediate, and high risk Decipher genomic classifier, respectively, and then adding these two values to obtain a clinical-genomic risk group (see Supplemental Figure S1). The Spratt

Score can be reported as either a six-tier or a three-tier risk stratification, with higher scores indicating higher risk.

2.8. Modeling and Statistical Analysis

To evaluate the contribution of radiomic variables to the predictive value of the clinical variables, we evaluated five models for predicting low-risk lesions/patients as defined by Spratt's criteria (Supplementary Figure S1). In Figure 2, the derivation of the outcome labels, model input variables and development, and the concept of future use are presented. The following models were generated:

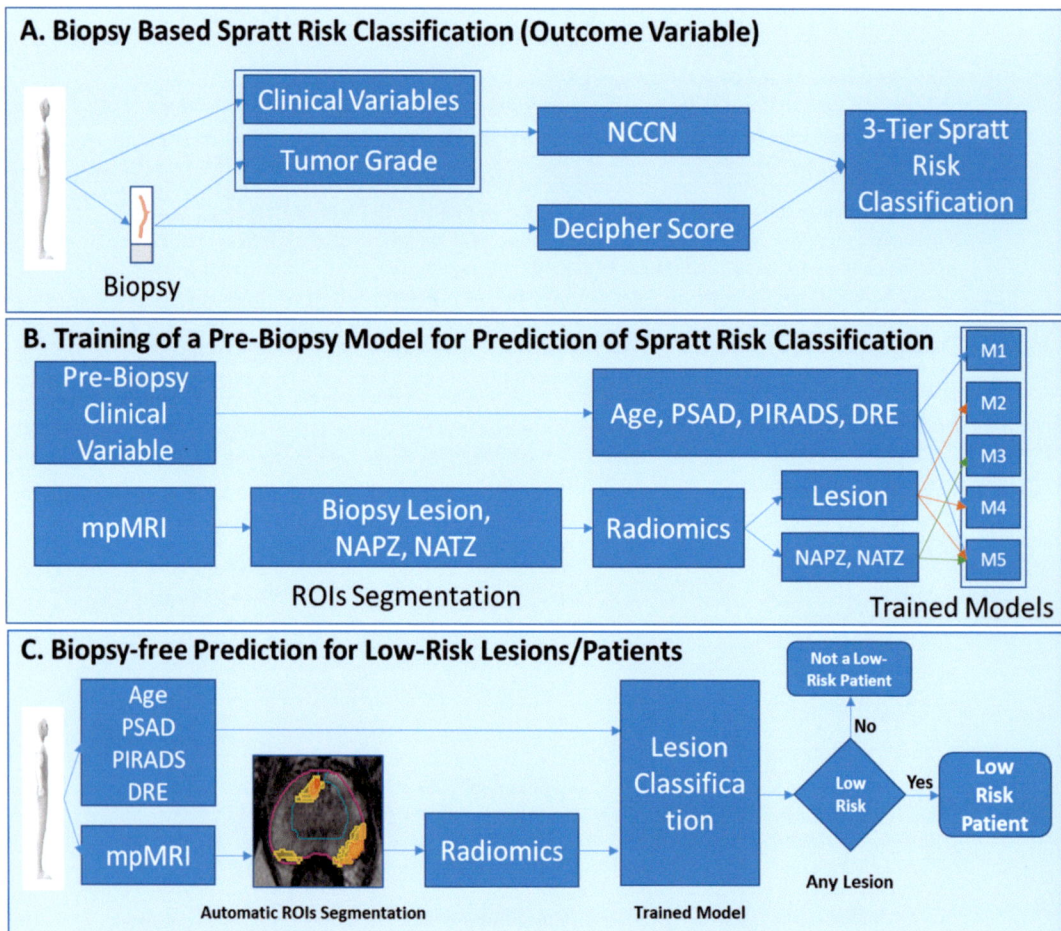

Figure 2. Modeling and analysis design. (**A**) Each biopsy is labeled using the Spratt criteria; (**B**) Five different models are trained, using the Spratt criteria's classification from (**A**) to predict low-risk disease. The input parameters to the models are minimal clinical variables subset and radiomic features from the lesion, NAPZ and NATZ; (**C**) The developed models will be used to classify patients at low risk. Abbreviations: NCCN = National Comprehensive Cancer Network; NAPZ = normally appearing peripheral zone; NATZ = normally appearing transition zone; ROI = Region of Interest; PSA = Prostate Specific Antigen, PSAD = PSA density; DRE = digital rectal exam.

Model 1: A clinical model using patient's age, PSA density (PSAD), digital rectal exam (DRE), and PI-RADS for input. Importantly, this model did not incorporate the results of biopsy tissue, as we wanted to simulate a pre-biopsy clinical scenario and limited the variables to the initial prostate exam.

Model 2: Lesion-based radiomics model.
Model 3: Lesion and NAPZ/NATZ radiomics model.
Model 4: A combined clinical and lesion radiomics model.
Model 5: A combined clinical and lesion/NAPZ/NATZ radiomics model.

For Model 1, all pre-biopsy clinical variables were used. For the radiomics models, since imaging data are highly correlated and multi-dimensional, we used a penalized logistic regression model (GLMNET) to select important imaging variables that predict low-risk lesions [30]. Radiomics imaging data were standardized for feature selection. The volume of HRS6 (tumor volume) was added to all radiomics models. The variables were selected based on the adaptive LASSO method. Logistic regression analysis, using all clinical variables for Model 1 and the selected radiomic variables for Model 2 and Model 3, was used to predict low-risk lesions. For patient-level prediction, we selected the lesion with the highest three-tier score and evaluated the models. The performance of the models was also evaluated on a subset of patients that had negative DRE. The rationale for this subgroup analysis was to eliminate patients that most likely are not at low-risk.

The area under the receiver operating characteristic (ROC) curve (AUC) is reported as a performance measure for each trained model. AUC comparison is performed using the Venkatraman and Begg method [31]. For each model, bootstrap-based optimism-corrected AUC was calculated using 1000 runs [32]. Analysis was performed using corresponding R 4.2.3 packages (R Foundation for Statistical Computing, www.R-project.org (accessed on 1 May 2023)).

3. Results

A total of 231 biopsy cores from 78 men were analyzed for this study, with 46 men coming from the MAST active surveillance trial and 32 from the BlaStM primary radiation trial. (Tables 2 and 3). As the patients in MAST were of low risk and in BlaStM of intermediate and high risk, the differences in the T-stage, PSA, DRE, GS/GG, Decipher, and the three-tier risk groups were statistically significant between the patients in the two trials.

A total of 83 mpMRI exams were analyzed. When available, both the diagnostic and protocol biopsies were matched with their corresponding mpMRIs. Thus, for five patients two mpMRI exams were analyzed. A detailed breakdown by MRI instruments is given in Table 2. The majority of the exams were acquired using Discovery, GE (50.6%), and Skyra, Siemens (39.8%) magnets.

In Table 4, the variables used for training each model are shown. All three pre-biopsy clinical variables were used in Model 1. Thirteen variables were selected for Model 2: Lesion Radiomics and 33 for Model 3: Lesion + NAPZ/NATZ Radiomics. The image intensity-based features (first-order radiomic features) were overrepresented (yellow highlight) in the lists of the significant variables; while they are one/sixth of all radiomic features, more than a third of the variables on both lists are related to image-intensities. For the lesion ROI, these variables are related to low T2 (L_t2_int_10) and high BVAL (L_b_int_75). In Supplementary Figure S2, four lesion imaging features used in the models: HRS6, L_t2_int_10, L_adc_int_50 and L_b_int_75 are displayed as box plots of the distribution of these features in low and intermediate/high-risk lesions. HRS6 (a surrogate of tumor volume) and BVAL were significantly higher, and T2 and ADC were significantly lower in intermediate/high risk in comparison with low-risk lesions.

Table 2. Patient characteristics for study cohort organized by the clinical trial.

Variable	TOTAL (N (%))	MAST (N (%))	BLASTM (N (%))	p-Value [a]
Patients	78	46	32	
Age (median, range) years	64.5 (44–82)	64.0 (44–82)	67.5 (44–79)	0.237
Age groups				0.559
≤44 years	2 (2.6)	1 (2.2)	1 (3.1)	
45 to 54 years	7 (9.0)	5 (10.9)	2 (6.3)	
55 to 64 years	30 (38.5)	20 (43.5)	10 (31.3)	
65 to 74 years	31 (39.7)	17 (37.0)	14 (43.8)	
≥75 years	8 (10.3)	3 (6.5)	5 (15.6)	
Race/ethnicity				0.218
Non-Hispanic White	37 (47.4)	25 (54.3)	12 (37.5)	
Non-Hispanic Black	11 (14.1)	6 (13.0)	5 (15.6)	
Hispanic/Latino	28 (35.9)	15 (32.6)	13 (40.6)	
Others	2 (2.6)	0 (0)	2 (6.3)	
PSA, ng/mL, median, range	6 (1.3–77.7)	4.7 (1.3–16.7)	9.7 (1.5–77.7)	0.0004
PSA groups, ng/mL				0.001
<10	57 (73.1)	40 (87.0)	17 (53.1)	
10–20	15 (19.2)	6 (13.0)	9 (21.8)	
>20	6 (7.7)	-	6 (18.8)	
Grade Group				<0.0001
1	40 (51.3)	36 (78.3)	4 (12.5)	
2	15 (19.2)	7 (15.2)	8 (25.0)	
3	10 (12.8)	3 (6.5)	7 (21.9)	
4–5	13 (16.7)	0 (0.0)	13 (40.6)	
T stage				<0.0001
T1	58 (74.4)	46 (100)	12 (37.5)	
T2–T3	20 (25.6)	0 (0)	20 (62.5)	
N of biopsy				0.3748
1	25 (32.1)	16 (34.8)	9 (28.1)	
2	10 (12.8)	7 (15.2)	3 (9.4)	
3	3 (25.6)	13 (28.3)	7 (21.9)	
4	9 (11.5)	5 (10.9)	4 (12.5)	
≥5	14 (17.9)	5 (10.9)	9 (28.1)	
DRE [b]				<0.0001
0	55 (70.5)	46 (100)	9 (28.1)	
1	18 (23.1)	0 (0.0)	18 (56.3)	
2	5 (6.4)	0 (0.0)	5 (15.6)	
PI-RADSv.2.1				0.0002
1–2	28 (35.9)	22 (47.8)	6 (18.8)	
3	8 (10.3)	7 (15.2)	1 (3.1)	
4	23 (29.5)	12 (26.1)	11 (34.3)	
5	19 (24.3)	5 (10.9)	14 (43.8)	
MRI scanner (Vendor)				0.2029
3T Discovery (GE)	42 (50.6)	21 (42.0)	21 (63.6)	
3T Skyra (Siemens)	33 (39.8)	24 (48.0)	9 (27.3)	
3T TimTrio (Siemens)	6 (7.2)	4 (8.0)	2 (6.1)	
1.5T Symphony (Siemens)	2 (2.4)	1 (2.0)	1 (3.0)	

Abbreviations: PSA = Prostate Specific Antigen; DRE = Digital Rectal Exam; T = Tesla. [a] p-values from t-test for continuous variables or Fisher's exact test for categorical variables; [b] DRE categories are: 0 = No palpable abnormality in the prostate or rectum; 1 = Palpable abnormality; 2 = Palpable abnormality, suggestive for extraprostatic extension.

Table 3. Biopsy characteristics for study cohort organized by clinical trial.

Variable	TOTAL (N (%))	MAST (N (%))	BLASTM (N (%))	p-Value [a]
Biopsy N	231	124	107	
Grade Group				<0.0001
1	123 (53.2)	102 (82.3)	21 (19.6)	
2	46 (19.9)	18 (14.5)	28 (26.2)	
3	21 (9.1)	4 (3.2)	17 (15.9)	
4–5	41 (17.7)	-	41 (38.3)	
Biopsy Type				0.656
Diagnostic	75 (32.5)	23 (18.5)	52 (48.6)	
Trial	156 (67.5)	101 (81.5)	55 (51.4)	
Decipher				<0.0001
Low risk	161 (69.7)	114 (91.9)	47 (43.9)	
Intermediate risk	23 (10.0)	7 (5.7)	16 (15.0)	
High Risk	47 (20.3)	3 (2.4)	44 (41.1)	
NCCN				<0.0001
Group 1	90 (39.0)	79 (63.7)	11 (10.3)	
Group 2	48 (20.8)	28 (22.6)	20 (18.7)	
Group 3	41 (17.7)	14 (11.3)	27 (25.2)	
Group 4	52 (22.5)	3 (2.4)	49 (45.8)	
3-tier classification system				<0.0001
Low risk	133 (57.6)	103 (83.1)	30 (28.0)	
Intermediate risk	61 (26.4)	21 (16.9)	40 (37.4)	
High Risk	37 (16.0)	-	37 (34.6)	

Abbreviations: MAST = "MIAMI MRI selection for Active surveillance versus Treatment" Clinical Trial; BlaStM = "MRI-Guided Prostate Boosts Via Initial Lattice Stereotactic versus Daily Moderately Hypo-fractionated Radiotherapy" Phase II clinical Trial. [a] p-values from t-test for continuous variables or Fisher's exact test for categorical variables.

ROC curves and AUCs for the five trained models in all patients and subset analysis for patients with negative DRE (DRE = 0) are shown in Figures 3 and 4. In each figure, the left panel shows the performance of the models on a biopsy level and on the right, it is shown on a patient level. In Figure 3, all lesions were analyzed: 133 low risk vs. 98 intermediate/high risk by the Spratt criteria. Interestingly, the clinical features performed similarly to the lesion radiomics. When the NAPZ/NATZ features were added to the model, there was a significant improvement in the performance, resulting in AUC of 0.95 for the best-performing Model 5. Similar patterns were observed on patient-level models (78 patients: 56 low-risk vs. 22 intermediate/high-risk). When only patients with DRE = 0 were considered, 149 lesions (110 low-risk vs. 39 intermediate/high risk) were analyzed (Figure 4). The prediction based on clinical variables degraded, indicating that positive DRE was a major driver in the performance in the previous models. The addition of the lesion radiomic features both in biopsy- and patient-level (55 patients: 48 low-risk vs. 7 intermediate/high-risk) significantly improved the classification.

Due to the high performance of the intensity's features, we tested the value of using only first-order radiomics by re-creating models Model 1–5. There is a major advantage of using only intensities, assuming that the resultant model is not substantially underperforming relative to the full variable selection. Intensity futures are easy to compute, and they are highly reproducible between groups and software. The results from the intensities-only analysis are given in the Supplement. In Supplemental Table S2, the variables used for training each model are shown. All three clinical variables were used in Model 1. Six variables were selected for Model 2, and three of these variables overlapped with the ones selected in Table 4. In addition, L_t2_int_25 is strongly correlated with L_t2_int_10 (Table 4). Thirteen variables were selected for Model 3 and the lesion features were >50% of the total; from the normal-appearing tissues, only TZ features were selected. ROC curves and AUCs for the five trained models in all patients and subset analysis for patients with negative DRE (DRE = 0) are shown in Supplemental Figures S3 and S4. The overall performance for lesion-classification was in the range of 0.727 to 0.884 and the radiomic models degraded relatively to full-variable selection in all instances. The addition of the radiomic variables to the clinical improved the prediction only in Model 5 in the subset analysis.

Table 4. Variables for the three models for prediction. Variables in yellow are image-intensity related.

Clinical Variables Model 1	Lesion Radiomic Variables Model 2	Lesion/NAPZ/NATZ Radiomic Variables Model 3
Age (continuous)	HRS6 (volume)	HRS6 (volume)
PSAD (continuous)	L_t2_int_10	L_t2_int_10 *
DRE (0 vs. 1–2)	L_adc_int_50	L_adc_int_Ske *
PI-RADS (1–2 vs. 3,4,5)	L_adc_int_Kur	L_adc_con_90 *
	L_adc_int_Ske	L_adc_cor_90
	L_b_int_75	L_adc_ene_25
	L_t2_con_25	L_adc_ene_SD *
	L_adc_con_90	L_b_ene_75
	L_t2_ene_SD	L_b_ent_10
	L_adc_ene_SD	L_t2_hom_90 *
	L_b_ene_25	NATZ_t2_int_SD
	L_b_ene_50	NATZ_t2_int_Ske
	L_adc_ent_10	NATZ_adc_int_90
	L_t2_hom_90	NATZ_b_int_90
		NATZ_b_int_SD
		NATZ_t2_con_SD
		NATZ_adc_con_10
		NATZ_adc_cor_50
		NATZ_t2_ene_SD
		NATZ_b_ene_75
		NATZ_t2_ent_50
		NATZ_b_hom_50
		NAPZ_t2_int_75
		NAPZ_t2_int_Kur
		NAPZ_t2_int_Ske
		NAPZ_b_int_90
		NAPZ_b_int_Kur
		NAPZ_t2_con_75
		NAPZ_adc_con_10
		NAPZ_b_con_10
		NAPZ_t2_cor_50
		NAPZ_adc_cor_25
		NAPZ_adc_ene_75
		NAPZ_t2_ent_90
		NAPZ_b_ent_10
		NAPZ_t2_hom_90
		NAPZ_t2_hom_SD
		NAPZ_b_hom_10
		NAPZ_b_hom_SD

Abbreviations: PSAD = Prostate Specific Antigen density; DRE = Digital Rectal Exam; NAPZ = Normal Appearing Peripheral Zone; NATZ = Normal Appearing Transition Zone; HRS6 = Volume defined by pixels with Habitat Risk Score = 6. * Variables that are on both "Lesion" and "Lesion and NAPZ/NATZ" lists.

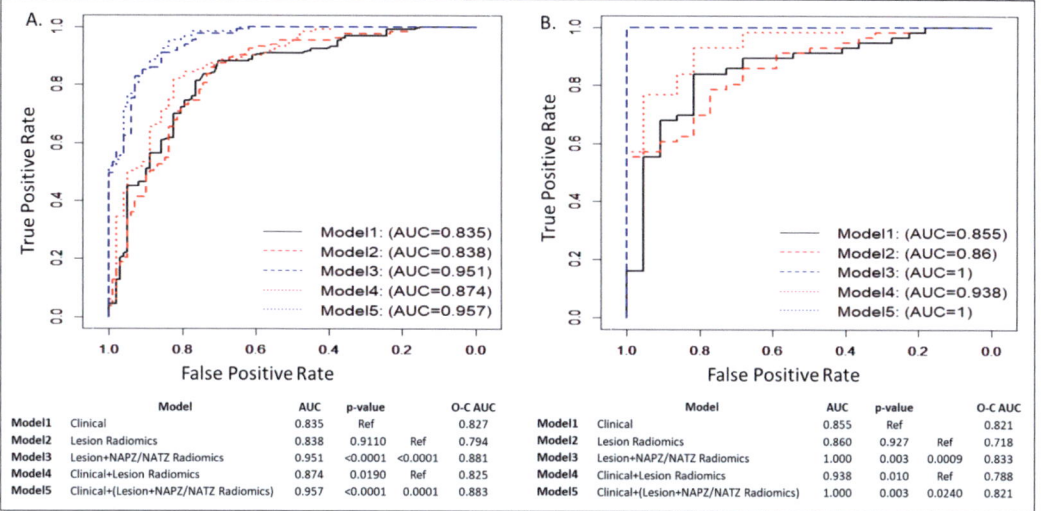

Figure 3. ROC curves and AUCs from five models: Model 1: Clinical model; Model 2: Lesion radiomics; Model 3: Lesion and NAPZ/NATZ radiomics; Model 4: Clinical variables with Lesion radiomics; Model 5: Clinical variables with Lesion and NAPZ/NATZ radiomics. (**A**) Lesion-based prediction for low risk, based on 231 lesions (133 low risk vs. 98 intermediate/high risk); (**B**) Patient-based prediction for low risk, based on 78 patients (56 low risk vs. 22 intermediate/high risk). The tables below the graphs show AUC, *p*-values and Optimism-Corrected (O-C) AUC.

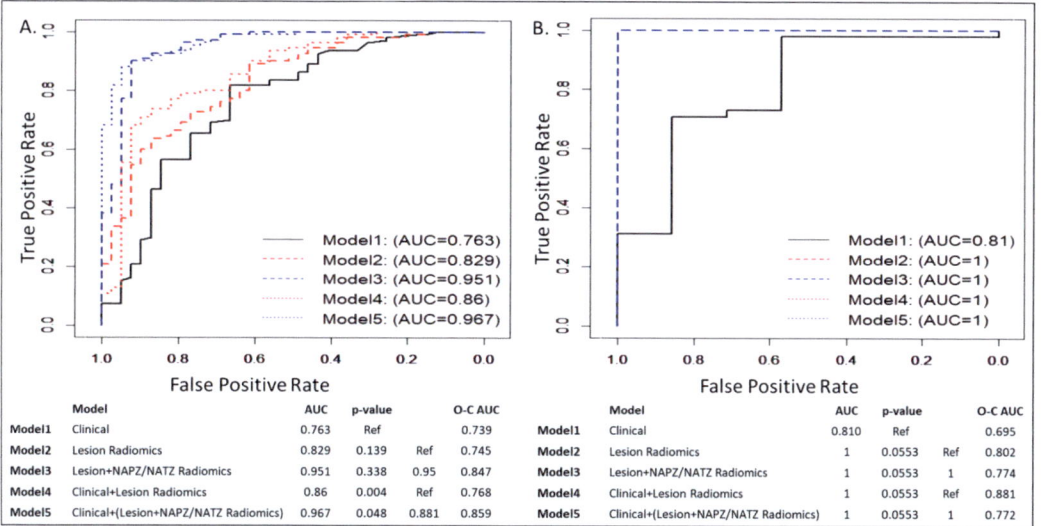

Figure 4. ROC curves and AUCs from five models in patients with negative DRE: Model 1: Clinical model; Model 2: Lesion radiomics; Model 3: Lesion and NAPZ/NATZ radiomics; Model 4: Clinical variables with Lesion radiomics; Model 5: Clinical variables with Lesion and NAPZ/NATZ radiomics. (**A**) Lesion-based prediction for low risk, based on 149 lesions (110 low risk vs. 39 intermediate/high risk); (**B**) Patient-based prediction for low risk, based on 55 patients (48 low risk vs. 7 intermediate/high risk). The tables below the graphs show AUC, *p*-values and Optimism-Corrected (O-C) AUC.

4. Discussion

Image-based automated prostate cancer classification is an area of active investigation. The standard underlying schema of the approach consists of feature extraction and classification. In the majority of radiomic applications, the goal is to predict the Gleason Score/Group Grade (see recent review by Castillo et al. [33]). Here, we investigated the ability of a radiomic model to predict the low-risk group of patients based on a novel clinical-genomic classifier that is increasingly relevant to making clinical decisions. Such a model can prospectively improve patients' selection for prostate biopsy and potentially tailor individual treatment decisions.

The main finding of our study is that it is feasible to build radiomics-based models that can predict the patient risk based on a clinical-genomic classifier. The performance of the lesion radiomics model (Model 2, AUC = 0.842) did not outperform the clinical Model 1, AUC = 0.8353. We hypothesized that the DRE results are driving the high performance of the clinical factors because of the strong association with abnormal DRE in high-risk patients. In a subsequent subset analysis, only of patients with negative findings on DRE (DRE = 0), Model 2's AUC = 0.832 was markedly, albeit not significantly, higher than Model 1's AUC = 0.763. In both cases, the AUCs of the lesion radiomic variables were almost the same, indicating the robustness of the model, while the exclusion of the DRE deteriorated the performance of the clinical variables. The combined models based on radiomics and clinical characteristics in all comparisons improved the predictive performance. Interestingly, radiomic features of the lesion environment, NAPZ and NATZ, contributed significantly to the overall model performance. In particular, the AUC of Model 1 (clinical variables) increased modestly, albeit significantly, from 0.835 to 0.871 in Model 4 (clinical + lesion radiomics). However, when the radiomics of PZ/TZ was added (Model 5), the AUC markedly increased to 0.962. The same pattern was observed in the subset analysis of patients with DRE = 0. Clinical decisions, on the other hand, are made on a per-patient basis rather than per-lesion. The outlined trends in model improvement after combining radiomic and clinical variables in Model 5 is also evident in per-patient models (Figures 3 and 4, second panels).

As a topic of research interest, radiomics of prostate cancer has received increasing attention in recent years. The translation the identification of quantitative imaging features in the clinical workflow is the main driver for these developments. With this goal in mind, despite the promising results, these efforts largely have not been successful. One of the main challenges in our view is that the majority of the radiomic models are trained on predicating GS/GG. The histopathology cancer grade, although currently the best available predictor for disease outcome, is still a surrogate factor for the disease. Biopsies, and, hence GS/GG, are part of the clinical workflow; thus, an optimal radiomic model, fulfilling an unmet clinical need, should provide additional diagnostic/prognostic information. Finally, there is a serious problem with the reproducibility and generalizability of the radiomic features on images acquired under different acquisition sequence parameters and magnets.

To the best of our knowledge, this is the first report addressing the clinical decision-making related to biopsy for patients on active surveillance in the context of a clinical-genomic classifier. In realistic scenarios, we evaluated models, combining radiomics with the available clinical data after a mpMRI exam and before a biopsy. In Woznicki et al., a similar approach to the one used here for Model 4 was used to evaluate models based on clinical characteristics (PI-RADS, PSAD and DRE) and radiomics, and the reported results discriminated between (i) malignant vs. benign prostate lesion (AUC = 0.889) and (ii) clinically significant prostate cancer (csPCa) vs. clinically insignificant prostate cancer (cisPCa) (AUC = 0.844) [34] (csPCa is defined as GG grade 2 or higher [35]). They also conducted a subgroup analysis of patients with lesions <0.5 cc (of note, only the index lesion with the highest PI-RADS score or the biggest lesion volume was selected for analysis). The performance of the model for small lesions degraded: (i) malignant vs. benign prostate lesion (AUC = 0.678) and (ii) csPCa vs. cisPCa (AUC = 0.686). Here, we conducted a similar subgroup analysis but selected patients with negative DRE. DRE has low efficacy for prostate cancer detection with a pooled sensitivity of 0.51 and specificity of 0.59, as reported in a recent meta-analysis study [36]. However, a clearly abnormal DRE is highly associated with bulky and aggressive cancer and in the realistic scenario for selecting low-risk patients, patients with abnormal DRE will be excluded. In this sense, our subgroup analysis is more clinically relevant, as tumor volume is not readily available to be considered in patient management decisions.

The associations between prostate mpMRI features and gene expression have been investigated before [28]. We demonstrated that there are significant correlations between the quantitative imaging features and genes of three commercial signatures for prostate cancer assessment: Decipher®6, Prolaris® Cell Cycle Progression (CCP) (Myriad Genetics, Salt Lake City, UT, USA) [37] and Genomic Prostate Score (GPS®) (Genomic Health, Redwood City, CA, USA) [38]. The presence of prostate cancer genomic prognostic signal in imaging was confirmed by Beksac et al. [39] and Hectors et al. [40]. Both studies identify individual sets of radiomic features that significantly correlate with GS and genomic signatures. Here, we report on models that predict clinical and genomic risk simultaneously.

Similar to our previous work [28], we analyzed multiple lesions per patient. This approach remains unique in the field, where typically only the index lesion is considered. In light of the genomic heterogeneity from different biopsy cores [13], the individual imaging characteristics of the biopsy locations need to be investigated in order to guide the prostate sampling to the highest-grade core with the highest genomic risk level.

Another unique aspect of our approach is the inclusion of NAPZ and NATZ in the radiomics pipeline. This was motivated by our previous gene ontology analysis that identified specific radiomic features, including from the tumor micro-environment, associated with immune/inflammatory response, metabolism, cell, and biological adhesion [28]. Indeed, as discussed above, when the radiomics of NAPZ/NATZ was considered (Model 5), the performance of the model significantly increased.

Despite the large heterogeneity in terms of magnets and manufacturers, about one-third of the variables on both lists are related to image intensities (Table 4, yellow highlight). For the tumor ROI, these variables are related to low T2 (L_t2_int_10) and BVAL (L_b_int_75). These characteristics: low T2-weighted and high intensities on the high b-value images, are used routinely by the radiologist in evaluating prostate mpMRI. As these radiomic variables are clearly related to the current practice for prostate mpMRI evaluation, we believe that this will increase the confidence of clinicians to use our models. We also developed models using only first-order radiomic features, and while the performance was satisfactory, it degraded significantly from the full variable selection setting.

Radiomic features were not extracted from the DCE sequence in mpMRI. One of the reasons is the high variability in DCE acquisitions and subsequent analysis. Computer-Aided Diagnosis (CAD) systems are hindered by an absence of standardization for DCE-MRI analysis. The Quantitative Imaging Network (QIN) at the National Cancer Institute (NCI) conducted two challenges among premier academic medical centers, and the evaluated pharmaco-kinetic parameters K^{trans}, v_e and k_{ep} were quite variable [41,42]. However, the areas of relatively fast contrast wash-in and subsequent wash-out were utilized in the automatic tumor volume delineation (HRS6) [23]. In addition, there is a growing body of scientific articles reporting no performance difference for studies that included T2, diffusion-weighted imaging (DWI), and ADC images as compared to studies that added a DCE sequence. The DCE sequence is included in the PI-RADSv2; however, there is a debate about its added value [43]. In Monti et al. [44], radiomic models using T2W and ADC images performed better than an advanced model with additional diffusion kurtosis imaging and DCE for prostate cancer detection.

Our study has several limitations, including the relatively small sample size, precluding analysis of a separate validation set. Evaluation in a larger prospective cohort would be beneficial to validate these preliminary findings. This study was conducted within a single-institution academic setting with subspecialized multidisciplinary expertise and the performance of the created models may not be generalizable to community practice. In the analysis, we included only first- and second-order radiomic features to avoid overfitting.

5. Conclusions

In conclusion, our study demonstrated that a machine-learning radiomics-based model is capable of predicting novel clinical-genomic classifications. While there are several reports on the association of radiomic variables with GS/GG, to the best of our knowledge, this is the first report for predicting an integrated clinical-genomic classification.

Supplementary Materials: The following supporting information can be downloaded at: https://www.mdpi.com/article/10.3390/cancers15215240/s1, Figure S1: Clinic-genomic Classifier (Spratt criteria): Schema, modified from Spratt et al. [7], for combining National Comprehensive Cancer Network (NCCN) risk groups with Decipher groups to develop clinical-genomic point system, resulting in clinical-genomic 3-tier risk groups. The goal is to create clinical-radiomics model to predict lesions/patients at low risk. Figure S2: Significantly different quantitative imaging features in low vs intermediate/high risk lesions. Box and whisker plots comparing HRS6, T2-weighted, ADC, and high B-value features in low and intermediate/high risk. Abbreviations: a.u. = arbitrary units. Figure S3: ROC curves and AUCs from five models using intensities features only: Model 1: Clinical model; Model 2: Lesion radiomics; Model 3: Lesion and NAPZ/NATZ radiomics; Model 4: Clinical variables with Lesion radiomics; Model 5: Clinical variables with Lesion and NAPZ/NATZ radiomics. (A) Lesion-based prediction for low risk, based on 231 lesions (133 low risk vs 98 intermediate/high risk); (B) Patient-based prediction for low risk, based on 78 patients (56 low risk vs 22 intermediate/high risk). The tables below the graphs show AUC, p-values and Optimism-Corrected (O-C) AUC. Figure S4: ROC curves and AUCs from five models using intensities features only in patients with negative DRE: Model 1: Clinical model; Model 2: Lesion radiomics; Model 3: Lesion and NAPZ/NATZ radiomics; Model 4: Clinical variables with Lesion radiomics; Model 5: Clinical variables with Lesion and NAPZ/NATZ radiomics. (A) Lesion-based prediction for low risk, based on 149 lesions (110 low risk vs 39 intermediate/high risk); (B) Patient-based prediction for low risk, based on 55 patients (48 low risk vs 7 intermediate/high risk). The tables below the graphs show AUC, p-values and Optimism-Corrected (O-C) AUC. Table S1: MRI acquisition parameters for mpMRI sequences. Table S2: Variables for the three models using only intensity-based radiomics features for prediction.

Author Contributions: R.S. and A.P. contributed to the conception and design of the study. B.N., S.P., D.J.P., B.S., M.C.A., A.D.P. and A.P. conducted the clinical trials and provided patient clinical and imaging data for use in the study. P.C. reviewed imaging studies and provided PIRADS scoring and biopsy targets. O.N.K. and S.M.G. reviewed and scored biopsy tissues. E.D. provided genomic analysis. R.S. and A.L.B. used software to identify biopsy locations on imaging. O.Z.-R., A.L.B. and I.R.X. performed radiomics features extraction. O.Z.-R. and R.S. organized the patient database. D.K., A.A. and M.A. performed statistical analysis. R.S. wrote the first draft of the manuscript. A.A. and S.M.G. provided substantial review and editing. All authors have read and agreed to the published version of the manuscript.

Funding: The research reported in this publication was supported by the National Cancer Institute of the National Institutes of Health under Award Number P30CA240139, R01CA189295, R01CA190105, and U01CA239141. The content is solely the responsibility of the authors and does not necessarily represent the official views of the National Institutes of Health.

Institutional Review Board Statement: The study was conducted in accordance with the Declaration of Helsinki, and the clinical trials were approved by the Institutional Review Board (or Ethics Committee) of The University of Miami (The Miami MAST Trial: IRB #20140372, Approval date: 5 September 2014; The Miami BLaStM Trial: IRB# 20140627, Approval date: 4 November 2014).

Informed Consent Statement: Informed consent was obtained from all subjects involved in the study.

Data Availability Statement: Restrictions apply to the availability of these data. Data were obtained from [third party] and are available [from the authors] with the permission of [third party].

Acknowledgments: The authors would like to thank the Non-therapeutic Trials Arm of the Biospecimen Shared Resource at the Sylvester Comprehensive Cancer Center.

Conflicts of Interest: The authors declare no conflict of interest.

References

1. Siegel, R.L.; Miller, K.D.; Fuchs, H.E.; Jemal, A. Cancer Statistics. *CA Cancer J. Clin.* **2021**, *71*, 7–33. [CrossRef] [PubMed]
2. Kryvenko, O.N.; Epstein, J.I. Prostate Cancer Grading: A Decade After the 2005 Modified Gleason Grading System. *Arch. Pathol. Lab. Med.* **2016**, *140*, 1140–1152. [CrossRef] [PubMed]
3. Vince, R.A., Jr.; Jiang, R.; Qi, J.; Tosoian, J.J.; Takele, R.; Feng, F.Y.; Linsell, S.; Johnson, A.; Shetty, S.; Hurley, P.; et al. Impact of Decipher Biopsy testing on clinical outcomes in localized prostate cancer in a prospective statewide collaborative. *Prostate Cancer Prostatic Dis.* **2021**, *25*, 677–683. [CrossRef]
4. Berlin, A.; Murgic, J.; Hosni, A.; Pintilie, M.; Salcedo, A.; Fraser, M.; Kamel-Reid, S.; Zhang, J.; Wang, Q.; Ch'Ng, C.; et al. Genomic classifier for guiding treatment of intermediate-risk prostate cancers to dose-escalated image guided radiation therapy without hormone therapy. *Int. J. Radiat. Oncol. Biol. Phys.* **2019**, *103*, 84–91. [CrossRef] [PubMed]
5. Mohler, J.L.; Armstrong, A.J.; Bahnson, R.R.; D'Amico, A.V.; Davis, B.J.; Eastham, J.A.; Enke, C.A.; Farrington, T.A.; Higano, C.S.; Horwitz, E.M.; et al. Prostate Cancer, Version 1. *J. Natl. Compr. Cancer Netw.* **2016**, *14*, 19–30. [CrossRef] [PubMed]
6. Erho, N.; Crisan, A.; Vergara, I.A.; Mitra, A.P.; Ghadessi, M.; Buerki, C.; Bergstralh, E.J.; Kollmeyer, T.; Fink, S.; Haddad, Z.; et al. Discovery and Validation of a Prostate Cancer Genomic Classifier that Predicts Early Metastasis Following Radical Prostatectomy. *PLoS ONE* **2013**, *8*, e66855. [CrossRef] [PubMed]
7. Spratt, D.E.; Zhang, J.; Santiago-Jiménez, M.; Dess, R.T.; Davis, J.W.; Den, R.B.; Dicker, A.P.; Kane, C.J.; Pollack, A.; Stoyanova, R.; et al. Development and validation of a novel integrated clinical-genomic risk group classification for localized prostate cancer. *J. Clin. Oncol.* **2018**, *36*, 581–590. [CrossRef]
8. Wilt, T.J.; Brawer, M.K.; Jones, K.M.; Barry, M.J.; Aronson, W.J.; Fox, S.; Gingrich, J.R.; Wei, J.T.; Gilhooly, P.; Grob, B.M.; et al. Radical Prostatectomy versus Observation for Localized Prostate Cancer. *N. Engl. J. Med.* **2012**, *367*, 203–213. [CrossRef]
9. Hamdy, F.C.; Donovan, J.L.; Lane, J.A.; Mason, M.; Metcalfe, C.; Holding, P.; Davis, M.; Peters, T.J.; Turner, E.L.; Martin, R.M.; et al. 10-Year Outcomes after Monitoring, Surgery, or Radiotherapy for Localized Prostate Cancer. *N. Engl. J. Med.* **2016**, *375*, 1415–1424. [CrossRef]
10. Klotz, L.; Zhang, L.; Lam, A.; Nam, R.; Mamedov, A.; Loblaw, A. Clinical Results of Long-Term Follow-Up of a Large, Active Surveillance Cohort with Localized Prostate Cancer. *J. Clin. Oncol.* **2010**, *28*, 126–131. [CrossRef]
11. Cooperberg, M.R.; Cowan, J.E.; Hilton, J.F.; Reese, A.C.; Zaid, H.B.; Porten, S.P.; Shinohara, K.; Meng, M.V.; Greene, K.L.; Carroll, P.R. Outcomes of Active Surveillance for Men With Intermediate-Risk Prostate Cancer. *J. Clin. Oncol.* **2011**, *29*, 228–234. [CrossRef] [PubMed]
12. Yamamoto, T.; Musunuru, H.B.; Vesprini, D.; Zhang, L.; Ghanem, G.; Loblaw, A.; Klotz, L. Metastatic Prostate Cancer in Men Initially Treated with Active Surveillance. *J. Urol.* **2015**, *195*, 1409–1414. [CrossRef] [PubMed]
13. Punnen, S.; Stoyanova, R.; Kwon, D.; Reis, I.M.; Soodana-Prakash, N.; Ritch, C.R.; Nahar, B.; Gonzalgo, M.L.; Kava, B.; Liu, Y.; et al. Heterogeneity in Genomic Risk Assessment from Tissue Based Prognostic Signatures Used in the Biopsy Setting and the Impact of MRI Targeted Biopsy. *J. Urol.* **2020**, *205*, 1344–1351. [CrossRef]
14. Ahmed, H.U.; El-Shater Bosaily, A.; Brown, L.C.; Gabe, R.; Kaplan, R.; Parmar, M.K.; Collaco-Moraes, Y.; Ward, K.; Hindley, R.G.; Freeman, A.; et al. Diagnostic accuracy of multi-parametric MRI and TRUS biopsy in prostate cancer (PROMIS): A paired validating confirmatory study. *Lancet* **2017**, *389*, 815–822. [CrossRef] [PubMed]
15. Barentsz, J.O.; Richenberg, J.; Clements, R.; Choyke, P.; Verma, S.; Villeirs, G.; Rouviere, O.; Logager, V.; Fütterer, J.J. ESUR prostate MR guidelines 2012. *Eur. Radiol.* **2012**, *22*, 746–757. [CrossRef]
16. Barentsz, J.O.; Weinreb, J.C.; Verma, S.; Thoeny, H.C.; Tempany, C.M.; Shtern, F.; Padhani, A.R.; Margolis, D.; Macura, K.J.; Haider, M.A.; et al. Synopsis of the PI-RADS v2 Guidelines for Multiparametric Prostate Magnetic Resonance Imaging and Recommendations for Use. *Eur. Urol.* **2016**, *69*, 41–49. [CrossRef]
17. Kwak, J.T.; Xu, S.; Wood, B.J.; Turkbey, B.; Choyke, P.L.; Pinto, P.A.; Wang, S.; Summers, R.M. Automated prostate cancer detection using T2-weighted and high-b-value diffusion-weighted magnetic resonance imaging. *Med. Phys.* **2015**, *42*, 2368–2378. [CrossRef]
18. Turkbey, B.; Mani, H.; Shah, V.; Rastinehad, A.R.; Bernardo, M.; Pohida, T.; Pang, Y.; Daar, D.; Benjamin, C.; McKinney, Y.L.; et al. Multiparametric 3T Prostate Magnetic Resonance Imaging to Detect Cancer: Histopathological Correlation Using Prostatectomy Specimens Processed in Customized Magnetic Resonance Imaging Based Molds. *J. Urol.* **2011**, *186*, 1818–1824. [CrossRef]
19. Khalvati, F.; Wong, A.; Haider, M.A. Automated prostate cancer detection via comprehensive multi-parametric magnetic resonance imaging texture feature models. *BMC Med. Imaging* **2015**, *15*, 27. [CrossRef]
20. Haider, M.A.; van der Kwast, T.H.; Tanguay, J.; Evans, A.J.; Hashmi, A.-T.; Lockwood, G.; Trachtenberg, J. Combined T2-Weighted and Diffusion-Weighted MRI for Localization of Prostate Cancer. *Am. J. Roentgenol.* **2007**, *189*, 323–328. [CrossRef]
21. Litjens, G.; Debats, O.; Barentsz, J.; Karssemeijer, N.; Huisman, H. Computer-Aided Detection of Prostate Cancer in MRI. *IEEE Trans. Med. Imaging* **2014**, *33*, 1083–1092. [CrossRef] [PubMed]
22. Litjens, G.J.S.; Huisman, H.J.; Elliott, R.M.; Shih, N.N.; Feldman, M.D.; Viswanath, S.; Fütterer, J.J.; Bomers, J.G.R.; Madabhushi, A. Quantitative identification of magnetic resonance imaging features of prostate cancer response following laser ablation and radical prostatectomy. *J. Med. Imaging* **2014**, *1*, 035001. [CrossRef] [PubMed]
23. Stoyanova, R.; Chinea, F.; Kwon, D.; Reis, I.M.; Tschudi, Y.; Parra, N.A.; Breto, A.L.; Padgett, K.R.; Pra, A.D.; Abramowitz, M.C.; et al. An Automated Multiparametric MRI Quantitative Imaging Prostate Habitat Risk Scoring System for Defining External Beam Radiation Therapy Boost Volumes. *Int. J. Radiat. Oncol.* **2018**, *102*, 821–829. [CrossRef] [PubMed]

24. Kwon, D.; Reis, I.M.; Breto, A.L.; Tschudi, Y.; Gautney, N.; Zavala-Romero, O.; Lopez, C.; Ford, J.C.; Punnen, S.; Pollack, A.; et al. Classification of suspicious lesions on prostate multiparametric MRI using machine learning. *J. Med. Imaging* **2018**, *5*, 034502.
25. Stoilescu, L.; Huisman, H. *Feasibility of Multireference Tissue Normalizaton of T2-Weighted Prostate MRI*; RSNA: Chicago, IL, USA, 2017.
26. Haralick, R.M. Statistical and structural approaches to texture. *Proc. IEEE* **1979**, *67*, 786–804. [CrossRef]
27. Fehr, D.; Veeraraghavan, H.; Wibmer, A.; Gondo, T.; Matsumoto, K.; Vargas, H.A.; Sala, E.; Hricak, H.; Deasy, J.O. Automat classification of prostate cancer Gleason scores from multiparametric magnetic resonance images. *Proc. Natl. Acad. Sci. USA* **201** *112*, E6265–E6273. [CrossRef] [PubMed]
28. Stoyanova, R.; Pollack, A.; Takhar, M.; Lynne, C.; Parra, N.; Lam, L.L.; Alshalalfa, M.; Buerki, C.; Castillo, R.; Jorda, M.; et al. Association of multiparametric MRI quantitative imaging features with prostate cancer gene expression in MRI-targeted prosta biopsies. *Oncotarget* **2016**, *7*, 53362–53376. [CrossRef]
29. Ross, A.E.; Johnson, M.H.; Yousefi, K.; Davicioni, E.; Netto, G.J.; Marchionni, L.; Fedor, H.L.; Glavaris, S.; Choeurng, V.; Buerki, C et al. Tissue-based Genomics Augments Post-prostatectomy Risk Stratification in a Natural History Cohort of Intermediate- an High-Risk Men. *Eur. Urol.* **2016**, *69*, 157–165. [CrossRef]
30. Friedman, J.; Hastie, T.; Tibshirani, R. Regularization Paths for Generalized Linear Models via Coordinate Descent. *J. Stat. Soft* **2010**, *33*, 1–22. [CrossRef]
31. Venkatraman, E.S.; Begg, C.B. A distribution-free procedure for comparing receiver operating characteristic curves from a paire experiment. *Biometrika* **1996**, *83*, 835–848. [CrossRef]
32. Harrell, F.E.; Lee, K.L.; Mark, D.B. Multivariable prognostic models: Issues in developing models, evaluating assumptions an adequacy, and measuring and reducing errors. *Stat. Med.* **1996**, *15*, 361–387. [CrossRef]
33. Castillo T, J.M.; Arif, M.; Niessen, W.J.; Schoots, I.G.; Veenland, J.F. Automated Classification of Significant Prostate Cancer c MRI: A Systematic Review on the Performance of Machine Learning Applications. *Cancers* **2020**, *12*, 1606. [CrossRef] [PubMed]
34. Woźnicki, P.; Westhoff, N.; Huber, T.; Riffel, P.; Froelich, M.F.; Gresser, E.; von Hardenberg, J.; Mühlberg, A.; Michel, M.S Schoenberg, S.O.; et al. Multiparametric MRI for Prostate Cancer Characterization: Combined Use of Radiomics Model wit PI-RADS and Clinical Parameters. *Cancers* **2020**, *12*, 1767. [CrossRef] [PubMed]
35. Carter, H.B.; Partin, A.W.; Walsh, P.C.; Trock, B.J.; Veltri, R.W.; Nelson, W.G.; Coffey, D.S.; Singer, E.A.; Epstein, J.I. Gleason score adenocarcinoma: Should it be labeled as cancer? *J. Clin. Oncol.* **2012**, *30*, 4294–4296. [CrossRef]
36. Naji, L.; Randhawa, H.; Sohani, Z.; Dennis, B.; Lautenbach, D.; Kavanagh, O.; Bawor, M.; Banfield, L.; Profetto, J. Digital Rect Examination for Prostate Cancer Screening in Primary Care: A Systematic Review and Meta-Analysis. *Ann. Fam. Med.* **2018**, *1* 149–154. [CrossRef]
37. Cuzick, J.; Berney, D.M.; Fisher, G.; Mesher, D.; Møller, H.; Reid, J.E.; Perry, M.; Park, J.; Younus, A.; Gutin, A.; et al. Prognost value of a cell cycle progression signature for prostate cancer death in a conservatively managed needle biopsy cohort. *Br. Cancer* **2012**, *106*, 1095–1099. [CrossRef]
38. Klein, E.A.; Cooperberg, M.R.; Magi-Galluzzi, C.; Simko, J.P.; Falzarano, S.M.; Maddala, T.; Chan, J.M.; Li, J.; Cowan, J.E.; Tsiat A.C.; et al. A 17-gene Assay to Predict Prostate Cancer Aggressiveness in the Context of Gleason Grade Heterogeneity, Tum Multifocality, and Biopsy Undersampling. *Eur. Urol.* **2014**, *66*, 550–560. [CrossRef]
39. Beksac, A.T.; Cumarasamy, S.; Falagario, U.; Xu, P.; Takhar, M.; Alshalalfa, M.; Gupta, A.; Prasad, S.; Martini, A.; Thulasidas H.; et al. Multiparametric Magnetic Resonance Imaging Features Identify Aggressive Prostate Cancer at the Phenotypic an Transcriptomic Level. *J. Urol.* **2018**, *200*, 1241–1249. [CrossRef]
40. Hectors, S.J.; Cherny, M.; Yadav, K.K.; Beksaç, A.T.; Thulasidass, H.; Lewis, S.; Davicioni, E.; Wang, P.; Tewari, A.K.; Taou B. Radiomics Features Measured with Multiparametric Magnetic Resonance Imaging Predict Prostate Cancer Aggressivenes *J. Urol.* **2019**, *202*, 498–505. [CrossRef]
41. Huang, W.; Li, X.; Chen, Y.; Li, X.; Chang, M.-C.; Oborski, M.J.; Malyarenko, D.I.; Muzi, M.; Jajamovich, G.H.; Fedorov, A.; et Variations of Dynamic Contrast-Enhanced Magnetic Resonance Imaging in Evaluation of Breast Cancer Therapy Response: Multicenter Data Analysis Challenge. *Transl. Oncol.* **2014**, *7*, 153–166. [CrossRef]
42. Huang, W.; Chen, Y.; Fedorov, A.; Li, X.; Jajamovich, G.H.; Malyarenko, D.I.; Aryal, M.P.; LaViolette, P.S.; Oborski, M.J.; O'Sulliva F.; et al. The Impact of Arterial Input Function Determination Variations on Prostate Dynamic Contrast-Enhanced Magnet Resonance Imaging Pharmacokinetic Modeling: A Multicenter Data Analysis Challenge. *Tomography* **2016**, *2*, 56–66. [CrossRe [PubMed]
43. Padhani, A.R.; Schoots, I.; Villeirs, G. Contrast Medium or No Contrast Medium for Prostate Cancer Diagnosis. That Is th Question. *J. Magn. Reson. Imaging* **2020**, *53*, 13–22. [CrossRef] [PubMed]
44. Monti, S.; Brancato, V.; Di Costanzo, G.; Basso, L.; Puglia, M.; Ragozzino, A.; Salvatore, M.; Cavaliere, C. Multiparametric MRI f Prostate Cancer Detection: New Insights into the Combined Use of a Radiomic Approach with Advanced Acquisition Protoc *Cancers* **2020**, *12*, 390. [CrossRef] [PubMed]

Disclaimer/Publisher's Note: The statements, opinions and data contained in all publications are solely those of the individu author(s) and contributor(s) and not of MDPI and/or the editor(s). MDPI and/or the editor(s) disclaim responsibility for any injury people or property resulting from any ideas, methods, instructions or products referred to in the content.

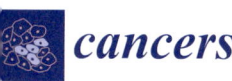

Article

Comparing Two Targeted Biopsy Schemes for Detecting Clinically Significant Prostate Cancer in Magnetic Resonance Index Lesions: Two- to Four-Core versus Saturated Transperineal Targeted Biopsy

Juan Morote [1,2,3,*], Nahuel Paesano [2,4], Natàlia Picola [5], Berta Miró [6], José M. Abascal [7,8], Pol Servian [9], Enrique Trilla [1,2,3,†] and Olga Méndez [3,†]

1. Department of Urology, Vall d'Hebron University Hospital, 08035 Barcelona, Spain; enrique.trilla@vallhe-bron.cat
2. Department of Surgery, Universitat Autònoma de Barcelona, 08193 Bellaterra, Spain; npaesa@gmail.com
3. Research Group in Urology, Vall d'Hebron Research Institute, 08035 Barcelona, Spain; olga.mendez@vhir.org
4. Clinica Creu Blanca, 08018 Barcelona, Spain
5. Department of Urology, Bellvitge University Hospital, Hospitalet de Llobregat, 08907 Barcelona, Spain; npicola.bellvitge@gencat.cat
6. Statistics Unit, Vall d'Hebron Research Institute, 08035 Barcelona, Spain; berta.miro@vhir.org
7. Department of Urology, Parc de Salut Mar, 08003 Barcelona, Spain; jabascal@psmar.cat
8. Department of Health Sciences, Universitat Pompeu Fabra, 08003 Barcelona, Spain
9. Department of Urology, Hospital Germans Trias I Pujol, 08916 Badalona, Spain; pservian.germanstrias@gencat.cat
* Correspondence: juan.morote@uab.cat; Tel.: +34-629-011-936
† These authors contributed equally to this work.

Simple Summary: Targeted biopsies of suspicious lesions detected in magnetic resonance imaging are crucial to discover clinically significant prostate cancer, especially those corresponding to index lesions. However, the optimal scheme for targeted biopsies remains unclear, despite the fact that a two- to four-core scheme is usually recommended. Saturated biopsies of the prostate gland have shown high efficiency in detecting significant PCa. In this article, we report a better efficacy for mapping using a 0.5 mm core biopsy scheme than that using the two- to four-core scheme for detecting clinically significant prostate cancer in magnetic resonance index lesions.

Abstract: Since the optimal scheme for targeted biopsies of magnetic resonance imaging (MRI) suspicious lesions remains unclear, we compare the efficacy of two schemes for these index lesions. A prospective trial was conducted in 1161 men with Prostate Imaging Reporting and Data System v 2.1 3–5 undergoing targeted and 12-core systematic biopsy in four centers between 2021 and 2023. Two- to four-core MRI-transrectal ultrasound fusion-targeted biopsies via the transperineal route were conducted in 900 men in three centers, while a mapping per 0.5 mm core method (saturated scheme) was employed in 261 men biopsied in another center. A propensity-matched 261 paired cases were selected for avoiding confounders other than the targeted biopsy scheme. CsPCa (grade group $\geq$ 2) was identified in 125 index lesions (41.1%) when the two- to four-core scheme was employed, while in 187 (71.9%) when the saturated biopsy ($p < 0.001$) was used. Insignificant PCa (iPCa) was detected in 18 and 11.1%, respectively ($p = 0.019$). Rates of csPCa and iPCa remained similar in systematic biopsies. CsPCa detected only in systematic biopsies were 5 and 1.5%, respectively ($p = 0.035$) in each group. The saturated scheme for targeted biopsies detected more csPCa and less iPCa than did the two- to four-core scheme in the index lesions. The rate of csPCa detected only in the systematic biopsies decreased when the saturated scheme was employed.

Keywords: prostate cancer; targeted biopsy; index lesion; number of cores

1. Introduction

Risk-stratified prostate cancer (PCa) screening, based on serum prostate-specific antigen (PSA) testing and magnetic resonance imaging (MRI) scanning as a follow-up measure, is currently recommended by the European Union [1]. This new paradigm of PCa screening is focused on maximizing the early detection of clinically significant PCa (csPCa), while minimizing the number of prostate biopsies and the over-detection of insignificant prostate cancer (iPCa) [2–5].

The Prostate Imaging Reporting and Data System (PI-RADS) predicts the risk of csPCa according to the imaging characteristics of lesions detected in MRI scans [6–8]. Men with PI-RADS < 3 have a very low probability of csPCa, and consequently, in this case, prostate biopsies can usually be avoided [9,10]. MRI can visualize most lesions containing csPCa, reporting them as PI-RADS 3 to 5, with an intermediate, high, and very high-risk of csPCa, respectively [11]. PI-RADS 3 is considered the gray zone of a PI-RADS score, since the csPCa detection rate is 18.5%, with a 95% confidence interval between 16.6 and 20.3%, but a range between 3.4 and 46.5% [12]. A significant contribution of MRI is the possibility of conducting targeted biopsies for suspicious lesions through MRI-transrectal ultrasound (TRUS) fusion images [13]. However, a small percentage of csPCa are not visualized in MRI scans and are detected only in systematic biopsies, which is the reason why these biopsies are still recommended [14].

The recommendation for changing the approach of prostate biopsies from the classic transrectal to the transperineal route has reduced the infrequent but dangerous infectious complications and the inappropriate use of antibiotics [15,16] accompanying this method. It is known that a prostate biopsy scheme for avoiding the upgrading of csPCa in radical prostatectomy specimens requires a mapping biopsy per 0.5 mm, with additional targeted biopsies of suspicious lesions detected by MRI [17]. However, systematic biopsies complementing targeted biopsies for suspicious lesions causes significant over-detection of iPCa [18].

The currently recommended prostate biopsy scheme suggests obtaining a two- to four-core targeted biopsy of suspicious lesions and a 12-core systematic biopsy [14,19–21]. However, the appropriate number of cores obtained from targeted biopsies remains unclear. Two studies have examined the correlation between the PCa grade groups detected in prostate biopsies and those observed in radical prostatectomy specimens, suggesting that obtaining more cores from suspicious lesions reduces the likelihood of upgrading [22,23]. Other studies, conducted in men undergoing transperineal prostate biopsies, suggest the improved detection of csPCa when a saturation scheme for targeted biopsies is employed; however, the results are not uniform [24–27]. The potential of the index lesion, defined from MRI as the largest lesion with the highest PI-RADS score, for defining the aggressiveness of PCa is known [28–30]. However, an appropriate biopsy scheme for the index lesion could minimized unnecessary biopsies from other areas of the prostate gland, as well as systematic biopsies [31]. Mainly, the specifics regarding the differences between the two- to four-core and the saturated scheme for targeted biopsies is the rationale of mapping each 0.5 mm, which has been shown to be the most appropriate scheme for avoiding upgrading in radical prostatectomy specimens [13,22–27].

We hypothesize than the saturated scheme for targeted biopsies detects more csPCa in the index lesions than does the recommended two- to four-core scheme. The objectives of this study are to compare the rates of csPCa and iPCa detection in both targeted biopsy schemes and to assess the rates of csPCa detected only in systematic biopsies.

2. Materials and Methods
2.1. Design, Setting, and Participants

A prospective non-randomized trial including 1161 consecutive men suspected of having PCa, based on a serum PSA > 3.0 ng/mL, was conducted in four centers participating in the csPCa opportunistic early detection program of Catalonia (Spain) between 1 January 2021 and 30 June 2023. All included men exhibited PI-RADS v 2.1 lesions 3 to 5 in pre-biopsy multiparametric MRI (mpMRI), undergoing targeted biopsy of suspicious lesions and 12-core systematic biopsy. Three participant centers, always obtaining two- to four-cores from each suspicious lesion, reported 900 cases, while 261 cases were reported in another center, where a mapping per 0.5 mm core scheme was always employed. Due to the possible influence on csPCa detection, men undergoing treatment with 5-alpha reductase inhibitors and those with prior history of PCa, atypical small acinar proliferation, or multifocal high-grade prostatic intraepithelial neoplasia were not included in this study.

2.2. Diagnostic Approach for csPCa Detection

MpMRI using a 3 Tesla scan was performed in each participant center using a pelvic phased-array surface coil. The acquisition protocol included T2-weighted imaging (T2W), diffusion-weighted imaging (DWI), and dynamic contrast-enhanced (DCE) imaging, according to the guidelines of the European Society of Urogenital Radiology [6]. MpMRI exams were reported by local expert radiologists using the PI-RADS v 2.1 [8]. Local experienced operators performed prostate biopsies using the Koelis Trinity® hands-free MRI/TUS prostate biopsy system (Koelis Inc., Grenoble, France) in the centers conducting targeted biopsies with the two- to four-core scheme, while the Artemis® hands-free MRI/TUS prostate biopsy system (Eigen Inc., Grass Valley, CA, USA) was used in the center performing the mapping per 0.5 mm core scheme. Experienced local uropathologists exa-mined the biopsy material in each pathology department, reporting PCa using the International Society of Urologic Pathology grade group (GG) classification. CsPCa was considered when the GG was ≥2 [32]. Baseline characteristics of the study cohort are summarized in Table 1.

Table 1. Characteristics of cohort study.

Characteristic	Measurement
Number of men	1161
Median age, years (IQR)	67 (61–73)
Median serum PSA, ng/mL (IQR)	6.7 (5.1–9.9)
Abnormal DRE, n (%)	200 (25.8)
Median prostate volume, ml (IQR)	50 (36–70)
Prior negative prostate biopsy, n (%)	403 (34.7)
Family history of PCa, n (%)	96 (8.3%)
Median suspicious lesions, n (IQR)	1 (1–2)
Median length of suspicious lesions, mm (IQR)	11 (5–17)
Localization of the index lesion, n (%)	
Peripheral zone	835 (71.9)
Central-transition zone	278 (23.9)
Anterior zone	48 (4.2)
PI-RADS score of the index lesion, n (%)	
3	260 (22.4)
4	587 (50.4)
5	315 (27.1)
Median cores obtained in targeted biopsy, n (IQR) index lesion, n (IQR)	3 (1–7)
Overall PCa detection, n (%)	815 (70.2)
csPCa	601 (51.8)
iPCa	241 (18.4)

IQR = interquartile range; n = number; PCa = prostate cancer; csPCa = clinically significant PCa; iPCa = insignificant PCa.

2.3. Variables in the Study and Outcome Variables

Age (years), first degree PCa family history (no vs. yes), type of prostate biopsy (initial vs. repeated), serum PSA (ng/mL), DRE (normal vs. suspicious), MRI-prostate volume (mL), PI-RADS score v 2.1 (3 to 5), size and localization of the index lesion, targeted biopsy scheme (two- to four-core vs. mapping per 0.5-core) were predictive variables in the study. Outcome variables were csPCa and iPCa detection.

2.4. Statistical Analysis

Statistical analysis was conducted after harmonization of the anonymized datasets. Data were prospectively collected and reported according to the Standards of Reporting for MRI-Targeted Biopsy Studies (START) to describe the study population [33]. Quantitative variables are described using medians and interquartile ranges (IQR: 25th–75th percentile), while qualitative variables are described using numbers and percentages. Quantitative variables were compared between groups using the Mann–Whitney U test. Qua-litative variables were compared between groups using Pearson's chi-square test. Relative risk (RR) of csPCa and 95% confidence intervals (CI) were assessed. A logistic regression analysis conducted for detecting independent predictive variables of csPCa, in addition to the targeted biopsy scheme, showed that PI-RADS score, prostate volume, age, serum PSA, location, and size of the index lesion were independent predictors of csPCa and were potential confounders for csPCa detection (Table 2).

Table 2. Multivariate analysis searching confounder variables for csPCa detection in the index lesion, in addition to the targeted biopsy scheme employed.

Predictive Variable	Odds Ratio (95% CI)	*p* Value
Age, Ref. year	1.061 (1.036–1.086)	<0.001
Serum PSA, Ref. ng/mL	1.062 (1.027–1.099)	<0.001
DRE, Ref. normal	1.154 (0.775–1.718)	=0.481
Type of biopsy, Ref. initial	0.960 (0.695–1.429)	=0.841
PCa family history, Ref. no	1.258 (0.749–2.111)	=0.386
Prostate volume, Ref. mL	0.972 (0.065–0.979)	<0.001
Number of suspicious lesions, Ref. one	1.387 (0.863–2.231)	=0.177
PI-RADS score of the index lesion, Ref. 3	2.718 (2.032–3.365)	<0.001
Size of the index lesion. Ref. mm	1.071 (1.030–1.113)	<0.001
Localization of the index lesion, Ref. peripheral zone	0.611 (0.438–0.852)	=0.004
Targeted prostate biopsy scheme, Ref. 2- to 4-core	2.137 (1.869–3.439)	<0.001

CI = confidence interval; PSA = prostate specific antigen; DRE = digital rectal examination; PCa = prostate cancer; PI-RADS = Prostate Imaging Reporting and Data System.

A randomized 1:1 matched group from all predictive variables was selected using the R package matching v 4.10, a multivariate and propensity score matching software with automated balance optimization (R Foundation for Statistical Computing, Vienna, Austria). In a subset of 522 men, the two- to four-core scheme was employed, and the mapping per 0.5 mm core scheme was used in the other 261 men. Table 3 shows the sui-tability of this matched paired group for analysis, since all baseline confounder characte-ristics for csPCa detection were equally distributed in both study subsets. A *p* value of <0.05 was considered statistically significant. The data were analyzed using the Statistical Package for the Social Sciences (version 29.0; IBM Corp., Armonk, NY, USA).

Table 3. Baseline characteristics of the paired matched study group and a comparative analysis between them, according to biopsy scheme applied for targeted biopsy of the index lesions.

Baseline Characteristic	Biopsy Scheme of the Index Lesion		*p* Value
	Two- to Four-Core	Mapping × 0.5 mm Core	
Number of men, *n* (%)	261 (50.0)	261 (50.0)	-
Median age, years (IQR)	67 (61–73)	67 (61–73)	=1.000
Median serum PSA, ng/mL (IQR)	6.7 (5.0–9.6)	6.7 (5.0–9.6)	=1.000
Abnormal DRE, *n* (%)	65 (24.9)	67 (25.7)	=0.678
Median prostate volume, ml (IQR)	45 (33–62)	45 (33–62)	=1.000
Prior negative prostate biopsy, *n* (%)	63 (24.1)	68 (26.0)	=0.357
Family history of PCa, *n* (%)	30 (11.5%)	28 (10.7)	=0.419
Median suspicious lesions, *n* (IQR)	1 (1–2)	1 (1–2)	=1.000
Median length of the index lesion, mm (IQR)	12 (9–18)	12 (9–18)	=1.000

Table 3. Cont.

Baseline Characteristic	Biopsy Scheme of the Index Lesion		p Value
	Two- to Four-Core	Mapping × 0.5 mm Core	
Index lesion localization, n (%)			
Peripheral zone	179 (68.6)	179 (68.6)	=1.000
Central/transition zone	62 (23.8)	62(23.8)	=1.000
Anterior zone	20 (7.7)	20 (7.7)	=1.000
PI-RADS score of index lesion, n (%)			
3	71 (27.2)	71 (27.2)	=1.000
4	118 (45.2)	118 (45.2)	=1.000
5	72 (27.6)	72 (27.6)	=1.000
Median number of cores in the index lesion, n (IQR) obtained, n (IQR)	2 (1–3)	9 (5–12)	=0.016
Overall PCa detection, n (%)	328 (63.9)	216 (82.7)	<0.001
csPCa, n (%)	235 (45.8)	187 (71.6)	<0.001
iPCa, n (%)	93 (18.1)	29 (11.1)	=0.012

IQR = interquartile range; n = number; PI-RADS = Prostate Imaging Reporting and Data System; PCa = prostate cancer; csPCa = clinically significant PCa; iPCa = insignificant PCa.

3. Results

3.1. Baseline Characteristics of the Study Population

The baseline characteristics of the propensity-matched group comprising 522 men, including 261 men who underwent targeted biopsies employing the two- to four-core scheme and 261 who underwent the mapping per 0.5 mm core scheme, were similar except in regards to the median number of cores utilized in each targeted biopsy scheme, which were 2 (IQR 1–2) and 9 (IQR 5–12), respectively ($p = 0.016$). The detection rate of PCa in the index lesion and the 12-core systematic biopsies, according to the employed scheme, were 63.6 and 82.7%, respectively ($p < 0.001$), with 45.8 and 71.6% csPCa, and 18.1 and 11.1% iPCa, respectively ($p = 0.012$), Table 3.

3.2. CsPCa Detection in the Index Lesions according to the PI-RADS Score and the Biopsy Scheme

Among 142 men with a PI-RADS score of 3, csPCa was identified in 13 of 71 (18.3%) index lesions biopsied using the two- to four-core scheme, while in 26 of 71 (26.8%) when the mapping per 0.5 mm core scheme was employed, with an RR of 1.298 (95% CI 0.824–2.045), $p = 0.158$. Among 236 men with a PI-RADS score of 4, these rates were 47.4% and 87.3%, respectively, with an RR of 2.286 (95% CI 1.802–2.900), $p = 0.001$. Among 144 men with a PI-RADS score of 5, the rates were 77.8% and 90.3%, respectively, with an RR of 1.503 (95% CI 1.079–2.094), $p < 0.001$ (Figure 1).

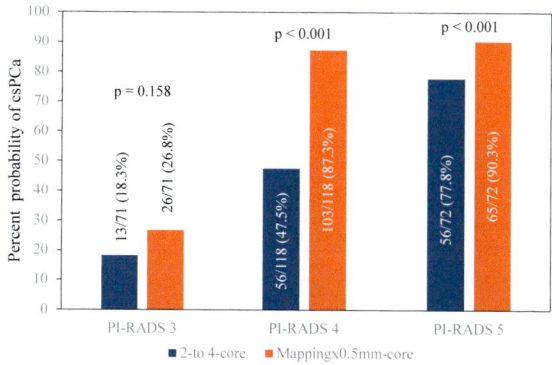

Figure 1. CsPCa detection in the index lesion targeted biopsies, according to the employed two- to four-core and mapping × 0.5 mm core schemes and the PI-RADS score.

3.3. Detection of csPCa and iPCa in the Index Lesions, According to the Employed Biopsy Scheme and Those Detected in Systematic Biopsies

Figure 2 summarizes the csPCa and iPCa detection in the targeted biopsies of the index lesions and systematic biopsies, according to the employed targeted biopsy scheme. CsPCa detection in the index lesions was 47.9% when two- to four-core scheme was applied, while 71.9% when mapping per 0.5 mm core scheme was used, with an RR of 1.616 (95% CI 1.366–1.913), $p < 0.001$. IPCa detected in the index lesions were 18.8 and 11.1%, respectively, with an RR of 0.760 (9% CI 0.624–0.925), $p = 0.006$. The csPCa detection rates in systematic biopsies, according to the biopsy scheme employed in the targeted biopsies, corresponded to 28.0%, when the two- to four-core scheme was used, and 26.8%, when the mapping per 0.5 mm core scheme was employed, with an RR of 0.829 (95% CI 0.789–1.121), $p = 0.228$. The IPCa detection rates in systematic biopsies were 19.2% and 21.5%, respectively, with an RR of 1.191 (95% CI 0.940–1.909), $p = 0.187$.

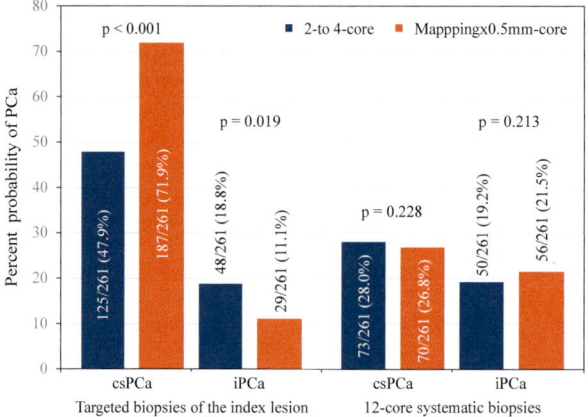

Figure 2. Detection of csPCa and iPCa in the index lesion targeted biopsies and the 12-core syste-matic biopsies, according to the two- to four-core and mapping × 0.5 mm core schemes employed in the targeted biopsies.

CsPCa was detected only in 12-core systematic biopsies in 5.0% of cases when the two- to four-core scheme was applied in the targeted biopsies, while it decreased to 1.5% when the mapping per 0.5 mm core scheme was employed, with an RR of 0.642 (95% CI 0.486–0.848), $p = 0.213$ (Figure 3).

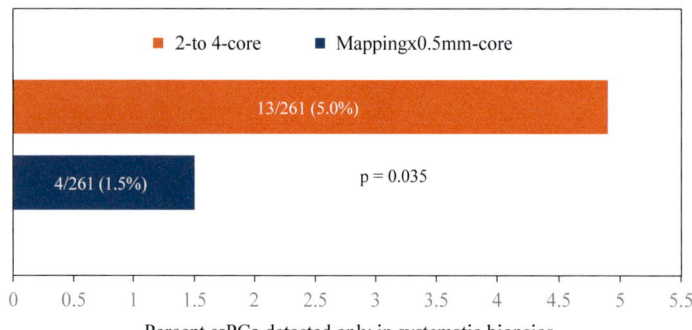

Figure 3. CsPCa detection in only the 12-core systematic biopsies, according to the two- to four-core and mapping × 0.5 mm core schemes employed in the targeted biopsies.

4. Discussion

The analysis of this prospective and multicenter trial was conducted in a propensity-paired matched group to avoid the influence of existing confounder variables for csPCa detection other than the targeted biopsy scheme. Our main findings were, (i) the csPCa detection in the index lesions improved when the saturated mapping per 0.5 mm core targeted biopsy scheme was employed, compared with the results for the currently recommended two- to four-core scheme; (ii) this improvement was observed in all PI-RADS categories, although it was significant only in categories 4 and 5; (iii) the iPCa detection rates in the index lesions decreased when the saturated scheme was employed, compared with the results for the two- to four-core scheme; (iv) the percentage of csPCa detected only in systematic biopsies decreased when the saturated scheme was employed compared to the results for the two- to four-core scheme.

In 2013, the Ginsburg Study Group first proposed obtaining two to four cores in targeted biopsies of suspicious lesions in MRI-TRUS fusion prostate biopsies conducted via the transperineal route. This group also proposed at least 4-core biopsies of the anterior, mid, posterior, and basal sectors of the right and left prostate lobules, resulting in 24 cores for prostate glands of less than 30 mL, 32 cores for those of 30 to 50 mL, and 38 additional cores for prostate glands of more than 50 mL [17]. In 2016, Radtke et al. observed that the Ginsburg approach was able to identify 97% of csPCa detected in 120 radical prostatectomy specimens, while only 79% of them were identified in systematic biopsies, and 88% were found in targeted biopsies alone [22]. In 2018, Calio et al. examined 122 men who underwent targeted MRI-TRUS index lesion biopsies employing a two-core scheme and 86 men who underwent a mapping per 0.6 mm core scheme. Additionally, all men underwent a 12-core systematic biopsy. The authors observed a surgical specimen upgrading of 40.9% with systematic biopsies, 23.6% with two-core targeted biopsies, and 13.8% with mapping per 0.6 mm core targeted biopsies [23]. Many studies have focused their attention on the findings in the index lesions, due to its high predictive power for defining PCa aggressiveness [28–30].

It is difficult to compare our results with those observed in previous reports due to the variability of study designs. In 2020, Hansen et al. analyzed 487 men who underwent transperineal MRI-TRUS prostate biopsies following the Ginsburg approach. Targeted biopsies of suspicious lesions using the two-core scheme only detected 67% of csPCa. In contrast, extended targeted biopsies obtaining two additional cores from sectors adjacent to the index lesion detected 76% of csPCa, and targeted biopsies using a six-core scheme detected 91% of csPCa [24]. This study suggested that obtaining more cores from targeted biopsies of the index lesion improved csPCa detection. In 2021, Tschirdewahn et al. reported a study conducted in 213 men who underwent targeted biopsies of suspicious MRI lesions, employing the Ginsburg approach, between 2016 and 2018. Targeted biopsies were collected using a four-core scheme. Targeted biopsies involved collecting 4 cores from suspicious lesions and additional cores from adjacent sectors, and systematic biopsies obtained 9 to 10 cores. Targeted saturated biopsies detected 99% of 134 csPCa, while non-saturated targeted biopsies detected 87%, and systematic biopsies detected 82% [25]. This study also confirms that greater core obtention in targeted biopsies increases csPCa detection.

In 2023, Cetin et al. reported an analysis of 167 men in whom targeted biopsies obtained two cores from the center of the suspicious lesions and two additional cores from the periphery. One central core identified 65.6% of csPCa, two central cores identified 92.2%, two central cores and one peripheral core identified 96.9%, and two central cores and two peripheral cores identified 100% of csPCa. These authors concluded that the two central cores scheme was sufficient to detect the vast majority of csPCa because the diffe-rence between two and four cores was non-significant [25].

Finally, in 2023, Sanner et al. reported a prospective single-center trial randomizing 170 men who underwent transperineal targeted biopsy of suspicious lesions employing a four-core scheme compared to targeted saturated biopsies using a nine-core scheme. Both schemes were complemented with a 24-core systematic biopsy. Targeted biopsies detected 91.7% of csPCa, while targeted saturated biopsies detected 100%. Because this difference was non-significant, the authors concluded that csPCa detection did not differ between targeted and saturated targeted biopsies [27]. The results of this prospective and randomized trial contradict the previous retrospective study reported by the same authors [24]. A recently reported study has noted the importance of only biopsying the index lesion with an appropriate scheme for avoiding targeted biopsies of secondary lesions and systematic biopsies [31]. Additionally, our results suggest that saturated targeted biopsies reduce the rate of csPCa detected only in systematic biopsies. This finding requires confirmation in additional studies.

Our study is limited by its non-randomized design, although the propensity-matched paired group selection minimized the effect of confounder variables for csPCa detection. The utilization of different devices for MRI-TRUS biopsies and the level of experience of the surgeon performing the two different types of prostate biopsies can influence the results, as can the inter-variability between pathologists. The csPCa outcome va-riable detected in prostate biopsies does not represent the true csPCa detected in the radical prostatectomy specimens. Since we decided to conduct this study using the index lesions, a limitation exists in regards to recommending the saturated targeted biopsy scheme for all suspicious lesions. A limitation exists for recommending a prostate biopsy approach based only on a saturated targeted scheme of the index lesion, since the current knowledge suggests the importance of perilesional biopsies for avoiding ipsilateral systematic biopsies [34–37].

One of the strengths of this study is that it is conducted using matched pairs of men suspected of having PCa in order to avoid the influence of confounders for csPCa detection. One of the study's weakness is that it is retrospective, with a non-randomized design. However, new evidence is generated for recommending saturated targeted biopsies, possibly without systematic biopsies, if perilesional biopsies are obtained. Well-designed prospective and multicenter randomized trials identifying the most effective and least aggressive prostate biopsy scheme for transperineal prostate biopsy are needed for maximizing the detection of csPCa, minimizing the over-detection of iPCa, and reducing prostate biopsy site effects.

5. Conclusions

Saturated targeted biopsies, using a mapping per 0.5 mm core scheme, were able to detect more csPCa and less iPCa than the recommended two- to four-core scheme in the index lesions. This advantage was particularly notable in individuals with PI-RADS scores above 3. The rate of csPCa detected only in 12-core systematic biopsies decreased when the mapping per 0.5 mm core scheme for targeted biopsies was employed.

Author Contributions: Conceptualization, J.M. and N.P. (Nahuel Paesano).; methodology, J.M.; formal analysis, B.M. and J.M.; resources, J.M.; data curation, N.P. (Nahuel Paesano), N.P. (Natàlia Picola), J.M.A. and P.S.; writing—original draft preparation, J.M.; writing—review and editing, N.P., O.M. and E.T.; supervision, E.T. and O.M.; project administration, J.M.; funding acquisition, J.M. All authors have read and agreed to the published version of the manuscript.

Funding: This research was funded by the Ministerio de Asuntos Económicos y Transformación Digital (SP) (MIA.2021.M02.0005) and the Instituto de Salut Carlos III (SP) through the project "PI20/01666" (Co-funded by European Regional Development Fund "A way to make Europe").

Institutional Review Board Statement: The study was conducted in accordance with the Declaration of Helsinki and approved by the Institutional Ethics Committee of Vall d'Hebron University Hospital (PRAG21/0002, approved on 12 February 2021).

Informed Consent Statement: Informed consent was obtained from all subjects involved in the study.

Data Availability Statement: Datasets from this study are available upon request from the corresponding author.

Conflicts of Interest: The authors declare no conflicts of interest.

References

1. Van Poppel, H.; Roobol, M.J.; Chandran, A. Early Detection of Prostate Cancer in the European Union: Combining Forces with PRAISE-U. *Eur. Urol.* **2023**, *84*, 519–522. [CrossRef]
2. Van Poppel, H.; Hogenhout, R.; Albers, P.; van den Bergh, R.C.N.; Barentsz, J.O.; Roobol, M.J. Early Detection of Prostate Cancer in 2020 and Beyond: Facts and recommendations for the European Union and the European Commission. *Eur. Urol.* **2020**, *79*, 327–329. [CrossRef]
3. Van Poppel, H.; Hogenhout, R.; Albers, P.; van den Bergh, R.C.N.; Barentsz, J.O.; Roobol, M.J. A European Model for an Organised Risk-stratified Early Detection Programme for Prostate Cancer. *Eur. Urol. Oncol.* **2021**, *4*, 731–739. [CrossRef] [PubMed]
4. Van Poppel, H.; Roobol, M.J.; Chapple, C.R.; Catto, J.W.F.; N'Dow, J.; Sønksen, J.; Stenzl, A.; Wirth, M. Prostate-specific Antigen Testing as Part of a Risk-Adapted Early Detection Strategy for Prostate Cancer: European Association of Urology Position and Recommendations for 2021. *Eur. Urol.* **2021**, *80*, 703–711.
5. Van Poppel, H.; Albreht, T.; Basu, P.; Hogenhout, R.; Collen, S.; Roobol, M. Serum PSA-based early detection of prostate cancer in Europe and globally: Past, present and future. *Nat. Rev. Urol.* **2022**, *19*, 562–572. [CrossRef] [PubMed]
6. Barentsz, J.O.; Richenberg, J.; Clements, R.; Choyke, P.; Verma, S.; Villeirs, G.; Rouviere, O.; Logager, V.; Futterer, J.J. ESUR prostate MR guidelines 2012. *Eur. Radiol.* **2012**, *22*, 746–757. [CrossRef]
7. Weinreb, J.C.; Barentsz, J.O.; Choyke, P.L.; Cornud, F.; Haider, M.A.; Macura, K.J.; Margolis, D.; Schnall, M.D.; Shtern, F.; Tempany, C.M.; et al. PI-RADS Prostate Imaging–Reporting and Data System: 2015, Version 2. *Eur. Urol.* **2016**, *69*, 16–40. [CrossRef]
8. Turkbey, B.; Rosenkrantz, A.B.; Haider, M.A.; Padhani, A.R.; Villeirs, G.; Macura, K.J.; Tempany, C.M.; Choyke, P.L.; Cornud, F.; Margolis, D.J.; et al. Prostate Imaging Reporting and Data System Version 2.1: 2019 Update of Prostate Imaging Reporting and Data System Version 2. *Eur. Urol.* **2019**, *76*, 340–351. [CrossRef]
9. Moldovan, P.C.; Van den Broeck, T.; Sylvester, R.; Marconi, L.; Bellmunt, J.; van den Bergh, R.C.; Bolla, M.; Briers, E.; Cumberbatch, M.G.; Fossati, N.; et al. What Is the Negative Predictive Value of Multiparametric Magnetic Resonance Imaging in Excluding Prostate Cancer at Biopsy? A Systematic Review and Meta-analysis from the European Association of Urology Prostate Cancer Guidelines Panel. *Eur. Urol.* **2017**, *71*, 618–629.
10. Wagaskar, V.G.; Levy, M.; Ratnani, P.; Moody, K.; Garcia, M.; Pedraza, A.M.; Parekh, S.; Pandav, K.; Shukla, B.; Prasad, S.; et al. Clinical Utility of Negative Multiparametric Magnetic Resonance Imaging in the Diagnosis of Prostate Cancer and Clinically Significant Prostate Cancer. *Eur. Urol. Open Sci.* **2021**, *28*, 9–16. [PubMed]
11. Oerther, B.; Engel, H.; Bamberg, F.; Sigle, A.; Gratzke, C.; Benndorf, M. Cancer detection rates of the PI-RADSv2.1 assessment categories: Systematic review and meta-analysis on lesion level and patient level. *Prostate Cancer Prostatic Dis.* **2022**, *25*, 256–263. [CrossRef]
12. Maggi, M.; Panebianco, V.; Mosca, A.; Salciccia, S.; Gentilucci, A.; Di Pierro, G.; Busetto, G.M.; Barchetti, G.; Campa, R.; Sperduti, I.; et al. Prostate Imaging Reporting and Data System 3 Category Cases at Multiparametric Magnetic Resonance for Prostate Cancer: A Systematic Review and Meta-Analysis. *Eur. Urol. Focus* **2020**, *6*, 463–478. [CrossRef]
13. Ahmed, H.U.; El-Shater Bosaily, A.; Brown, L.C.; Gabe, R.; Kaplan, R.; Parmar, M.K.; Collaco-Moraes, Y.; Ward, K.; Hindley, R.G.; Freeman, A.; et al. Diagnostic accuracy of multi-parametric MRI and TRUS biopsy in prostate cancer (PROMIS): A paired validating confirmatory study. *Lancet* **2017**, *389*, 815–822. [CrossRef]
14. Drost, F.H.; Osses, D.; Nieboer, D.; Bangma, C.H.; Steyerberg, E.W.; Roobol, M.J.; Schoots, I.G. Prostate Magnetic Resonance Imaging, with or Without Magnetic Resonance Imaging-targeted Biopsy, and Systematic Biopsy for Detecting Prostate Cancer: A Cochrane Systematic Review and Meta-analysis. *Eur. Urol.* **2020**, *77*, 78–94. [CrossRef]
15. Hu, J.C.; Assel, M.; Allaf, M.E.; Ehdaie, B.; Vickers, A.J.; Cohen, A.J.; Ristau, B.T.; Green, D.A.; Han, M.; Rezaee, M.E.; et al. Transperineal Versus Transrectal Magnetic Resonance Imaging-targeted and Systematic Prostate Biopsy to Prevent Infectious Complications: The PREVENT Randomized Trial. *Eur. Urol.* **2024**. [CrossRef]
16. Connor, M.J.; Gorin, M.A.; Eldred-Evans, D.; Bass, E.J.; Desai, A.; Dudderidge, T.; Winkler, M.; Ahmed, H.U. Landmarks in the evolution of prostate biopsy. *Nat. Rev. Urol.* **2023**, *20*, 241–258. [CrossRef]
17. Kuru, T.H.; Wadhwa, K.; Chang, R.T.; Echeverria, L.M.; Roethke, M.; Polson, A.; Rottenberg, G.; Koo, B.; Lawrence, E.M.; Seidenader, J.; et al. Definitions of terms, processes and a minimum dataset for transperineal prostate biopsies: A standardization approach of the Ginsburg Study Group for Enhanced Prostate Diagnostics. *BJU Int.* **2013**, *112*, 568–577.
18. Hugosson, J.; Månsson, M.; Wallström, J.; Axcrona, U.; Carlsson, S.V.; Egevad, L.; Geterud, K.; Khatami, A.; Kohestani, K.; Pihl, C.G.; et al. Prostate Cancer Screening with PSA and MRI Followed by Targeted Biopsy Only. *N. Engl. J. Med.* **2022**, *387*, 2126–2137. [CrossRef]
19. Gandaglia, G.; Pellegrino, A.; Montorsi, F.; Briganti, A. Prostate Cancer: Is There Still a Role for Systematic Biopsies? Yes. *Eur. Urol. Open Sci.* **2022**, *38*, 10–11.
20. EAU-EANM-ESTRO-ESUR-ISUP-SIOG Guidelines on Prostate. Cancer. 2024. Available online: http://uroweb.org/guidelines/compilations-of-all-guidelines/ (accessed on 5 June 2024).
21. Wei, J.T.; Barocas, D.; Carlsson, S.; Coakley, F.; Eggener, S.; Etzioni, R.; Fine, S.W.; Han, M.; Kim, S.K.; Kirkby, E.; et al. Early Detection of Prostate Cancer: AUA/SUO Guideline Part II: Considerations for a Prostate Biopsy. *J. Urol.* **2023**, *210*, 154–163.
22. Radtke, J.P.; Schwab, C.; Wolf, M.B.; Freitag, M.T.; Alt, C.D.; Kesch, C.; Popeneciu, I.V.; Huettenbrink, C.; Gasch, C.; Klein, T.; et al. Multiparametric Magnetic Resonance Imaging (MRI) and MRI-Transrectal Ultrasound Fusion Biopsy for Index Tumor Detection: Correlation with Radical Prostatectomy Specimen. *Eur. Urol.* **2016**, *70*, 846–853. [CrossRef]

23. Calio, B.P.; Sidana, A.; Sugano, D.; Gaur, S.; Maruf, M.; Jain, A.L.; Merino, M.J.; Choyke, P.L.; Wood, B.J.; Pinto, P.A.; et al. Risk of Upgrading from Prostate Biopsy to Radical Prostatectomy Pathology-Does Saturation Biopsy of Index Lesion during Multiparametric Magnetic Resonance Imaging-Transrectal Ultrasound Fusion Biopsy Help. *J. Urol.* **2018**, *199*, 976–982. [CrossRef]
24. Hansen, N.L.; Barrett, T.; Lloyd, T.; Warren, A.; Samel, C.; Bratt, O.; Kastner, C. Optimising the number of cores for magnetic resonance imaging-guided targeted and systematic transperineal prostate biopsy. *BJU Int.* **2020**, *125*, 260–269. [CrossRef]
25. Tschirdewahn, S.; Wiesenfarth, M.; Bonekamp, D.; Püllen, L.; Reis, H.; Panic, A.; Kesch, C.; Darr, C.; Heß, J.; Giganti, F.; et al. Detection of Significant Prostate Cancer Using Target Saturation in Transperineal Magnetic Resonance Imaging/Transrectal Ultrasonography-fusion Biopsy. *Eur. Urol. Focus* **2021**, *7*, 1300–1307. [CrossRef]
26. Cetin, S.; Huseyinli, A.; Koparal, M.Y.; Bulut, E.C.; Ucar, M.; Gonul, I.I.; Sozen, S. How many cores should be taken from each region of interest when performing a targeted transrectal prostate biopsy. *Prostate Int.* **2023**, *11*, 122–126. [CrossRef]
27. Saner, Y.M.; Wiesenfarth, M.; Weru, V.; Ladyzhensky, B.; Tschirdewahn, S.; Püllen, L.; Bonekamp, D.; Reis, H.; Krafft, U.; Heß, et al. Detection of Clinically Significant Prostate Cancer Using Targeted Biopsy with Four Cores Versus Target Saturation Biopsy with Nine Cores in Transperineal Prostate Fusion Biopsy: A Prospective Randomized Trial. *Eur. Uro.l Oncol.* **2023**, *6*, 49–5. [CrossRef]
28. Ahmed, H.U. The index lesion and the origin of prostate cancer. *N. Engl. J. Med.* **2009**, *361*, 1704–1706. [CrossRef]
29. Valerio, M.; Anele, C.; Freeman, A.; Jameson, C.; Singh, P.B.; Hu, Y.; Emberton, M.; Ahmed, H.U. Identifying the index lesion with template prostate mapping biopsies. *J. Urol.* **2015**, *193*, 1185–1190. [CrossRef]
30. Russo, F.; Regge, D.; Armando, E.; Giannini, V.; Vignati, A.; Mazzetti, S.; Manfredi, M.; Bollito, E.; Correale, L.; Porpiglia, Detection of prostate cancer index lesions with multiparametric magnetic resonance imaging (mp-MRI) using whole-mount histological sections as the reference standard. *BJU Int.* **2016**, *118*, 84–94. [CrossRef]
31. Paesano, N.; Catalá, V.; Tcholakian, L.; Alomar, X.; Barranco, M.; Trilla, E.; Morote, J. The effectiveness of mapping-targeted biopsies on the index lesion in transperineal prostate biopsies. *Int. Braz. J. Urol.* **2024**, *50*, 119–131. [CrossRef]
32. Epstein, J.I.; Egevad, L.; Amin, M.B.; Delahunt, B.; Srigley, J.R.; Humphrey, P.A.; Grading, C. The 2014 International Society of Urological Pathology (ISUP) Consensus Conference on Gleason Grading of Prostatic Carcinoma: Definition of Grading Patterns and Proposal for a New Grading System. *Am. J. Surg Pathol.* **2016**, *40*, 244–252. [CrossRef]
33. Moore, C.M.; Kasivisvanathan, V.; Eggener, S.; Emberton, M.; Fütterer, J.J.; Gill, I.S.; Grubb Iii, R.L.; Hadaschik, B.; Klotz, L.; Margolis, D.J.; et al. Standards of reporting for MRI-targeted biopsy studies (START) of the prostate: Recommendations from a International Working Group. *Eur. Urol.* **2013**, *64*, 544–552. [CrossRef]
34. Raman, A.G.; Sarma, K.V.; Raman, S.S.; Priester, A.M.; Mirak, S.A.; Riskin-Jones, H.H.; Dhinagar, N.; Speier, W.; Felker, E.; Sisk, A.E.; et al. Optimizing Spatial Biopsy Sampling for the Detection of Prostate Cancer. *J. Urol.* **2021**, *206*, 595–603. [CrossRef]
35. Brisbane, W.G.; Priester, A.M.; Ballon, J.; Kwan, L.; Delfin, M.K.; Felker, E.R.; Sisk, A.E.; Hu, J.C.; Marks, L.S. Targeted Prostate Biopsy: Umbra, Penumbra, and Value of Perilesional Sampling. *Eur. Urol.* **2022**, *82*, 303–310. [CrossRef]
36. Tomioka, M.; Seike, K.; Uno, H.; Asano, N.; Watanabe, H.; Tomioka-Inagawa, R.; Kawase, M.; Kato, D.; Takai, M.; Iinuma, K.; et al. Perilesional Targeted Biopsy Combined with MRI-TRUS Image Fusion-Guided Targeted Prostate Biopsy: An Analysis According to PI-RADS Scores. *Diagnostics* **2023**, *13*, 2608. [CrossRef] [PubMed]
37. Lombardo, R.; Tema, G.; Nacchia, A.; Mancini, E.; Franco, S.; Zammitti, F.; Franco, A.; Cash, H.; Gravina, C.; Guidotti, A.; et al. Role of Perilesional Sampling of Patients Undergoing Fusion Prostate Biopsies. *Life* **2023**, *13*, 1719. [CrossRef] [PubMed]

Disclaimer/Publisher's Note: The statements, opinions and data contained in all publications are solely those of the individual author(s) and contributor(s) and not of MDPI and/or the editor(s). MDPI and/or the editor(s) disclaim responsibility for any injury to people or property resulting from any ideas, methods, instructions or products referred to in the content.

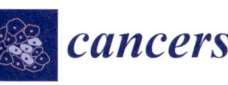

Article

Quantitative Multi-Parametric MRI of the Prostate Reveals Racial Differences

Aritrick Chatterjee [1,2,*], Xiaobing Fan [1], Jessica Slear [1], Gregory Asare [1], Ambereen N. Yousuf [1,2], Milica Medved [1,2], Tatjana Antic [3], Scott Eggener [4], Gregory S. Karczmar [1,2] and Aytekin Oto [1,2]

[1] Department of Radiology, University of Chicago, Chicago, IL 60637, USA; xfan@uchicago.edu (X.F.); ayousuf@uchicagomedicine.org (A.N.Y.); mmedved@uchicago.edu (M.M.); gskarczm@uchicago.edu (G.S.K.); aoto@bsd.uchicago.edu (A.O.)
[2] Sanford J. Grossman Center of Excellence in Prostate Imaging and Image Guided Therapy, University of Chicago, Chicago, IL 60637, USA
[3] Department of Pathology, University of Chicago, Chicago, IL 60637, USA; tatjana.antic@bsd.uchicago.edu
[4] Section of Urology, University of Chicago, Chicago, IL 60637, USA; seggener@bsd.uchicago.edu
* Correspondence: aritrick@uchicago.edu; Tel.: +1-773-702-4467

Simple Summary: This study investigated whether quantitative MRI and histology of the prostate reveal differences between races that can affect diagnosis. The cancer signal enhancement rate (α) on dynamic contrast-enhanced MRI (DCE-MRI) was significantly higher for African Americans (AAs) compared to Caucasian Americans (CAs). The signal washout rate (β) was significantly lower in benign tissue in AAs and significantly elevated in cancers in AAs. However, no significant differences were found for ADC and T2. The ROC analysis showed that the apparent diffusion coefficient (ADC) and T2 are slightly less effective in AAs compared to CAs. DCE significantly improves the differentiation of PCa from benign in AAs (α: 52%, β: 62% more effective in AAs compared to CAs). Histologic analysis showed that cancers have a greater proportion of epithelium and lower lumen in AAs compared to CAs. This study shows that the different races have different quantitative MRI values and histologic makeup. Quantitative DCE-MRI is highly effective and improves PCa diagnosis in African Americans.

Abstract: Purpose: This study investigates whether quantitative MRI and histology of the prostate reveal differences between races, specifically African Americans (AAs) and Caucasian Americans (CAs), that can affect diagnosis. **Materials and Methods:** Patients (98 CAs, 47 AAs) with known or suspected prostate cancer (PCa) underwent 3T MRI (T2W, DWI, and DCE-MRI) prior to biopsy or prostatectomy. Quantitative mpMRI metrics: ADC, T2, and DCE empirical mathematical model parameters were calculated. **Results:** AAs had a greater percentage of higher Gleason-grade lesions compared to CAs. There were no significant differences in the quantitative ADC and T2 values between AAs and CAs. The cancer signal enhancement rate (α) on DCE-MRI was significantly higher for AAs compared to CAs (AAs: 13.3 ± 9.3 vs. CAs: 6.1 ± 4.7 s^{-1}, $p < 0.001$). The DCE signal washout rate (β) was significantly lower in benign tissue of AAs (AAs: 0.01 ± 0.09 s^{-1} vs. CAs: 0.07 ± 0.07 s^{-1}, $p < 0.001$) and significantly elevated in cancer tissue in AAs (AAs: 0.12 ± 0.07 s^{-1} vs. CAs: 0.07 ± 0.08 s^{-1}, $p = 0.02$). DCE significantly improves the differentiation of PCa from benign in AAs (α: 52%, β: 62% more effective in AAs compared to CAs). Histologic analysis showed cancers have a greater proportion ($p = 0.04$) of epithelium (50.9 ± 12.3 vs. 44.7 ± 12.8%) and lower lumen (10.5 ± 6.9 vs. 16.2 ± 6.8%) in CAs compared to AAs. **Conclusions:** This study shows that AAs have different quantitative DCE-MRI values for benign prostate and prostate cancer and different histologic makeup in PCa compared to CAs. Quantitative DCE-MRI can significantly improve the performance of MRI for PCa diagnosis in African Americans but is much less effective for Caucasian Americans.

Keywords: prostate cancer; MRI; racial differences; quantitative; DCE-MRI; African Americans; Caucasian Americans

1. Introduction

Prostate cancer (PCa) is the second most commonly diagnosed cancer in men, with 1 in 8 men diagnosed with it, and is one of the leading causes of cancer-related deaths worldwide [1,2]. PCa incidence and mortality are strongly associated with age, with an average age of diagnosis at 67 years old [3]. In addition to age, there are inherited and genetic risk factors for prostate cancer. Men with a family history of prostate cancer (inherited risk factors), genetic risk factors (germline mutations—BRCA2 gene), and specific race (African ancestry) have an elevated risk for developing prostate cancer [3–6].

Race is an important factor in prostate cancer risk and incidence. African Americans (AAs) have a higher risk and incidence for prostate cancer compared to Caucasian Americans (CAs), while PCa occurs less often in Asian Americans, Hispanics, and Latino men than in non-Hispanic Caucasian men. Specifically for AAs, this higher risk for PCa is likely due to a combination of factors, including underlying tumor differences (aggressiveness), genetic factors, and racial disparities in access to healthcare [5,7–9]. This is a critical problem, especially because PCa detected in AAs is typically more aggressive and advanced compared to PCa in CAs, and the mortality rate for AAs with PCa compared to CAs is significantly higher, even after adjusting for prognostic factors (PSA level, age, clinical stage, and Gleason score) [10,11]. A recent study found that racial disparities were greatest in non-clinically significant low-grade Gleason 6 disease, in which AA men were twice as likely to die of Gleason 6 tumors compared to men from other ethnicities [5]. There are no studies that have clearly established racial differences in prostate cancer biology and physiology that could affect diagnosis using imaging methods.

MRI can play an important role in the diagnosis and management of PCa because it is non-invasive, can reliably detect clinically significant tumors, and can provide information regarding tumor size, location, and grade [12]. The current diagnostic radiology guideline for prostate MRI is the Prostate Imaging—Reporting and Data System (PI-RADS v2.1) [13]. This system utilizes T2-weighted (T2W) imaging and diffusion-weighting imaging (DWI) as the primary sequences, while there is less emphasis on dynamic contrast-enhanced (DCE) MRI, which is used as a secondary sequence. It is also important to note that the PI-RADS guidelines were recommended by a steering committee that is almost entirely comprised of experts from the US and Europe, and most of the published prostate MRI research has been carried out predominantly on Caucasian populations [14]. While the PI-RADS guidelines may provide accurate diagnoses for certain populations (Caucasians), we should not assume that the same solution will work for other patient populations as well, such as African Americans who are at a higher risk for PCa [15] and Asians who are at a lower risk for PCa [16]. This is especially important, as physician decision bias and disparities in access to healthcare exist for AA patients. AAs are less likely to undergo MRI imaging following an elevated prostate-specific antigen (PSA) compared to CAs [17].

A recent study by Mahran et al. [18] showed a racial disparity in the utility of qualitative multi-parametric MRI for the diagnosis of PCa. It is likely that the poor performance in PCa diagnosis is due, in part, to the failure to account for racial differences in prostate and PCa biology and physiology. However, no studies have evaluated the racial differences in biomarkers/parameters from quantitative MRI. Whether PCas have different MR characteristics in AA versus CA men has yet to be determined. MRI-based quantitative biomarkers that account for racial differences could be used to create MRI protocols specifically for different racial groups. Therefore, this study investigates whether quantitative MRI and quantitative histology of the prostate reveal differences between races, specifically African Americans and Caucasian Americans, that can affect diagnosis.

2. Materials and Methods

Study participants: This study involved retrospective analysis of prospectively acquired data. This study was approved by the institutional review board and conducted with informed patient consent, and was HIPPA compliant. Inclusion criteria for the study included patients with known or suspected PCa who underwent prostate mpMRI between

February 2014 and November 2021 at the MRI Research Center prior to undergoing prostatectomy or biopsy. Patients were excluded from the study if they had undergone radiation, chemotherapy, or hormonal therapy, as these therapies can alter the MRI signal. Patients self-reported their race. For further analysis, we chose the two races in this cohort with the largest sample size: Caucasian Americans and African Americans.

MRI Acquisition: Patients underwent a preoperative mpMRI scan on the 3T Philips Ingenia or Achieva MR scanners with the use of a 16-channel phased array coil around their pelvis (Philips, Eindhoven, The Netherlands) and an endorectal coil (Medrad, Warrendale, PA, USA). The MR protocol included T2-weighted images (axial, coronal) and axial multi-echo T2-weighted, diffusion-weighted, and dynamic contrast-enhanced images (DCE). For DCE MR imaging, either gadobenate dimeglumine (Multihance, Bracco, Milan, Italy) or gadoterate meglumine (Dotarem, Guerbet, Paris, France) of 0.1 mmol/kg was injected, followed by a 20 mL saline flush. Since the quantitative MR parameters depend on imaging parameters (b-value, echo time, etc.) [19–21], we chose a cohort where all patients underwent a very similar MRI protocol so that the quantitative parameters could be compared. Typical imaging parameters for the cohort used in this study are described in Table 1.

Table 1. Typical MR imaging parameters.

Imaging Sequence	Pulse Sequence	FOV (mm)	Scan Matrix Size	In-Plane Resolution (mm)	TE (ms)	TR (ms)	Slice Thickness (mm)	Flip Angle (°)
Axial T2W	SE-TSE	180 × 180	450 × 450	0.4 × 0.4	115 or 150	4800	3	90
Multi-echo T2W (T2 mapping)	SE-TSE	160 × 160	212 × 212	0.75 × 0.75	30, 60, 90, 120, 150, 180, 210, 240, 270	7850	3	90
DWI [a]	SE-EPI	180 × 180	120 × 120	1.5 × 1.5	80	5000	3	90
DCE-MRI [b]	T1-FFE	220 × 260	148 × 171	1.5 × 1.5	1.5	3.1	3	10

SE—spin echo; TSE—turbo spin echo; EPI—echo planar imaging; FFE—fast field echo; DCE-MRI—dynamic contrast-enhanced MRI. [a] b-values used: 0, 50, 150, 990, and 1500 s/mm^2. [b] Contrast agent: gadoterate meglumine (Dotarem, Guerbet, France) or gadobenate dimeglumine (Multihance, Bracco, Minneapolis, MN, USA) was injected at a rate of 2.0 mL/s followed by a 20 mL saline flush. The contrast dose amount was based on the patient's weight (0.1 mmol/kg). DCE-MRI T1-weighted images were taken with a temporal resolution of ~6.4 s at 60 dynamic scan points over 6.4 min.

Reference standard: Post imaging, patients with known cancer underwent radical prostatectomy, and patients with suspected cancer underwent 12 core systematic biopsies along with MR-TRUS biopsies based on the assessment of radiologists using the PI-RADS guidelines. The prostatectomy samples were fixed overnight in 10% buffered formalin, transversally sectioned every 4 mm, and then used to create whole-mount histology slides. The biopsy samples from patients with suspected PCa were also processed to create histological slides. All slides were H&E stained and evaluated for cancer by an expert pathologist (TA, 18 years experience). Cancers were outlined, and the Gleason score for each lesion was assigned. The prostatectomy slides were also digitized at 20× magnification using a bright-field Olympus VS120 whole-mount digital microscope (Olympus, Waltham, MA, USA), which was to be used for the subsequent quantitative histologic analyses described later.

MRI analysis: Histology slides and MR images were correlated with the consensus of an expert radiologist, a pathologist, and a medical physicist (AO, TA, and AC with 20, 18, and 9 years of experience, respectively). Only cancers larger than the threshold 5 mm × 5 mm on the prostatectomy specimens and 5 mm on mpMRI for the biopsy cases were used for analysis. Using a custom PCampReviewer module on a 3D slicer [22] and T2-weighted images as a reference, the apparent diffusion coefficient (ADC) and DCE MR images were co-registered and matched with the corresponding histological portions. The axial T2-weighted images were marked by a radiologist (AO, 20 years experience) for sections with a pathologist-verified PCa and benign tissue. The radiologist used the pathology whole-mount histology cancer outlines as a guide to drawing ROIs on the T2-weighted MR images. These ROIs were then transferred to the other mpMRI sequences using 3D Slicer to maintain the same PCa shape and size.

Quantitative analysis of the mpMRI data was performed in MATLAB (MathWorks, Natick, MA, USA) using in-house programs. This code calculated the ADC and quantitative T2 (T2 relaxation or spin–spin relaxation time) maps using a mono-exponential signal decay model on a voxel-by-voxel basis using the diffusion-weighted and multi-echo T2-weighted images. Quantitative analysis of the DCE-MRI data was conducted using the empirical mathematical model (EMM) as described in Fan et al. [23]. The EMM makes no assumptions about the underlying physiology of a tumor and provides quantitative analysis of the kinetics that the radiologist sees on visual assessment. The percent signal enhancement (PSE) curve was calculated using the formula below where S_0 = the baseline signal intensity and $S(t)$ = the DCE signal at time 't'.

$$PSE(t) = \frac{S(t) - S_0}{S_0} \times 100$$

Then, PSE vs. the time curves were analyzed using the following equation

$$PSE(t) = A(1 - e^{-\alpha t})e^{-\beta t}$$

to estimate the amplitude of the relative percent signal enhancement or PSE curve or A, the signal enhancement rate or α, and the signal washout rate or β.

Quantitative histology: We used the digitized H&E stained prostatectomy samples for subsequent quantitative histologic analysis, similar to previous work that validated this approach [24,25]. ROIs were selected using ImageJ (National Institutes of Health, Bethesda, MD, USA) for the confirmed cancers and benign tissue in the peripheral and transition zones corresponding to the ROIs taken for quantitative MRI analysis earlier. Using the "Smart Segment" functionality in Image Pro (Media Cybernetics, Rockville, MD, USA), the images were segmented into the three constituents that make up prostate tissue: stroma, epithelium, and lumen on the basis of color, intensity, morphology, and background. The results were iteratively rectified semi-automatically by the consensus of a pathologist and medical physicist until the final segmented image was determined to have an error of less than 5%. Then, using the "Count" functionality, the percentage volumes of these prostatic tissue components were calculated.

Statistical analysis: Statistical analysis was performed using SPSS v29 (IBM Corporation, Armonk, NY, USA). The difference in measured mpMRI and quantitative histologyy parameters between AAs and CAs was assessed by t-test. The chi-squared test was used to test if the distribution was different between the two cohorts. Receiver operating characteristic (ROC) analysis was used to evaluate the performance of the quantitative mpMRI parameters in diagnosing PCa. The area under the ROC curve (AUC) and ideal cutoff point or the Youdens index with associated sensitivity and specificity were reported. The Z-score test was used to determine the significant difference in the AUC value between the two populations.

3. Results

Patient and lesion characteristics: The final cohort for this study included 47 African American and 98 Caucasian American subjects. No significant difference in age ($p = 0.29$) and PSA level ($p = 0.94$) was found between the AAs (age = 60 ± 7 years, PSA = 8.5 ± 5.9 ng/mL) versus CAs (age = 58 ± 8 years, PSA = 8.6 ± 9.9 ng/mL). The percentage of patients undergoing biopsy and prostatectomy were similar ($p = 0.89$) between the two groups, with 25 biopsies (53%) and 22 prostatectomy cases (47%) for AAs and 51 (52%) and 47 (48%), respectively, in CA patients. AAs (29% Gleason 3 + 3, 36% Gleason 3 + 4, 22% Gleason 4 + 3, 11% Gleason 4 + 4, 2% Gleason 4 + 5) had a greater ($p = 0.01$) percentage of higher Gleason-grade lesions compared to CAs (29% Gleason 3 + 3, 57% Gleason 3 + 4, 11% Gleason 4 + 3,

1% Gleason 4 + 4, 2% Gleason 4 + 5). Detailed patient and lesion characteristics can be found in Table 2.

Table 2. Patient characteristics.

		African Americans	Caucasian Americans	p
Age (years)		60 ± 7	58 ± 8	0.29
PSA (ng/mL)		8.5 ± 5.9	8.6 ± 9.9	0.94
Patients	Biopsy	25 (53%)	51 (52%)	0.89
	Prostatectomy	22 (47%)	47 (48%)	
	Total	47	98	-
ROIs	Cancer	45 (32%)	99 (34%)	0.81
	Benign	94 (68%)	196 (66%)	
	Total	139	295	-
ISUP grade group (Gleason score)	1 (Gleason 3 + 3)	13 (29%)	29 (29%)	0.01
	2 (Gleason 3 + 4)	16 (36%)	56 (57%)	
	3 (Gleason 4 + 3)	10 (22%)	11 (11%)	
	4 (Gleason 4 + 4)	5 (11%)	1 (1%)	
	5 (Gleason 4 + 5)	1 (2%)	2 (2%)	

Quantitative mpMRI results: Representative figures depicting prostate MRI for a typical AA and CA patient in this study are shown in Figures 1 and 2, respectively. We found no significant difference in the quantitative ADC values (Cancers: 1.03 ± 0.32 μm^2/ms in AA vs. 1.07 ± 0.34 μm^2/ms in CA, p = 0.75, Benign: 1.53 ± 0.37 in AA vs. 1.62 ± 0.37 μm^2/ms in CA, p = 0.12) and T2 values (Cancer: 107.5 ± 55.8 ms in AA vs. 99.7 ± 27.7 ms, in CA p = 0.25, Benign: 151.9 ± 96.5 ms for AA, 159.1 ± 73.2 ms for CA, p = 0.70) between AAs and CAs for cancer and benign tissue. However, the ADC and T2 values for cancers were nominally higher in AAs than in CAs despite the higher Gleason-grade cancers in the AA cohort. No significant difference was found between AAs and CAs for these metrics when compared for each Gleason score category. The detailed results for quantitative MRI metrics measured in this study can be found in Table 3.

However, significant differences were found in the quantitative DCE metrics between the two cohorts. The DCE signal enhancement rate (α) was significantly higher in cancerous tissue for AAs compared to CAs (AA: 13.3 ± 9.3 s^{-1} vs. CA: 6.1 ± 4.7 s^{-1}, p < 0.001). Similarly, differences were found across all Gleason scores (Gleason 3 + 3: 10.3 ± 4.4 vs. 4.9 ± 2.9 s^{-1}, p = 0.002; Gleason 3 + 4: 11.7 ± 6.5 vs. 6.7 ± 5.6 s^{-1}, p = 0.04; and Gleason ≥ 4 + 3: 15.6 ± 11.7 and 6.2 ± 2.9 s^{-1}, p = 0.02, respectively) where the signal enhancement rate was significantly higher in AAs than CAs. No significant differences in the signal enhancement rate were found in benign tissue (5.1 ± 4.6 for AA vs. 4.9 ± 2.9 s^{-1} for CA, p = 0.81).

The DCE signal washout rate (β) was significantly lower in the benign tissue of AAs (AA: 0.01 ± 0.09 s^{-1} vs. CA: 0.07 ± 0.07 s^{-1}, p < 0.001) and was significantly elevated in cancer tissue in AAs (AA: 0.12 ± 0.07 s^{-1} vs. CA: 0.07 ± 0.08 s^{-1}, p = 0.02). However, while these differences were found to be significant in cancer ROIs overall for AAs versus CAs, no significant differences were found across the Gleason score categories.

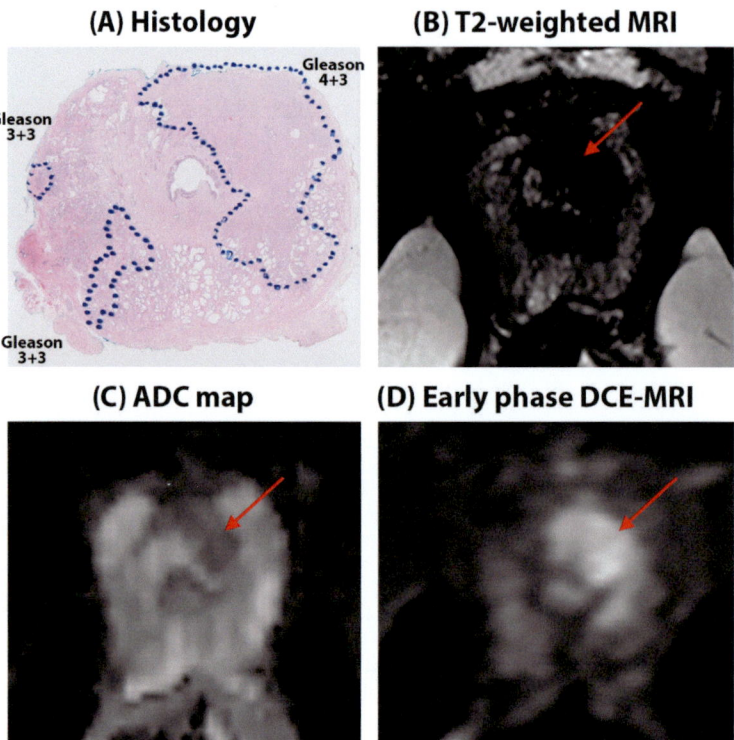

Figure 1. 52-year-old African American patient with Gleason 4 + 3 cancer in the left apex in the peripheral zone (red arrows on MRI). The lesion is seen as a hypo-intense region on the T2W image, T2 (87.9 ± 16.4 ms), and mildly hypo-intense on ADC (1.32 ± 0.20 μm²/ms) maps with early focal enhancement on DCE-MRI, evidenced by high signal enhancement rate (19.3 s^{-1}) and rapid washout rate (0.07 s^{-1}). Surrounding benign tissue in the peripheral zone had ADC = 2.05 ± 0.10 μm²/ms, T2 = 308.9 ± 62.6 ms, α = 2.87 s^{-1}, and β = 0.04 s^{-1}. Another relevant finding is the presence of Gleason 3 + 3 cancers in the right apex. Cancers are outlined in blue on histology sections.

Significant differences in the DCE signal enhancement amplitude (A) were found between different Gleason grades between AAs and CAs, except for Gleason 3 + 4 tumors. In the cancer ROIs overall, the AA signal enhancement amplitude (181.1 ± 44.8%) was significantly higher ($p < 0.001$) compared to CAs (120.2 ± 47.4%). In benign tissue, the amplitude was also significantly higher ($p < 0.001$) for AAs (157.6 ± 82.6%) compared to CAs (126.1 ± 51.2%) for CAs.

Diagnostic performance: The diagnostic performance, as evidenced by the area under the ROC curve, showed that ADC (AA = 0.79 vs. CA = 0.87, $p = 0.21$) and T2 (AA = 0.68 vs. CA = 0.79, $p = 0.15$) were statistically equally effective in differentiation between the benign and cancer tissues in both CAs and AAs. However, it should be noted that the ADC (AUC 10% lower in AAs) and T2 (AUC 16% lower in AAs) were nominally less effective in AAs compared to CAs for the diagnosis of PCa in CAs despite a higher proportion of high-grade cancer in the AA cohort. DCE, on the other hand, significantly improved the differentiation of PCa from benign in AAs but was found to be ineffective in CAs. The area under the ROC curve showed that the DCE signal enhancement rate (AUC for AAs = 0.88 vs. CAs = 0.58, $p < 0.001$) and signal washout rate (AUC for AAs = 0.81 vs. CAs = 0.50, $p < 0.001$) were 52% and 62% significantly more effective ($p < 0.001$), respectively, in diagnosing PCa in AA patients. In addition, the cutoff values based on the Youdens index for the quantitative mpMRI parameters were different for the two cohorts. This leads to a different sensitivity and specificity measured using these cutoffs (the detailed results are in Table 4).

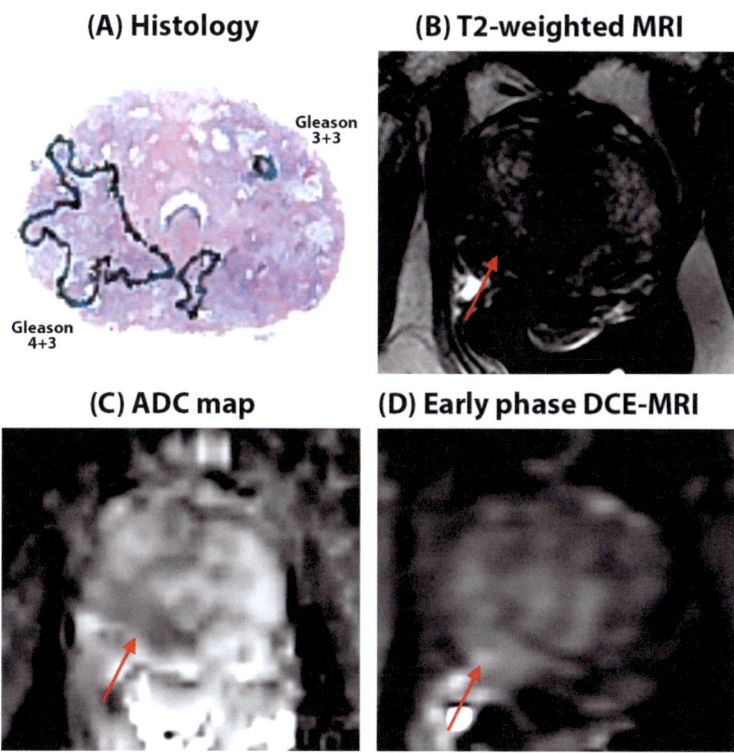

Figure 2. 52-year-old Caucasian American patient with Gleason 3 + 4 cancer in the right apex in the peripheral zone (red arrows on mpMRI). The lesion is seen as a hypo-intense region on the T2W image, T2 (112.4 ± 54.6 ms), and mildly hypo-intense on ADC (0.86 ± 0.12 μm^2/ms) maps with only diffuse early enhancement on DCE-MRI, evidenced by low signal enhancement rate (3.50 s^{-1}) and washout rate (0.03 s^{-1}). Surrounding benign tissue in the peripheral zone had ADC = 1.16 ± 0.19 μm^2/ms, T2 = 125.1 ± 34.5 ms, α = 3.20 s^{-1}, and β = 0.01 s^{-1}. Cancers are outlined in blue on histology sections.

Quantitative histology: The histology analysis for prostate tissue composition showed a similar breakdown of tissue components between AAs (epithelium 28.7 ± 9.0%, lumen 28.8 ± 13.3%, stroma 42.3 ± 10.2%) and CAs (epithelium 29.6 ± 9.2%, lumen 27.4 ± 11.1%, stroma 43.1 ± 12.1%) for benign tissue. However, in cancerous tissue, there were greater proportions of epithelium and lower lumen (p = 0.04) in CAs (epithelium 50.9 ± 12.3%, lumen 10.5 ± 6.9%) compared to AAs (epithelium 44.7 ± 12.8%, lumen 16.2 ± 6.8%), suggesting differences in the histologic makeup and micro-anatomy of PCa in AAs versus CAs. No difference in stroma volume was found for cancer between the two groups. The detailed results are in Table 5.

Table 3. Quantitative mpMRI results from both populations.

		African Americans	Caucasian Americans	p-Value
ADC (μm^2/ms)	Benign	1.53 ± 0.37	1.62 ± 0.37	0.12
	Cancer	1.03 ± 0.32	1.07 ± 0.34	0.75
	Gleason 3 + 3	1.23 ± 0.27	1.22 ± 0.34	0.88
	Gleason 3 + 4	1.12 ± 0.29	1.06 ± 0.33	0.55
	Gleason ≥ 4 + 3	0.85 ± 0.28	0.81 ± 0.27	0.62
T2 (ms)	Benign	151.9 ± 96.5	159.1 ± 73.2	0.70
	Cancer	107.5 ± 55.8	99.8 ± 27.5	0.25
	Gleason 3 + 3	110.8 ± 40.2	112.7 ± 31.2	0.89
	Gleason 3 + 4	108.0 ± 26.5	96.9 ± 26.6	0.31
	Gleason ≥ 4 + 3	104.9 ± 74.5	85.7 ± 12.8	0.35
DCE Signal enhancement amplitude or A (%)	**Benign**	**157.6 ± 82.6**	**126.1 ± 51.2**	**0.01**
	Cancer	**181.1 ± 44.8**	**120.2 ± 47.4**	**<0.001**
	Gleason 3 + 3	**200.9 ± 64.1**	**114.8 ± 28.44**	**<0.001**
	Gleason 3 + 4	158.5 ± 28.2	123.3 ± 55.6	0.18
	Gleason ≥ 4 + 3	**179.1 ± 35.3**	**125.4 ± 35.6**	**0.03**
DCE Signal enhancement rate (s^{-1})	Benign	5.1 ± 4.6	4.9 ± 2.9	0.81
	Cancer	13.3 ± 9.3	6.1 ± 4.7	<0.001
	Gleason 3 + 3	10.3 ± 4.4	4.9 ± 2.9	0.002
	Gleason 3 + 4	11.7 ± 6.5	6.7 ± 5.6	0.04
	Gleason ≥ 4 + 3	15.6 ± 11.7	6.2 ± 2.9	0.02
DCE Signal washout rate (s^{-1})	Benign	0.01 ± 0.09	0.07 ± 0.07	<0.001
	Cancer	0.12 ± 0.07	0.07 ± 0.08	0.02
	Gleason 3 + 3	0.10 ± 0.09	0.04 ± 0.08	0.12
	Gleason 3 + 4	0.11 ± 0.07	0.09 ± 0.08	0.62
	Gleason ≥ 4 + 3	0.13 ± 0.07	0.08 ± 0.03	0.13

Table 4. ROC analysis for differentiating cancer from benign prostate tissue.

	African Americans	Caucasian Americans	p-Value [+]
ADC	AUC = 0.79 95% CI = [0.69, 0.88] Cutoff = 1.00 μm^2/ms Sensitivity = 93% Specificity = 56%	AUC = 0.87 95% CI = [0.81, 0.92] Cutoff = 1.23 μm^2/ms Sensitivity = 89% Specificity = 74%	0.06 *
T2	AUC = 0.68 95% CI = [0.56, 0.78] Cutoff = 136.2 ms Sensitivity = 45% Specificity = 88%	AUC = 0.79 95% CI = [0.72, 0.86] Cutoff = 116.9 ms Sensitivity = 67% Specificity = 80%	0.10 *
DCE Signal enhancement rate	AUC = 0.88 95% CI = [0.81, 0.96] Cutoff = 6.0 s^{-1} Sensitivity = 96% Specificity = 73%	AUC = 0.58* 95% CI = [0.48, 0.69] Cutoff = 6.3 s^{-1} Sensitivity = 38% Specificity = 79%	<0.001

Table 4. Cont.

	African Americans	Caucasian Americans	p-Value [+]
DCE Signal washout rate	AUC = 0.81 95% CI = [0.73, 0.91] Cutoff = 0.02 s^{-1} Sensitivity = 96% Specificity = 52%	AUC = 0.50* 95% CI = [0.39, 0.60] Cutoff = 0.10 s^{-1} Sensitivity = 38% Specificity = 69%	<0.001

* not significant ($p > 0.05$). [+] p-value comparing if performance is better in one population over the other.

Table 5. Quantitative histology results from both populations.

		African Americans	Caucasian Americans	p-Value
Stroma	Benign	42.3 ± 10.2	43.1 ± 12.1	0.44
	Cancer	39.1 ± 11.5	38.6 ± 12.4	0.46
Epithelium	Benign	28.7 ± 9.0	29.6 ± 9.2	0.41
	Cancer	44.7 ± 12.8	50.9 ± 12.3	0.04
Lumen	Benign	28.8 ± 13.3	27.4 ± 11.1	0.38
	Cancer	16.2 ± 6.8	10.5 ± 6.9	0.04

4. Discussion

The results of our study show that the cancer signal enhancement rate (α) of prostate cancer is significantly higher for AAs compared to CAs. The DCE signal washout rate (β) is significantly lower in the benign tissue of AAs and significantly elevated in the cancer tissue of AAs. Due to these differences, DCE significantly improves the differentiation of PCa from benign prostate tissue in AAs but not in CAs. There were no significant differences in the quantitative ADC and T2 values between AAs and CAs. The histologic analysis showed that cancers have a greater proportion of epithelium and lower lumen in CAs compared to AAs. These findings underscore the importance of considering racial differences when developing screening or diagnostic guidelines, especially as bi-parametric MRI is increasingly being proposed for population screening.

PCa detected in AAs tends to have higher Gleason score lesions (more aggressive and advanced, Gleason 4 + 3 and above) compared to sPCa in CAs [10,11]. We found a similar trend in our cohort. Despite having more high-grade lesions in AA, cancers in AAs tend to have very similar ADC and T2 values to CAs. The background benign tissue has a nominally lower T2 and ADC in AAs. This potentially decreases the contrast between the cancer and normal regions in the prostate and can make the cancer less conspicuous. [26] This is evidenced by the lower AUC values for cancer detection using ADC and T2 in AAs. This is consistent with the qualitative mpMRI results from Mahran et al., where the negative predictive value for AAs using mpMRI is lower than that for CAs [18]. Our quantitative histology results showed that cancer in AAs tend to be less dense cancers that have lower epithelium (epithelium is associated with lower ADC and T2 values) and higher lumen (lumen is associated with higher ADC and T2 values), making them less conspicuous on T2 and ADC. In addition, increased inflammation in the tumor microenvironment of prostate cancer in AA men has been noted; this is a driver of disparate clinical outcomes [27]. From the MRI literature, we also know that inflammation affects T2 relaxometry and diffusion measures and can mimic prostate cancer, making cancer diagnosis more difficult [28].

Quantitative DCE-MRI using EMM has been shown to be effective in the diagnosis of PCa [29,30]. The results of this study demonstrate that EMM is even more effective for differentiating PCa from benign tissue in AAs, with the AUCs for α and β being 52% and 62% greater, respectively, in AAs compared to CAs. Numerous studies have noted inherent molecular and biological differences in cancer of AA patients [31,32]. The observed difference in contrast uptake and washout can be attributed to the tumor microenvironment.

Most importantly, neo-angiogenesis or higher microvessel density (MVD) in cancer of AA subjects compared to CAs has been reported [32]. These blood vessels, produced by cancers, allow an increased blood flow, which results in rapid contrast uptake and quick washout. The increased blood flow brings increased oxygen and nutrients that support tumor growth, invasion, and metastatic progression. This is consistent with findings of increased tumor progression and worse clinical outcomes in AAs [33].

This study found that the ideal cutoff values (Youdens index) for the quantitative mpMRI parameters were very different for AAs vs. CAs, showing that the standard diagnostic model is not optimal for AAs. This also suggests the more general hypothesis that quantitative MRI protocols and thresholds for PCa diagnosis for different races should be determined independently. The current PI-RADS v2.1 guideline [13] utilizes T2-weighted (T2W) imaging and diffusion-weighting imaging (DWI) as the primary sequences while giving less emphasis to dynamic contrast-enhanced (DCE) MRI. The results showing that DCE-MRI is highly effective for PCa diagnosis in African Americans suggest that the PI-RADS guidelines should be modified to include a greater emphasis on DCE-MRI for AAs. However, the current results must be verified in a larger cohort in a multi-center setting.

There is growing interest in bi-parametric MRI, with T2-weighted images and DWI images only, leaving out DCE-MRI completely [34,35]. This would have advantages in terms of cost, efficiency, and accessibility [35]. However, the results of this study suggest that bi-parametric MRI would not produce optimal outcomes for African Americans and perhaps also be sub-optimal for other groups that are at risk for aggressive PCa. In addition, there is also increasing interest in quantitative MR imaging and analysis methods and artificial intelligence (AI) tools for PCa diagnosis [36,37]. Machine learning and other AI technologies can only perform well when constructed from representative and appropriate training sets. As such, training sets that do not include relevant information on potential confounding variables such as race may produce biased models. Therefore, bi-parametric MRI, quantitative MRI, and AI tools should be considered substitutes for conventional mpMRI and should account for the racial differences in prostate and PCa physiology and biology. Future studies should compare the current results with results for races or genetic sub-groups with lower incidences of PCa, e.g., the Asian population. MRI-based quantitative biomarkers that account for racial differences could be used to optimize the MRI protocols specifically for different racial groups. This will be a critical step towards personalized PCa screening.

There are a few limitations to this study. First, this study is a retrospective single-center study with a relatively small sample size. Therefore, these results should be validated in a multi-center setting with a large sample size. Second, we used equipment and software from a single MR vendor. Similar studies are needed using scanners from other vendors as hardware and imaging parameters have been shown to affect quantitative MRI results [19–21]. Third, quantitative histology was performed on a subset of patients undergoing prostatectomy. Therefore, due to the small sample size, a comparison of quantitative histology in the two populations stratified by the Gleason score could not be performed. Fourth, we did not have the histological specimens to confirm an increased vessel density in cancers in African Americans, where a DCE analysis suggests increased blood flow [38]. This should be tested in future studies. Fifth, the use of a combined cohort of prostatectomy and biopsy can introduce potential bias while comparing the two populations when stratifying cancers by the Gleason score. This is due to the fact that a significant number of cancers are upgraded when biopsy subjects undergo prostatectomy [39].

5. Conclusions

This study shows that AAs have different quantitative DCE-MRI values for benign prostate and prostate cancer compared to CAs. Quantitative DCE-MRI is highly effective and improves PCa diagnosis in African Americans. These findings should be confirmed in larger studies, but we believe they are particularly important to consider, especially as bi-parametric MRI, which excludes DCE, is attracting increasing interest as a replacement for mpMRI. There are also some quantitative histologic differences between the cancers in AAs and CAs. The results also suggest that other racial groups may have differing prostate biology and physiology and may require specialized MRI screening methods. Racial differences should be taken into account when creating screening or diagnostic guidelines, particularly as bi-parametric MRI is being increasingly suggested for population screening.

Author Contributions: Conceptualization, A.C., G.S.K. and A.O.; methodology, A.C., X.F., T.A., G.S.K. and A.O.; software, A.C. and X.F.; validation, A.C. and A.O.; formal analysis, A.C., X.F., J.S., G.A., M.M., T.A. and A.O.; investigation, A.C., J.S., G.A., A.N.Y., T.A. and A.O.; resources, M.M., T.A., S.E., G.S.K. and A.O.; data curation, A.C., X.F., J.S., G.A., A.N.Y. and T.A.; writing—original draft preparation, A.C. and J.S.; writing—review and editing, A.C., X.F., J.S., G.A., A.N.Y., M.M., T.A., S.E., G.S.K. and A.O; visualization, A.C., T.A., G.S.K. and A.O.; supervision, A.C., T.A., S.E., G.S.K. and A.O.; project administration, A.C., T.A., G.S.K. and A.O.; funding acquisition, G.S.K. and A.O. All authors have read and agreed to the published version of the manuscript.

Funding: This research was funded by the NIH (R01 CA227036, 1R41CA244056-01A1, R01 CA17280, 1S10OD018448-01) and Sanford J. Grossman Charitable Trust.

Institutional Review Board Statement: This study was conducted in accordance with the Health Insurance Portability and Accountability Act and approved by the Institutional Review Board of the University of Chicago.

Informed Consent Statement: The institutional review board approved the study, which involved retrospective analysis of prospectively acquired data. It was conducted with prior informed patient consent and was HIPAA compliant.

Data Availability Statement: In accordance with the institutional review board, the data acquired in this study contain person-sensitive information, which can be shared only in the context of scientific collaborations.

Acknowledgments: We would like to acknowledge and thank the MRI Research Center at the University of Chicago (MRIRC, RRID:SCR_024723) for their assistance in the MRI data acquisition of this study.

Conflicts of Interest: The authors state that they have no conflicts of interest related to the material discussed in this article. Drs. Chatterjee, Oto, and Karczmar have equity in QMIS, LLC, which is unrelated to this study.

References

Siegel, R.L.; Giaquinto, A.N.; Jemal, A. Cancer statistics, 2024. *CA A Cancer J. Clin.* **2024**, *74*, 12–49. [CrossRef] [PubMed]

Sung, H.; Ferlay, J.; Siegel, R.L.; Laversanne, M.; Soerjomataram, I.; Jemal, A.; Bray, F. Global Cancer Statistics 2020: GLOBOCAN Estimates of Incidence and Mortality Worldwide for 36 Cancers in 185 Countries. *CA A Cancer J. Clin.* **2021**, *71*, 209–249. [CrossRef] [PubMed]

American Cancer Society. Key Statistics for Prostate Cancer. Available online: https://www.cancer.org/cancer/types/prostate-cancer/about/key-statistics.html (accessed on 9 April 2024).

Mahal, B.A.; Alshalalfa, M.; Spratt, D.E.; Davicioni, E.; Zhao, S.G.; Feng, F.Y.; Rebbeck, T.R.; Nguyen, P.L.; Huang, F.W. Prostate Cancer Genomic-risk Differences Between African-American and White Men Across Gleason Scores. *Eur. Urol.* **2019**, *75*, 1038–1040. [CrossRef] [PubMed]

Mahal, B.A.; Berman, R.A.; Taplin, M.-E.; Huang, F.W. Prostate Cancer–Specific Mortality Across Gleason Scores in Black vs Nonblack MenProstate Cancer–Specific Mortality Across Gleason Scores in Black and Nonblack MenLetters. *JAMA* **2018**, *320*, 2479–2481. [CrossRef] [PubMed]

US Centers for Disease Control and Prevention (CDC). Prostate Cancer Risk Factors. Available online: https://www.cdc.gov/prostate-cancer/risk-factors/index.html (accessed on 9 May 2024).

Lillard, J.W.; Moses, K.A., Jr.; Mahal, B.A.; George, D.J. Racial disparities in Black men with prostate cancer: A literature review. *Cancer* **2022**, *128*, 3787–3795. [CrossRef]

Krimphove, M.J.; Cole, A.P.; Fletcher, S.A.; Harmouch, S.S.; Berg, S.; Lipsitz, S.R.; Sun, M.; Nabi, J.; Nguyen, P.L.; Hu, J.C.; et al. Evaluation of the contribution of demographics, access to health care, treatment, and tumor characteristics to racial differences in survival of advanced prostate cancer. *Prostate Cancer Prostatic Dis.* **2019**, *22*, 125–136. [CrossRef]

Sundi, D.; Ross, A.E.; Humphreys, E.B.; Han, M.; Partin, A.W.; Carter, H.B.; Schaeffer, E.M. African american men with very low-risk prostate cancer exhibit adverse oncologic outcomes after radical prostatectomy: Should active surveillance still be an option for them? *J. Clin. Oncol.* **2013**, *31*, 2991–2997. [CrossRef]

10. Tolcher, A.; Moinpour, C.M.; Tangen, C.M.; Crawford, E.D.; Thompson, I.M.; Eisenberger, M. Association of African-American Ethnic Background With Survival in Men With Metastatic Prostate Cancer. *JNCI J. Natl. Cancer Inst.* **2001**, *93*, 219–225.
11. Rebbeck, T.R. Prostate Cancer Genetics: Variation by Race, Ethnicity, and Geography. *Semin. Radiat. Oncol.* **2017**, *27*, 3–1 [CrossRef]
12. Bonekamp, D.; Jacobs, M.A.; El-Khouli, R.; Stoianovici, D.; Macura, K.J. Advancements in MR Imaging of the Prostate: From Diagnosis to Interventions. *RadioGraphics* **2011**, *31*, 677–703. [CrossRef]
13. Turkbey, B.; Rosenkrantz, A.B.; Haider, M.A.; Padhani, A.R.; Villeirs, G.; Macura, K.J.; Tempany, C.M.; Choyke, P.L.; Cornud, Margolis, D.J.; et al. Prostate Imaging Reporting and Data System Version 2.1: 2019 Update of Prostate Imaging Reporting and Data System Version 2. *Eur. Urol.* **2019**, *76*, 340–351. [CrossRef] [PubMed]
14. Davenport, M.S.; Shankar, P.R. Biparametric Prostate MRI Influencing Care Patterns in a Caribbean Population. *Radiol Imagin Cancer* **2020**, *2*, e200096. [CrossRef] [PubMed]
15. Powell, I.J. Epidemiology and pathophysiology of prostate cancer in African-American men. *J. Urol.* **2007**, *177*, 444–449. [CrossRef]
16. Chung, B.H.; Horie, S.; Chiong, E. The incidence, mortality, and risk factors of prostate cancer in Asian men. *Prostate Int.* **201** *7*, 1–8. [CrossRef]
17. Abashidze, N.; Stecher, C.; Rosenkrantz, A.B.; Duszak, R.; Hughes, D.R., Jr. Racial and Ethnic Disparities in the Use of Prosta Magnetic Resonance Imaging Following an Elevated Prostate-Specific Antigen Test. *JAMA Netw. Open* **2021**, *4*, 32388. [CrossRef]
18. Mahran, A.; Mishra, K.; Bukavina, L.; Schumacher, F.; Quian, A.; Buzzy, C.; Nguyen, C.T.; Gulani, V.; Ponsky, L.E. Observed raci disparity in the negative predictive value of multi-parametric MRI for the diagnosis for prostate cancer. *Int. Urol. Nephrol.* **201** *51*, 1343–1348. [CrossRef]
19. Peng, Y.; Jiang, Y.; Antic, T.; Sethi, I.; Schmid-Tannwald, C.; Eggener, S.; Oto, A. Apparent Diffusion Coefficient for Prosta Cancer Imaging: Impact of b Values. *Am. J. Roentgenol.* **2014**, *202*, W247–W253. [CrossRef]
20. Feng, Z.; Min, X.; Wang, L.; Yan, X.; Li, B.; Ke, Z.; Zhang, P.; You, H. Effects of Echo Time on IVIM Quantification of the Norm Prostate. *Sci. Rep.* **2018**, *8*, 2572. [CrossRef]
21. Chatterjee, A.; Nolan, P.; Sun, C.; Mathew, M.; Dwivedi, D.; Yousuf, A.; Antic, T.; Karczmar, G.S.; Oto, A. Effect of Echo Times o Prostate Cancer Detection on T2-Weighted Images. *Acad. Radiol.* **2020**, *27*, 1555–1563. [CrossRef]
22. Chatterjee, A.; Tokdemir, S.; Gallan, A.J.; Yousuf, A.; Antic, T.; Karczmar, G.S.; Oto, A. Multiparametric MRI Features an Pathologic Outcome of Wedge-Shaped Lesions in the Peripheral Zone on T2-Weighted Images of the Prostate. *Am. J. Roentgen* **2019**, *212*, 124–129. [CrossRef]
23. Fan, X.; Medved, M.; River, J.N.; Zamora, M.; Corot, C.; Robert, P.; Bourrinet, P.; Lipton, M.; Culp, R.M.; Karczmar, G.S. Ne model for analysis of dynamic contrast-enhanced MRI data distinguishes metastatic from nonmetastatic transplanted rode prostate tumors. *Magn. Reson. Med.* **2004**, *51*, 487–494. [CrossRef] [PubMed]
24. Chatterjee, A.; Gallan, A.; Fan, X.; Medved, M.; Akurati, P.; Bourne, R.M.; Antic, T.; Karczmar, G.S.; Oto, A. Prostate Cance Invisible on Multiparametric MRI: Pathologic Features in Correlation with Whole-Mount Prostatectomy. *Cancers* **2023**, *15*, 582 [CrossRef] [PubMed]
25. Chatterjee, A.; Mercado, C.; Bourne, R.; Yousuf, A.; Hess, B.; Antic, T.; Eggener, S.; Oto, A.; Karczmar, G.S. Validation of prosta tissue composition using Hybrid Multidimensional MRI: Correlation with histology. *Radiology* **2022**, *302*, 368–377. [CrossRef]
26. Hötker, A.M.; Dappa, E.; Mazaheri, Y.; Ehdaie, B.; Zheng, J.; Capanu, M.; Hricak, H.; Akin, O. The Influence of Background Sign Intensity Changes on Cancer Detection in Prostate MRI. *Am. J. Roentgenol.* **2019**, *212*, 823–829. [CrossRef]
27. Lowder, D.; Rizwan, K.; McColl, C.; Paparella, A.; Ittmann, M.; Mitsiades, N.; Kaochar, S. Racial disparities in prostate cance A complex interplay between socioeconomic inequities and genomics. *Cancer Lett.* **2022**, *531*, 71–82. [CrossRef]
28. Rourke, E.; Sunnapwar, A.; Mais, D.; Kukkar, V.; DiGiovanni, J.; Kaushik, D.; Liss, M.A. Inflammation appears as high Prosta Imaging-Reporting and Data System scores on prostate magnetic resonance imaging (MRI) leading to false positive MRI fusio biopsy. *Investig. Clin. Urol.* **2019**, *60*, 388–395. [CrossRef]
29. Chatterjee, A.; He, D.; Fan, X.; Wang, S.; Szasz, T.; Yousuf, A.; Pineda, F.; Antic, T.; Mathew, M.; Karczmar, G.S.; et al. Performanc of ultrafast DCE-MRI for diagnosis of prostate cancer. *Acad. Radiol.* **2018**, *25*, 349–358. [CrossRef]
30. Clemente, A.; Selva, G.; Berks, M.; Morrone, F.; Morrone, A.A.; Aulisa, M.D.C.; Bliakharskaia, E.; De Nicola, A.; Tartaro, A Summers, P.E. Comparison of Early Contrast Enhancement Models in Ultrafast Dynamic Contrast-Enhanced Magnetic Resonan Imaging of Prostate Cancer. *Diagnostics* **2024**, *14*, 870. [CrossRef]
31. Goswami, S.; Sarkar, C.; Singh, S.; Singh, A.P.; Chakroborty, D. Racial differences in prostate tumor microenvironment: Implic tions for disparate clinical outcomes and potential opportunities. *Cancer Health Disparities* **2022**, *6*, 31.
32. Gillard, M.; Javier, R.; Ji, Y.; Zheng, S.L.; Xu, J.; Brendler, C.B.; Crawford, S.E.; Pierce, B.L.; Griend, D.J.V.; Franco, O.E. Elevation Stromal-Derived Mediators of Inflammation Promote Prostate Cancer Progression in African-American Men. *Cancer Res.* **201** *78*, 6134–6145. [CrossRef]
33. Powell, I.J.; Bock, C.H.; Ruterbusch, J.J.; Sakr, W. Evidence supports a faster growth rate and/or earlier transformation to clinical significant prostate cancer in black than in white American men, and influences racial progression and mortality disparity. *J. Ur* **2010**, *183*, 1792–1796. [CrossRef] [PubMed]
34. Schieda, N.; Nisha, Y.; Hadziomerovic, A.R.; Prabhakar, S.; Flood, T.A.; Breau, R.H.; McGrath, T.A.; Ramsay, T.; Morash, C.; Go V. Comparison of Positive Predictive Values of Biparametric MRI and Multiparametric MRI–directed Transrectal US–guide Targeted Prostate Biopsy. *Radiology* **2024**, *311*, e231383. [CrossRef] [PubMed]

5. Greenberg, J.W.; Koller, C.R.; Casado, C.; Triche, B.L.; Krane, L.S. A narrative review of biparametric MRI (bpMRI) implementation on screening, detection, and the overall accuracy for prostate cancer. *Ther. Adv. Urol.* **2022**, *14*, 17562872221096377. [CrossRef]
6. Chatterjee, A.; Dwivedi, D.K. MRI-based virtual pathology of the prostate. *Magn. Reson. Mater. Phys. Biol. Med.* **2024**, *37*, 709–720. [CrossRef]
7. Saha, A.; Bosma, J.S.; Twilt, J.J.; van Ginneken, B.; Bjartell, A.; Padhani, A.R.; Bonekamp, D.; Villeirs, G.; Salomon, G.; Giannarini, G. Artificial intelligence and radiologists in prostate cancer detection on MRI (PI-CAI): An international, paired, non-inferiority, confirmatory study. *Lancet Oncol.* **2024**, *25*, 879–887. [CrossRef]
8. Singanamalli, A.; Rusu, M.; Sparks, R.E.; Shih, N.N.; Ziober, A.; Wang, L.P.; Tomaszewski, J.; Rosen, M.; Feldman, M.; Madabhushi, A. Identifying in vivo DCE MRI markers associated with microvessel architecture and gleason grades of prostate cancer. *J. Magn. Reson. Imaging* **2016**, *43*, 149–158. [CrossRef]
9. Epstein, J.I.; Feng, Z.; Trock, B.J.; Pierorazio, P.M. Upgrading and downgrading of prostate cancer from biopsy to radical prostatectomy: Incidence and predictive factors using the modified Gleason grading system and factoring in tertiary grades. *Eur. Urol.* **2012**, *61*, 1019–1024. [CrossRef]

Disclaimer/Publisher's Note: The statements, opinions and data contained in all publications are solely those of the individual author(s) and contributor(s) and not of MDPI and/or the editor(s). MDPI and/or the editor(s) disclaim responsibility for any injury to people or property resulting from any ideas, methods, instructions or products referred to in the content.

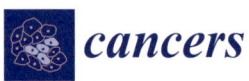

Article

A Deep Learning-Based Framework for Highly Accelerated Prostate MR Dispersion Imaging

Kai Zhao [1,*], Kaifeng Pang [2], Alex LingYu Hung [3], Haoxin Zheng [3], Ran Yan [4] and Kyunghyun Sung [1]

[1] Department of Radiological Sciences, University of California, Los Angeles, CA 92521, USA
[2] Department of Electrical and Computer Engineering, University of California, Los Angeles, CA 92521, USA; kaifengpang@mednet.ucla.edu
[3] Department of Computer Science, University of California, Los Angeles, CA 92521, USA; alexhung96@ucla.edu (A.L.H.); hzheng@mednet.ucla.edu (H.Z.)
[4] Department of Bioengineering, University of California, Los Angeles, CA 92521, USA; ranyan@mednet.ucla.edu
* Correspondence: kz@kaizhao.net

Simple Summary: Nonlinear curve fitting of the pharmacokinetic model to DCE-MRI concentration curves is highly time-consuming. The estimation of highly non-linear dispersion-related parameter in MR dispersion imaging (MRDI) makes the process even more tedious. The fast MRDI (fMRDI) model is proposed to simplify and accelerate the MRDI model by representing the dispersion-applied arterial input function (AIF) as the weighted-sum of a fast and a slow population-based AIFs. A deep learning-based two-stage inference method is proposed to accelerate quantitative MRDI. The deep learning model makes a initial estimation of the parameters directly from the concentration curves and the parameters is then refined by a number of iterative optimization.

Abstract: Dynamic contrast-enhanced magnetic resonance imaging (DCE-MRI) measures microvascular perfusion by capturing the temporal changes of an MRI contrast agent in a target tissue, and it provides valuable information for the diagnosis and prognosis of a wide range of tumors. Quantitative DCE-MRI analysis commonly relies on the nonlinear least square (NLLS) fitting of a pharmacokinetic (PK) model to concentration curves. However, the voxel-wise application of such nonlinear curve fitting is highly time-consuming. The arterial input function (AIF) needs to be utilized in quantitative DCE-MRI analysis. and in practice, a population-based arterial AIF is often used in PK modeling. The contribution of intravascular dispersion to the measured signal enhancement is assumed to be negligible. The MR dispersion imaging (MRDI) model was recently proposed to account for intravascular dispersion, enabling more accurate PK modeling. However, the complexity of the MRDI hinders its practical usability and makes quantitative PK modeling even more time-consuming. In this paper, we propose fast MR dispersion imaging (fMRDI) to effectively represent the intravascular dispersion and highly accelerated PK parameter estimation. We also propose a deep learning-based, two-stage framework to accelerate PK parameter estimation. We used a deep neural network (NN) to estimate PK parameters directly from enhancement curves. The estimation from NN was further refined using several steps of NLLS, which is significantly faster than performing NLLS from random initializations. A data synthesis module is proposed to generate synthetic training data for the NN. Two data-processing modules were introduced to improve the model's stability against noise and variations. Experiments on our in-house clinical prostate MRI dataset demonstrated that our method significantly reduces the processing time, produces a better distinction between normal and clinically significant prostate cancer (csPCa) lesions, and is more robust against noise than conventional DCE-MRI analysis methods.

Keywords: MRI; DCE-MRI; dispersion imaging; prostate cancer; deep learning; transformer

1. Introduction

Tumor development is associated with the growth of new irregular microvessels, a process known as angiogenesis [1]. The angiogenic microvessels are characterized by leaky vessel walls and, therefore, a high degree of permeability [2]. Increased microvascular density and permeability [3,4] have been reported in several studies to correlate with cancer aggressiveness [5,6]. In the prostate, increased microvascular density and permeability can be characterized by dynamic contrast-enhanced magnetic resonance imaging (DCE-MRI) [7–9]. Prostate DCE-MRI acquires a time series of T1-weighted images before, during, and after the injection of a contrast agent (CA, e.g., gadolinium-based contrast agents [10]). After the bolus injection, the CA leaks across the vascular wall to the extracellular extravascular space (EES), resulting in MR enhancement uptakes. The temporal variations in MRI signals provide information about permeability and angiogenesis, which can be quantified as the leakage from the vessel to EES [2,11]. As illustrated in Figure 1, there is a noticeable disparity in tissue-concentration curves between clinically significant prostate cancer (csPCa) and normal prostate tissue. The concentration curve in the tumor exhibits a significantly faster uptake compared to normal tissue, which could be attributed to leaky vascular walls in the tumor [1,12].

Quantitative DCE-MRI analysis aims to extract physiological parameters that reflect the permeability and microvascular density of the underlying tissue. This can be achieved by fitting a pharmacokinetic (PK) model to time-series concentration curves using nonlinear least square (NLLS) curve fitting. The standard Tofts model [10] is a widely used PK model for prostate DCE-MRI. It formulates the tissue concentration, $C_t(t)$, as the convolution of the plasma concentration (or arterial input function, AIF), $C_p(t)$, and the tissue impulse response. The tissue-imposed response is characterized by several PK parameters related to microvascular permeability, such as the forward volume transfer constant, K^{trans}, and the flux rate, k_{ep}.

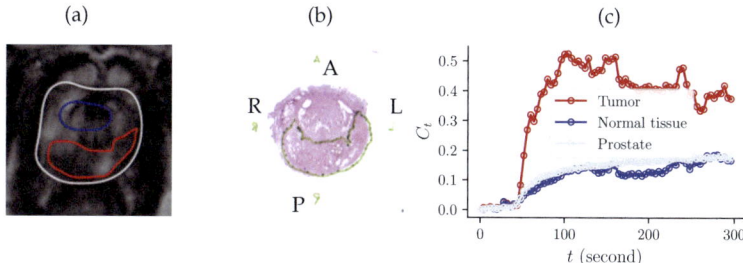

Figure 1. (a) T2-weighted MR slice with annotated prostate (gray), normal tissue (blue), and a tumor (red). (b) Corresponding histopathology image. (c) Concentration curves for the three regions demonstrate different contrast-agent concentrations, $C_t(t)$, in three different ROIs.

The accurate quantification of AIFs is critical to PK modeling [9,13–15]. Either the AIF can be measured [15,16] or a population-based AIF can be assumed [14,17,18]. Measuring the AIF necessitates a high temporal resolution [19] and a wide dynamic range [20], which is not always possible in clinical settings [21]. In practice, a population-based AIF is often assumed across patients [14,17,18]. In particular, a line of AIF models [14,22,23] has been proposed to achieve an analytical solution to the convolution in the Tofts model and, therefore, simplify the computation. However, the AIF has a significant impact on the estimated PK parameters [9,16], and location-specific AIFs can improve the estimation [15,16].

Recently, the MR dispersion imaging (MRDI) model [24] has been introduced to characterize the intravascular dispersion of the contrast agent. The quantification of intravascular dispersion inherently yields dispersion-related parameters, which were calculated by applying voxel-wise dispersion to AIFs within the prostate [8,24,25]. Adopting the dispersion-applied AIF in PK modeling is considered to improve the model and parameter estimation precision [8,24–28]. In addition, dispersion-related parameters can be used to identify clinically significant prostate cancer (csPCa) [26,29]. The dispersion-related parameters, either alone [8,24,26] or combined with other PK parameters [25,28], have been shown to be indicative of prostate cancer. In Turco's study [8], dispersion-related parameters were suggested to outperform other DCE parameters for prostate cancer detection.

The modified MRDI (mMRDI) model [25] simplified the dispersion-applied AIF as a convolution parameterized by a dispersion-related parameter. mMRDI effectively approximates the dispersion-applied AIFs with a reduced number of parameters. Additionally, the dispersion-related parameter in the mMRDI model can be used alongside the volume transfer constant (K^{trans}) for prostate cancer diagnosis [25]. However, mMRDI still requires an AIF estimation, and the high computation of MRDI and mMRDI limits their practical usability in prostate DCE-MRI.

Performing voxel-wise curve fitting of the nonlinear PK model can be time-consuming [30–32], particularly in prostate DCE-MRI, where a large number of voxels have to be processed in a multi-slice scan. Murase proposed using the simplex method [33] to efficiently fit the PK model, but this method requires a fixed AIF and low sampling interval, limiting its practical application. Moreover, the iterative fitting of a nonlinear PK model is susceptible to noise and initialization [34–37], and improper initializations could result in suboptimal results. Several workarounds have been used to find proper initializations [25,35]. Dikaios et al. [35] iteratively searched for the initialization values until convergence was achieved. Sung [25] repeated the optimization with ten different initializations and then selected the best results to avoid improper initializations. However, these workarounds introduced extra computation time.

Recently, a line of studies has demonstrated the advantages of using deep learning for fast PK parameter estimation [37–39]. Bliesener et al. [37] used deep Bayesian learning to estimate both PK parameters and uncertainty in longitudinal brain DCE-MRI. Ottens et al. [38] compared various deep-learning models for PK parameter estimation in pancreatic cancer detection. Witowski et al. [39] proposed a supervised method that directly localizes lesions from DCE-MRI data for breast cancer detection. These methods either rely on a particular AIF [37,38] or annotated data [38,39], making them less flexible. Directly estimating the parameters of a complicated PK model from noisy DCE-MRI data is challenging, and the estimations of these methods are less accurate [37,38].

In this paper, we introduce the fast MR dispersion imaging (fMRDI) model, which further simplifies the MRDI model and simulates the dispersion-applied AIF with the weighted sum of AIFs of different dispersion levels. An AIF with greater dispersion exhibits a slow uptake, and an AIF with less dispersion has a fast uptake [25]. Therefore, fMRDI can effectively account for voxel-wise AIFs with various dispersion levels, yielding estimates of the intravascular dispersion-related parameter. As shown in Figure 2, the weighted-sum AIF (Figure 2d) essentially mimics various dispersion levels in MRDI and mMRDI (Figure 2a,b) in a simple form.

The benefits of fMRDI are twofold. First, it resembles intravascular dispersion in a simpler form, making it easier to optimize and less computational. Second, as suggested by [8,24,25], the dispersion parameter λ can be used along with other pharmacokinetic (PK) parameters to differentiate between csPCa and normal tissue. Experiments on clinical prostate DCE-MRI data showed that λ improves the overall csPCa detection accuracy (see Section 3.2).

To accelerate the time-consuming NLLS while maintaining its accuracy, we propose a deep-learning-based, two-stage framework for PK parameter estimation. In particular, we used a transformer-based [40] deep neural network to achieve a coarse estimation of the PK parameters, which serve as the initializations of subsequent NLLS. With the coarse estimation as the initialization, the subsequent NLLS converges in a few steps, significantly reducing the iteration steps compared to plain NLLS. Our network is trained with synthetical DCE-MRI concentration curves. We also designed two data-preprocessing modules, the time series pyramid, and sinusoidal normalization, to improve the robustness of our model against the noise in DCE-MRI dynamic images.

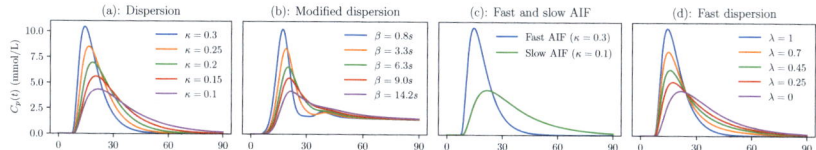

Figure 2. Various dispersion-applied AIFs in MRDI [24] (**a**) and mMRDI [25] (**b**) with different dispersion parameters, κ and λ. Our fMRDI model uses a weighted sum of slow and fast AIFs (**c**) to achieve similar AIFs of different dispersion levels (**d**).

We conducted experiments on our in-house clinical DCE-MRI dataset of 182 patients who underwent prostate MRI prior to radical prostatectomy. We used linear discriminant analysis (LDA) to test the precision of csPCa detection using PK parameters from different methods. Additionally, we experimented with digital reference objects (DROs) to test the quality and robustness of different fitting methods. The experimental results show that our fMRDI model produces PK parameters with high contrast between csPCa and normal tissue. Our method is significantly faster and more robust against noise compared to NLLS. In summary, our method enjoys the following favorable properties:

1. The fMRDI model resembles intravascular dispersion with a simple linear combination of slow and fast AIFs, which is easier to optimize and requires less computation.
2. The dispersion parameter in our fMRDI model can be used to differentiate csPCa from normal tissue and improve the overall performance of csPCa identification (Section 3.2).
3. The two-stage estimation framework is fast, accurate, flexible, and more robust against noise and initializations. It does not restrict the form of the AIF or the sampling interval. It operates significantly faster than NLLS and achieves more accurate fitting results.

The rest of this paper is organized as follows. Section 2.1 briefly reviews the standard Tofts model, as well as the MRDI and mMRDI models, and then it introduces our fast MRDI model. Section 2 systematically presents our deep learning-based framework for PK parameter estimation. Section 2.6 outlines the clinical DCE-MRI data used in our experiments. Section 3 reports and analyzes the experimental results and makes comparisons against other methods. Sections 4 and 5 examine the motivation and background context of our study, discusses potential limitations and areas for future work, and presents concluding remarks.

2. Methods and Materials

2.1. From Tofts Model to Fast MRDI Model

We first review the classical Tofts PK model, the modified MRDI model, and our fast MRDI model.

2.1.1. The Tofts Model

In the classical Tofts model [10], the tissue contrast agent (CA) concentration, denoted as C_t, is represented by the convolution of the plasma CA concentration, also known as arterial input function (AIF), denoted as C_p, and the tissue impulse response:

$$C_t(t) = \int_0^t \underbrace{C_p(\tau - t_0)}_{\text{AIF}} \cdot \underbrace{K^{trans} e^{-k_{ep} \cdot (t-\tau)}}_{\text{impulse response}} d\tau, \tag{1}$$

where t_0 is the bolus arrival time. The tissue impulse response, $K^{trans} e^{-k_{ep} \cdot t}$, is characterized by a few PK parameters, such as the volume-transfer constant (K^{trans}, measured in $\min^{-1}$) and the rate constant (k_{ep}, measured in $\min^{-1}$), that are relevant to tissue perfusion and permeability. K^{trans} and k_{ep}, which measure the CA wash-in and wash-out, are commonly associated with csPCa, as indicated by studies such as those of Fütterer et al. [41],

Kuenen et al. [24], and Sung et al. [25]. They can enhance lesion visibility, according to the Prostate Imaging Reporting and Data System (PI-RADS) [7].

The classical Tofts model assumes that the intravascular contribution to the measured MR signal is negligible, and constant population-averaged AIFs [17,18,20,38,42] are often used for PK modeling. A recent work [38] assumed an exponential-based AIF obtained from [42] so that the convolution in Equation (1) could be analytically expressed and the estimation could be simplified. However, assuming a constant AIF across all patients is not accurate because AIFs may vary across patients or locations within the same patient.

2.1.2. MRDI and mMRDI: Dispersion-Applied AIFs

The MR dispersion model [24] considered the intravascular dispersion in the prostate and, therefore, characterized location-specific AIFs within the prostate. In particular, the dispersion-applied AIF is formulated as follows:

$$C_p(t)^{MRDI} = \alpha \sqrt{\frac{\kappa}{2\pi(t-t_0)}} \exp\left(\frac{-\kappa(t-t_0-\mu)^2}{2(t-t_0)}\right) \quad (2)$$

where κ (s^{-1}) is the dispersion parameter, μ is the average transit time from the injection site to the detection site, and α is the integral of C_t.

In the modified MRDI (mMRDI) model [25], the dispersion-applied AIF is formulated as the convolution of a vascular transport function:

$$C_p^{mMRDI} = C_p(t) \otimes \frac{1}{\lambda} e^{-\frac{t}{\lambda}} \quad (3)$$

where $C_p(t)$ is a population-based AIF and λ is the dispersion coefficient, (e.g., the larger the λ, the larger the dispersion). mMRDI characterizes intravascular dispersion with a simpler formulation and improves practical usability.

However, the convolution in Equation (3) is nonlinear, and the dispersion parameter λ in the denominator typically makes optimization more challenging. This is because the denominator introduces nonlinearity and discontinuity, which can complicate and destabilize the optimization process [43].

To address optimization instability, mMRDI [25] repeatedly performed NLLS with various initializations and selected the best fit for each voxel. This process can be very tedious, and it takes hours to process a patient.

2.1.3. fMRDI: Fast MRDI Model

To simplify the formulation and ease the optimization, we propose the fast MRDI (fMRDI) model, which represents dispersion-applied AIF as the weighted sum of two AIFs of different dispersion levels.

$$\tilde{C}_p^{fMRDI} = \lambda C_p^1(t-t_0) + (1-\lambda) C_p^2(t-t_0), \quad (4)$$

where C_p^1 is the 'fast' AIF with less dispersion, and C_p^2 is the 'slow' AIF with greater dispersion. $\lambda \in [0,1]$ is the intravascular dispersion parameter balancing the summation. To achieve AIFs of different dispersion levels, we used the dispersion-applied AIF (C_p^{MRDI} in Equation (2)) with $\kappa = 0.3$ s^{-1}, $\mu = 10$ s as the fast AIF (C_p^1), and $\kappa = 0.1$ s^{-1}, $\mu = 20$ s as the slow AIF (C_p^2). The two bases were selected according to the distribution of the two parameters in our dataset. Specifically, we calculated μ and κ using the MRDI model on our dataset, and we chose $\kappa = 0.3$ s^{-1}, $\mu = 10$ s and $\kappa = 0.1$ s^{-1}, $\mu = 20$ s because more than 99% of the voxel parameters fell within this range. Figure 2a,b,d demonstrate various dispersion-applied AIFs in MRDI [24], mMRDI [25], and our fMRDI model. Figure 2c shows the slow and fast AIFs in fMRDI. Figure 2d shows that the AIFs with various dispersion factors can be similarly achieved using fMRDI with different λ parameters.

As per previous studies [8,25], AIFs in csPCa exhibit lower dispersion levels and faster uptakes, whereas the AIFs of normal tissue have higher dispersion levels and slower uptakes. Therefore, λ is close to 1 in csPCa and close to 0 in normal tissue. This is verified by the results in Figures 11, 13 and 14.

With the simplified dispersion-applied AIF, we can derive the fast MRDI model by substituting Equation (4) for Equation (1):

$$C_t(t) = \int_0^t \underbrace{\left(\lambda C_p^1 + (1-\lambda)C_p^2\right)}_{\text{weighted-sum AIF}} \cdot K^{trans} e^{-k_{ep}(t-\tau)} d\tau, \tag{5}$$

The derivation of Equation (5) is similar to Equation (4) in [8]. The fMRDI model in Equation (5) provides an assessment of the microvascular architecture using the dispersion parameter λ and of microvascular permeability using K^{trans} and k_{ep}.

For simplicity of notation, we will refer to the fast MRDI model as follows:

$$C_t = \text{fMRDI}(P) \tag{6}$$

where $P = \{K^{trans}, k_{ep}, t_0, \lambda\} \in \mathbb{R}_+^4$ are the PK parameters to be estimated. The PK parameter estimation from DCE-MRI data is essentially the reverse of Equation (6), which estimates P from C_t.

We introduce our deep learning-based framework for PK parameter estimation. In Section 2.2, we introduce our overall pipeline, including training and inference workflows. Then, we describe how we synthesize data for model training in Section 2.3. Section 2.4 provides a brief description of the model architecture and training procedure. And finally, we introduce two novel data-preprocessing modules, sinusoidal normalization and time series pyramid, in Section 2.4.2. The overall workflows are illustrated in Figure 3.

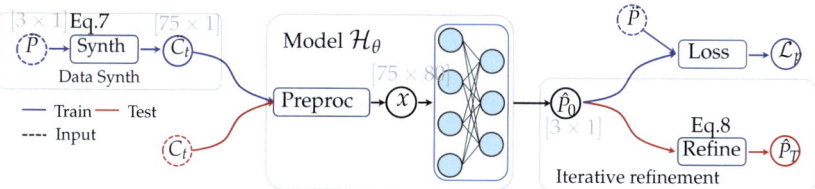

Figure 3. The overall workflow of our proposed method for PK parameter estimation. Circles represent the processed data, and the shape of the data is indicated near each circle. In training, the random PK parameter P is sampled to synthesize the training data, C_t. After preprocessing, the data are fed into the neural network, and the estimated parameter $\hat{P}_0$ is compared against P for loss computation. In testing, the model takes clinical DCE-MRI concentration curves, C_t, as input, and the subsequent 'iterative refinement' takes $\hat{P}_0$ as the starting point of the iteration and refines the initial estimation with NLLS.

2.2. Overall Workflows

Our overall workflows are illustrated in Figure 3. In general, there are three key components in our framework: a data synthesis module, the neural network (NN), and iterative refinement. During training, the data synthesis module synthesizes the training curves $\ddot{C}_t$ for the NN. The NN takes the synthetical data $\ddot{C}_t$ as input and predicts the initial coarse estimation $\hat{P}_0$, which is then compared against the randomly sampled parameter $\ddot{P}$ that was used for data synthesis. There are two crucial preprocessing modules in the neural network model that will be described in detail in Section 2.4.2. During inference, the model takes clinical concentration curves as input and produces the initial estimation of the PK parameters, $\hat{P}_0$, which is then refined via iterative curve fitting. The final PK parameters after iterative refinement are denoted as $\hat{P}_T$, where $T = 20$ is the number of iterations.

2.3. Training Data Synthesis

Let $C_t \in \mathbb{R}_+^L$ be the time-series DCE-MRI data, where L is the length of the time series ($L = 75$ in our case). Our model learns a mapping from the time series to the PK parameters:

$$P = \mathcal{H}(C_t)$$

where $\mathcal{H}(\cdot) : \mathbb{R}_+^L \to \mathbb{R}_+^4$ is our model, which learns to reverse Equation (6). To train such a model, we need the pairwise training datasets $\{(C_t^1, P^1), (C_t^2, P^2), ..., (C_t^N, P^N)\}$. Instead of collecting training datasets from clinical scans, we designed a data synthesis framework to generate unlimited training data for our neural network. A similar synthesis process was also used in [38,44] for model training. In general, the data synthesis module is composed of three steps.

1. Sample random PK parameters K^{trans}, k_{ep}, t_0, and λ from designated distributions.
2. Synthesize smooth time series using the fMRDI formulated in Equation (5).
3. Add Gaussian noise to the smooth time series to close the gap between synthetical and real data.

The overall pipeline of data synthesis is illustrated in Figure 4, the distributions used to sample PK parameters are shown in Figure 5, and some examples of synthetical and real data can be found in Figure 6.

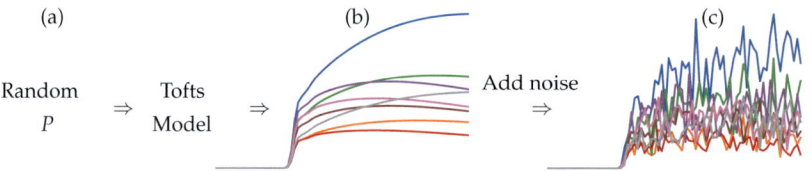

Figure 4. The pipeline of concentration-curve synthesis. (**a**) random PK parameters are sampled to synthesize smooth curves (**b**). (**c**) noise is added to the smooth curves to simulate the real cases.

(1) Sample PK parameters As a statistical model, the predictions from neural networks are highly related to the statistics of the training data. To mimic the statistics of real DCE-MRI data, we first analyzed the PK parameters of clinical DCE-MRI cases. Specifically, we estimated the PK parameters of 20 patients using conventional nonlinear least square (NLLS) curve fitting and then constructed their histograms. As shown in Figure 5 (top), the histograms closely resemble specific beta distributions. Then, we used beta distributions, to sample PK parameters for data synthesis. The beta distributions used for data synthesis are shown in Figure 5 (bottom). t_0 is sampled from a uniform distribution, $U(0, 0.1)$.

(2) Synthesize smooth time series Let $\dot{P}$ be the randomly sampled PK parameter from designated distributions. We synthesized a smooth time series using the fMRDI model defined in Equation (6). Example smooth curves are demonstrated in Figure 4.

(3) Add Gaussian noise In order to close the gap between real and synthetical time series, we added random Gaussian noise to the smooth time series. The data synthesis can be formulated as follows:

$$\ddot{C}_t(t) = \left\lfloor \text{fMRDI}(\dot{P}) \times (1 + \mathcal{N}(0, \gamma)) \right\rfloor, \quad (7)$$

where $\mathcal{N}(0, \gamma) \in \mathbb{R}^L$ is the Gaussian noise with zero mean, and the standard deviation of the noise is randomly sampled to achieve synthetical data with a signal-to-noise ratio (SNR) between 4 and 32. $\lfloor \cdot \rfloor$ is the rectification operator that rectifies all values less than zero as zero because the DCE-MRI data are always greater than zero. Example noisy synthetical curves are demonstrated in Figure 6.

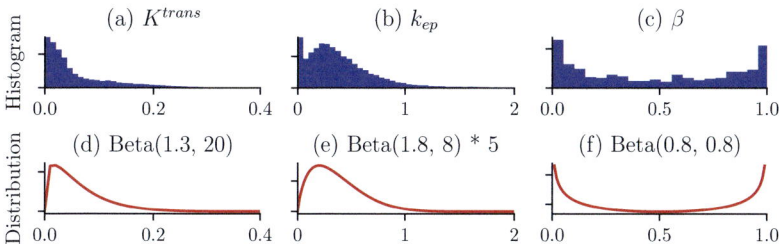

Figure 5. Histograms of pharmacokinetic parameters (**top**) and distributions used for data synthesis (**bottom**).

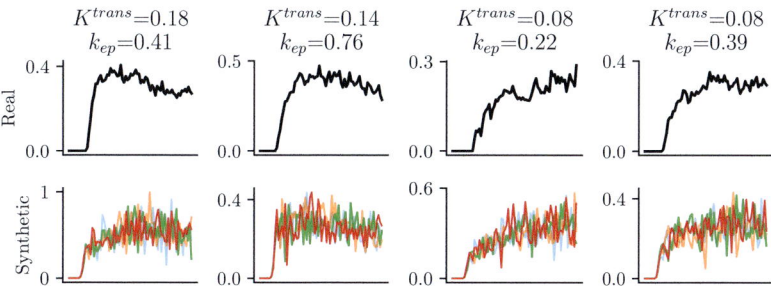

Figure 6. Real (**top**) and synthetic concentration curves (**bottom**). Curves of each column share the same PK parameters.

2.4. Model Training Workflow

2.4.1. Model Architecture

We utilized the transformer architecture, which is renowned for its outstanding performance using sequential data. We used a three-layer transformer network, and a similar network has been widely used in computer vision [45] and natural language processing [40]. As shown in Figure 7, the input time-series C_t first passes through preprocessing modules, which is detailed in Section 2.4.2, after which the position embedding is added. Afterward, three transformer layers process the high-dimensional inputs, and then a feedforward network produces the predictions. Rectified linear unit (ReLU) activation is used in the end to ensure positive predictions. ReLU is an activation function that retains positive input values while setting negative inputs to zero. The detailed architecture of a transformer layer is illustrated on the left side of Figure 7.

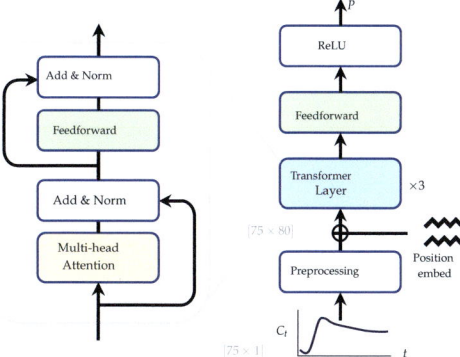

Figure 7. The architecture of the transformer neural network used in our experiments. ReLU activation was used in the last of the network to ensure positive estimations.

2.4.2. Preprocessing for Robust Neural Networks

The time-series dynamic images are noisy, unnormalized, and presented as one-dimensional time series, posing challenges in training deep neural networks. We propose two crucial data preprocessing modules to stabilize the training process and enhance the model's performance. The purposes of the two preprocessing modules are threefold:

1. To enhance the model's robustness against the noise and capture information at various scales.
2. To increase the data dimension and project the one-dimensional time series into high-dimensional space.
3. To normalize the time series data into a fixed range with zero mean and constant variance.

The experimental results in Table 1 demonstrate that the proposed preprocessing modules improve the estimation accuracy.

Table 1. Squared errors are assessed by incrementally adding model components. The baseline model, labeled 'NN + Parker', represents the NN model without the proposed preprocessing or WS AIF.

NN + Parker AIF	0.6681 ± 2.2015
+WS AIF	0.5982 ± 1.9383
+Pyramid	0.5892 ± 1.9012
+Sinusoidal	0.5801 ± 1.8729
+Refine	0.4114 ± 1.5181

Without a loss of generality, let $\mathbb{R}^{L \times D}$ be the shape of input to each preprocessing module, where L is the length of the time series and D is the feature dimension (which is one for C_t). The preprocessing modules process each row of the input independently and generate N rows based on a single input row, leading to output data with the shape of $\mathbb{R}^{L \times (D \cdot N)}$. N is the scaling factor, which means that the module increases the feature dimension of the input by a certain factor.

The scaling factor is set to $N = 5$ in the time series pyramid, and $N = 16$ is used in the sinusoidal normalization. In general, the DCE-MRI time series has a shape of $L \times 1$ and will be sequentially processed through the time-series pyramid and the sinusoidal normalization. The data shape after the time-series pyramid is $L \times 5$, and after sinusoidal normalization, the shape becomes $L \times 80$.

Time series pyramid Our first preprocessing module is the *time series pyramid*, which convolves C_t with kernels of different scales to depress the noise and capture information at various contextual scales. This operation draws deep inspiration from the seminal concept of an image pyramid [46] in image processing and computer vision. The image pyramid provides a flexible and convenient multiresolution format that closely resembles the multi-scale processing in the human perceptual system.

We construct the time series pyramid, similar to the image pyramid, by convolving the original time series with Gaussian kernels of different variances (sigmas). Let K^σ be the Gaussian kernel, where σ is the variance of the kernel, and $2\sigma + 1$ is the kernel size. The convolved time series is denoted as $C_t^\sigma = C_t \otimes K^\sigma$. We construct the time series pyramid by stacking several convolutions. Let N be the number of Gaussian kernels used to construct the pyramid. For arbitrary input $C_t \in \mathbb{R}+^{L \times D}$, where L is the length of the time series, and D is the feature dimension, the dimension of the pyramid would be $C_t \in \mathbb{R}+^{L \times (D \times N)}$.

In practice, we used $N = 5$ different kernels with $\sigma = 0, 2, 4, 8, 10$, where $\sigma = 0$ corresponds to the original signal. The time series pyramid takes raw DCE-MRI data as input (with shape $L \times 1$), and the output shape is $L \times 5$. Example pyramids and corresponding Gaussian kernels can be found in Figure 8.

Sinusoidal normalization Data normalization is critical to deep neural networks. Normalization techniques rescale input data in a fixed range with zero mean and constant variance, which accelerates the convergence and improves the performance [47,48] of deep neural networks.

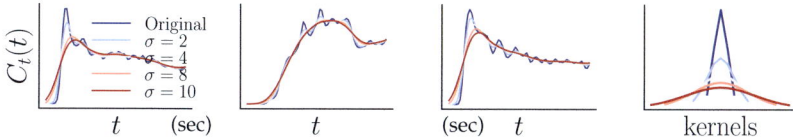

Figure 8. The time series pyramid with different σ and respective Gaussian kernels.

In DCE-MRI, the magnitude range exhibits significant variations among time series from different locations. Additionally, the intensity values are highly biased and follow a long-tail distribution. We employ simple sinusoidal functions to normalize the input data into a fixed range of $[-1, 1]$. To normalize the input data while maintaining an injective mapping between the input and output, we utilize a series of sinusoidal functions with different frequencies: $[\sin(1w_0 x), \cos(1w_0 x), ..., \sin(8w_0 x), \cos(8w_0 x)]$. where $w_0 = 2\pi/100$ is the fundamental frequency. The sinusoidal functions project the input into higher-dimensional spaces and ensure a one-to-one mapping between the input and output. The signals after the sinusoidal functions fall within a fixed range and possess a zero mean with constant variance. The input to sinusoidal normalization is the output of the time series pyramid, which has a shape of $L \times 5$. The output of sinusoidal normalization has a shape of $L \times 80$.

2.4.3. Model Training

Let $\mathcal{H}_\theta(\cdot)$ be our model parameterized by θ. Our model is trained with synthetical data introduced in Section 2.3. Suppose $(\ddot{C}_t, \ddot{P})$ is the training data pair; the model takes $\ddot{C}_t$ as input and predicts $\hat{P}_0$, as shown in Figure 3. Our model is trained by minimizing the L_1 discrepancy between the estimated PK parameter $\hat{P}_0$ and the one used for data synthesis $\ddot{P}$: $\mathcal{L} = |\hat{P} - \ddot{P}|$, where $\mathcal{L}$ is the training loss. The loss is computed separately for each sample (concentration curve) and then averaged across the batch. We use the ADAM algorithm to optimize the neural network. The model is trained for 100,000 iterations with a fixed learning rate of 10^{-4} and a batch size of 256.

2.5. Model Inference Workflow

2.5.1. From MRI Signal to CA Concentration

Before any pharmacokinetic analysis can take place, the CA concentration, C_t, has to be calculated from the MRI signal enhancement. T_1 is reduced from the pre-contrast value T_{10} by the presence of CA: $\frac{1}{T_1} = \frac{1}{T_{10}} + r_1 C$, where r_1 is the relaxivity, and usually an in vitro value of $4.5 \text{ L} \times \text{mmol}^{-1} \times \text{s}^{-1}$ is used. The CA concentration C_t can be expressed as $C_t(t) = (\frac{1}{T_1(t)} - \frac{1}{T_{10}})/r_1$, where T_{10} is the precontrast T_1 that can be obtained from the variable flip-angle method [25,49].

2.5.2. Initial Coarse Estimation

Given the CA concentration curve, $C_t(t)$, the initial estimation of the PK parameters is made via the neural network: $\hat{P}_0 = \mathcal{H}(C_t)$.

2.5.3. Coarse-to-Fine via Iterative Fitting

We refine the initial estimation, $\hat{P}_0$, with iterative curve fitting. Specifically, we use the square of the residual as the objective and iteratively update $\hat{P}_\tau$ to minimize the discrepancy between fitting and the observation using gradient descent. The PK parameter $\hat{P}_\tau$ is updated based on the following rule:

$$\hat{P}_{\tau+1} = \hat{P}_\tau - \gamma \frac{\partial \left| \text{fMRDI}(\hat{P}_\tau) - C_t \right|^2}{\partial \hat{P}_\tau} \tag{8}$$

where τ is the step index, and $\gamma = 0.01$ is the learning rate (or step size). In our experiments, Equation (8) converges significantly faster than starting from scratch. The running time, starting from the initial estimation and starting from scratch, can be found in Table 2.

Table 2. Squared errors, iterations required to converge, and per-patient times of different fitting methods and PK models. fMRDI achieves significantly lower errors compared to the Tofts model, and the two-stage fitting method also outperforms NLLS in both fitting errors and running time.

Fitting Method	Ottens	NLLS			NN + NLLS Refine		
PK Model	Tofts + Exp	Tofts + Parker	MRDI	fMRDI	Tofts + Parker	MRDI	fMRDI
Error	0.6723 ±2.2209	0.6184 ±1.9867	0.4272 ±1.6618	0.4261 ±1.5687	0.5917 ±2.1221	0.4175 ±1.5212	0.4114 ±1.5181
Iterations	N/A	200	300	200	20	50	30
Time (per-patient)	109 s	480 s	644 s	480 s	71 s	115 s	176 s

2.6. Study Population and DCE-MRI Data

Our retrospective study was conducted in compliance with the 1996 Health Insurance Portability and Accountability Act (HIPAA) and approved by the Institutional Review Board (IRB) of the University of California, Los Angeles, with a waiver of the requirement for informed consent. All methods were performed in accordance with the relevant guidelines and regulations.

The study cohort was derived from patients who underwent 3T mpMRI exams prior to robotic-assisted radical prostatectomy at a single academic center between December 2010 and July 2019. Patients with prior radiotherapy or partial prostate resection, and those with technical limitations, were excluded from the study. The complete dataset comprised 182 patients who had whole-mount histopathology (WMHP) conformed with prostate cancer lesions (PCa). Patient-specific, 3D-printed prostate molds were used to hold the surgically excised prostate glands in the same orientation observed in vivo MRI.

All imaging, including T2W, DWI, and DCE-MRI, was performed on several 3T MRI scanners using a pelvic phased-array coil. The DCE-MRI protocol consisted of precontrast T1(T10) mapping and dynamic imaging. The variable flip angle (VFA) imaging was used for T10 mapping for the conversion of signal intensity to contrast agent concentration. With a temporal resolution of 4~5 s, dynamic 3D images were acquired before, during, and after a single-dose injection of gadopentetate dimeglumine (Magnevist; Bayer, Wayne, NJ, USA) at a dose of 0.1 mmol/kg through an eripheral vein at a rate of 2 mL/s via a mechanical injector. Additionally, 6~10 precontrast frames (total acquisition time to be around 24~50 s), and a total of 75 frames were acquired sequentially without a delay between acquisitions. The last frame of precontrast acquisitions was located by searching for the largest gradient concentration curves in the first 15 frames. All concentration values in precontrast acquisitions were set to zero for ease of optimization. A total of 1500 images were acquired, and the dimension of the DCE-MRI data was $160 \times 160 \times 20 \times 75$, where 160×160 is the in-plane resolution, 20 is the number of slices, and 75 is the number of frames.

Each prostate MRI scan was reviewed by genitourinary (GU) radiologists (10+ years of clinical prostate MRI reading experience) as part of the standard clinical care, following the PI-RADS v2.1 guideline. All clinically significant PCa (csPCa) lesions were initially annotated on T2-weighted MRI, and later, research fellows (K.Z. and K.P.) supervised by an MRI scientist (K.S. with 15+ years of experience analyzing DCE-MRI) refined the regions of interest (ROIs) on DCE-MRI using MRI and WMHP as references.

3. Experiments and Results

We compared our method with conventional NLLS and a deep learning-based method [38]. We used the CNN architecture for the baseline deep learning-based method [38] due to its simplicity and higher performance. For NLLS, we used the trust region-refective algorithm with a step tolerance of 10^{-2}, a function tolerance of 10^{-3}, and a minimum gradient change of 0.1. All implementations were based on the PyTorch framework.

3.1. Running Time and Quality of Fitting

3.1.1. Running Time and Fitting Errors

We first compared the quantitative fitting errors and running time. Let $\hat{P}$ be the estimated PK parameter; then, we used Equation (6) to get the fitting curves, $\hat{C}_t = \text{MRDI}(\hat{P})$. The fitting quality was quantified according to the squared error between the reconstructed and the original concentration curves: $error = |C_t - \hat{C}_t|^2$. We measured the per-patient processing time on an Intel(R) Xeon(R) W-2123 CPU@3.60GHz CPU. For each iterative method, we stopped the iteration if the loss reduction was less than 0.5% for five consecutive iterations. The fitting error, average number of iterations, and running time are summarized in Table 2.

In Table 2, 'NLLS', 'NN', and 'NN + NLLS refine' denote different curve-fitting methods, where 'NN' denotes the direct estimation of PK parameters with neural networks, and 'NN + NLLS refine' denotes our proposed two-stage method that refines the NN estimation with subsequent NLLS iterations. When starting from scratch, NLLS was performed for 240 iterations. When using 'NN + NLLS', we ran 20 iterations.

In general, with the same fitting method, such as NLLS, our fMRDI model significantly reduced the fitting error compared to the Tofts model with the Parker AIF. Furthermore, using the same PK model, such as Tofts + Parker, the two-stage 'NN + NLLS' fitting method significantly reduced the running time by a factor of more than four while achieving a lower fitting error. These results demonstrate the strong efficiency and accuracy of our method in PK modeling.

The running time and fitting error are summarized in Table 2, and some example fitting results are in Figure 9.

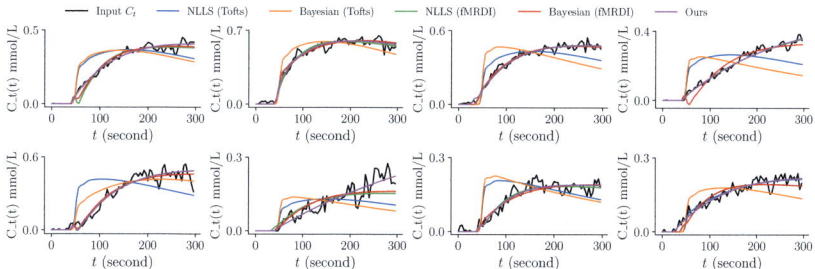

Figure 9. Example fitting results of different methods. Methods with Parker AIF do not fit data with slow uptakes well. fMRDI model achieves the best overall fittings that match the data points the best.

We also tested the fitting error with different components: the *fMRDI model*, the *NN inference + iterative refinement pipeline*, and the two *preprocessing modules*. The results in Table 1 clearly demonstrate that each individual component contributes incrementally to the quality of fitting and plays a role in our method. The results in Table 1 were confirmed with the paired *t*-test with $p < 0.01$ to verify the effectiveness of each component.

3.1.2. Compared with MRDI and mMRDI

We compared the fitting quality of our method with MRDI and mMRDI and evaluated their robustness. In particular, we fit our fMRDI, MRDI [24], and mMRDI [25] models with NLLS and various numbers of random initializations. For each model, we repeated NLLS with different random initializations and then selected the best fitting for each voxel. The model is considered more stable if it achieves higher performance with fewer repeats.

As shown in Figure 10, fMRDI is more stable and less susceptible to initialization, as it achieves a lower error with fewer repeats. This is because the linear weighted sum AIF is much simpler than MRDI and mMRDI, making it easier to optimize. When a saturated number of repeats is performed, the three models perform similarly, with MRDI slightly better than the other two, as MRDI has more free parameters.

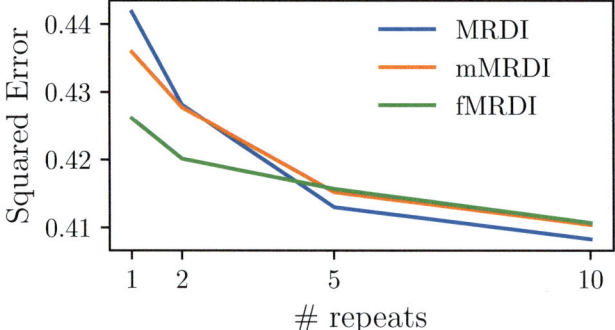

Figure 10. The squared error of fitting with different numbers of repeats. We performed NLLS fitting various times with random initializations and then picked the best fitting for each voxel.

3.2. csPCa Lesions with K^{trans}

We compared PK parametric maps derived from different methods and evaluated the contrast of PK parameters in csPCa and normal tissue. Both the conventional NLLS and the baseline deep learning-based method with exponential AIF [38] were included for comparison. We first visualized different parametric maps and then quantitatively compared the parameter values in csPCa and normal tissue. Linear discrimination analysis (LDA) was lastly performed to quantitatively evaluate the discrimination of csPCa from normal tissue.

Since the volume-transfer constant (K^{trans}, min^{-1}) [7] and the dispersion parameter λ [8,24,25] were considered to be indicative of csPCa, we only visualized K^{trans} and λ.

3.2.1. Qualitative Visualization of K^{trans} Maps.

Figure 11 displays several exemplary K^{trans} maps (1–5 columns), along with corresponding histopathological maps (last column) that indicate the tumor locations. 'Ours' represents the fMRDI model with the *NN+refine* fitting method. Each row represents maps of the same patient generated using different methods. Since the tumor spans across multiple slices, we visualized the maximum intensity projection (MIP) of two to five consecutive slices. The specific number of slices in MIP varies among patients. As shown in Figure 11, our K^{trans} maps generally have better contrast in identifying csPCa lesions and are less noisy than other methods.

3.2.2. Quantitative Comparison of Tissue Contrast

In addition to qualitative visualization, we quantitatively analyzed the contrast between the csPCa and normal tissue. The quantitative analysis was conducted on the ROI-averaged parametric maps.

Due to severe misalignment in the prostate tumor delineation between T2W images and DCE [50], the annotations on T2W could not be propagated to K^{trans}. Instead, we annotated csPCa lesions on K^{trans} maps with histopathological images as a reference. As shown in Figure 12, we first annotated hyperintensity regions as lesions (red ROIs) with T2W and histopathological images as references. To ensure a fair comparison that did not favor our method, the ROIs were annotated on K^{trans} maps derived from NLLS with the standard Tofts model and Parker AIF and then propagated to other parameter maps (e.g., $ktrans$, k_{ep}, and λ maps derived from different methods). In addition to lesions, we also annotated the corresponding ROI of normal tissue (blue ROIs in Figure 12) in the same zone (transitional zone or peripheral zone) for contrast analysis. The ROI annotation could be biased due to being annotated on Ktrans maps. However, it is not biased toward any specific DCE-MRI analysis method, ensuring that the comparisons are fair.

After the annotation, ROI-averaged PK parameters are calculated for ROI-wise quantitative evaluations. For each patient, we annotate a representative lesion and a corresponding normal tissue. There are 135 lesions in the peripheral zone (PZ) and 47 lesions in the transitional zone (TZ).

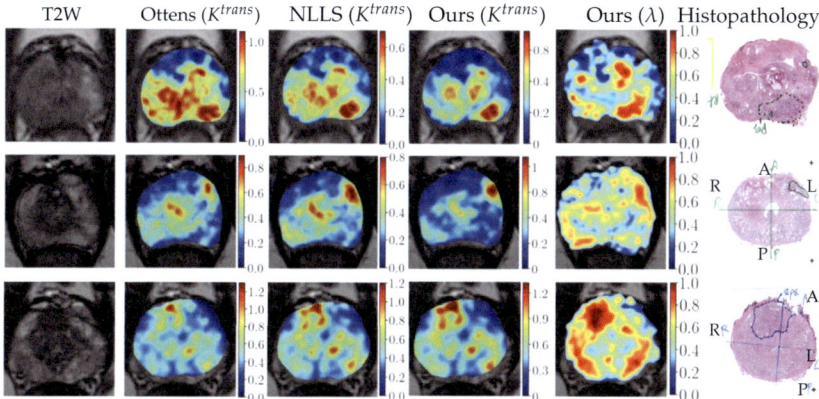

Figure 11. Visualization of PK parametric maps generated using different methods and the beta K^{trans} maps proposed in our study. The T2-weighted images are used as a background, and corresponding histopathological images are provided in the right-most column for reference to identify the location of the lesion.

The scatter plot in Figure 13 depicts the K^{trans} and λ values of csPCa and normal tissue in PZ and TZ. Not unexpectedly, as demonstrated in Figure 13a,b, csPCa ROIs generally have larger values for both K^{trans} and λ. csPCa and normal tissue are more separable when simultaneously considering K^{trans} and λ, as demonstrated in Figure 13c.

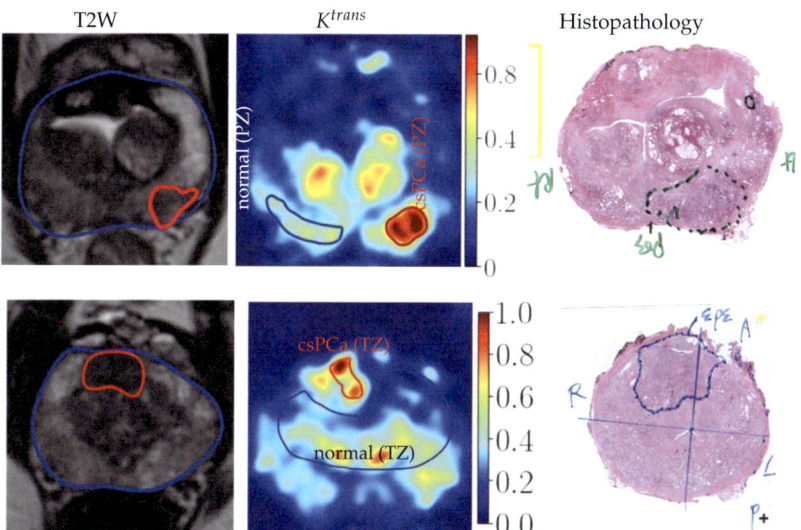

Figure 12. Illustration of how we annotated csPCa and normal tissue ROIs on K^{trans} maps. Using the T2W annotations and the histopathological images as references, we annotated hyperintensity areas on K^{trans} maps as lesions, and then we annotated normal tissue in the same zone on the K^{trans} maps.

We applied the linear discriminant analysis (LDA) to quantitatively analyze the discrimination of csPCa from normal tissue in PZ and TZ. The ROI-averaged PK parameters (K^{trans}, k_{ep}, t_0, and λ) values derived from different methods were used for the classification of csPCa from normal tissue. The performance of each DCE-MRI analysis model was evaluated using 5-fold cross-validation, and the average results are reported. Sensitivity and specificity values were calculated from the cut-off points on the ROC curves by maximizing Youden's index. The specificity-0sensitivity curves are shown in Figure 14, and the specificity, sensitivity, and AUC values are summarized in Table 3. In particular, in Figure 14, for 'NLLS', we employed the Tofts model with K^{trans}, k_{ep}, t_0 as the input to the LDA model. For 'Ours', we used our fMRDI model and K^{trans}, k_{ep}, t_0 as the input. And for 'Ours (with λ)', we used the fMRDI model with K^{trans}, k_{ep}, t_0, and λ as the input.

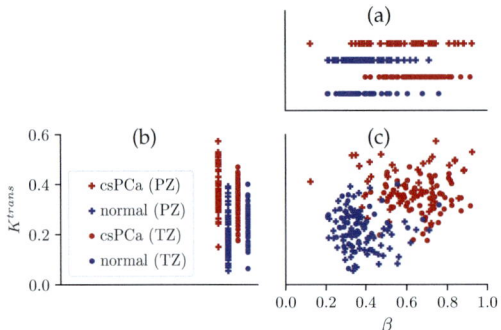

Figure 13. Scatter plot of ROI-averaged K^{trans} and λ values in TZ and PZ. When applied individually, both λ (**a**) and K^{trans} (**b**) can differentiate csPCa lesions from normal tissue, while K^{trans} performs better. When applied jointly (**c**), the lesions and normal tissue can be better separated.

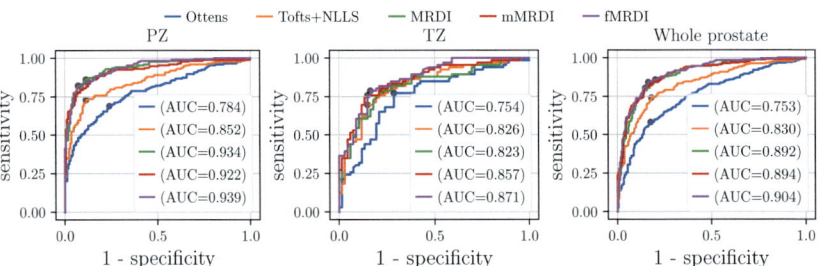

Figure 14. Specificity–sensitivity curves of csPCa detection in the peripheral zone (PZ), the transitional zone (TZ), and the whole prostate (PZ+TZ). Different colors represent different pharmacokinetic models. 'Ours' represents the fMRDI model with NN + refine curve fitting.

Table 3. Sensitivity, specificity, and AUC values of different methods in the PZ, the TZ, and the whole prostate. The sensitivity and specificity values are calculated by maximizing Youden's index.

Method	Ottens [38]			NLLS+Tofts+Parker			MRDI			fMRDI (Ours)		
Zone	PZ	TZ	PZ+TZ	PZ	TZ	PZ+TZ	PZ	TZ	PZ+TZ	PZ	TZ	PZ+TZ
AUC	0.784	0.754	0.753	0.852	0.826	0.830	0.934	0.823	0.892	0.939	0.871	0.904
1 - specificity	0.236	0.288	0.179	0.109	0.152	0.183	0.109	0.227	0.204	0.069	0.167	0.167
Sensitivity	0.690	0.773	0.583	0.730	0.697	0.742	0.862	0.788	0.858	0.822	0.788	0.842

The results in Figure 14 and Table 3 demonstrate the following: (1) using the same PK parameters, our fMRDI model ('Ours') improves the csPCa detection performance compared to Ottens and NLLS. (2) the detection performance is further improved by using λ as additional input ('Ours (with λ)'). The AUCs in Table 3 were compared via DeLong's test with a 95% confidence interval, and the specificity and sensitivity were compared via the Chi-squared test ($p < 0.05$).

Figure 15 demonstrates the ROCs of different combinations of PK parameters. When applied individually, K^{trans} performed the best, followed by λ and k_{ep}. And t_0 can barely differentiate csPCa from normal tissue. When applied individually, the inclusion of λ noticeably improved the performance.

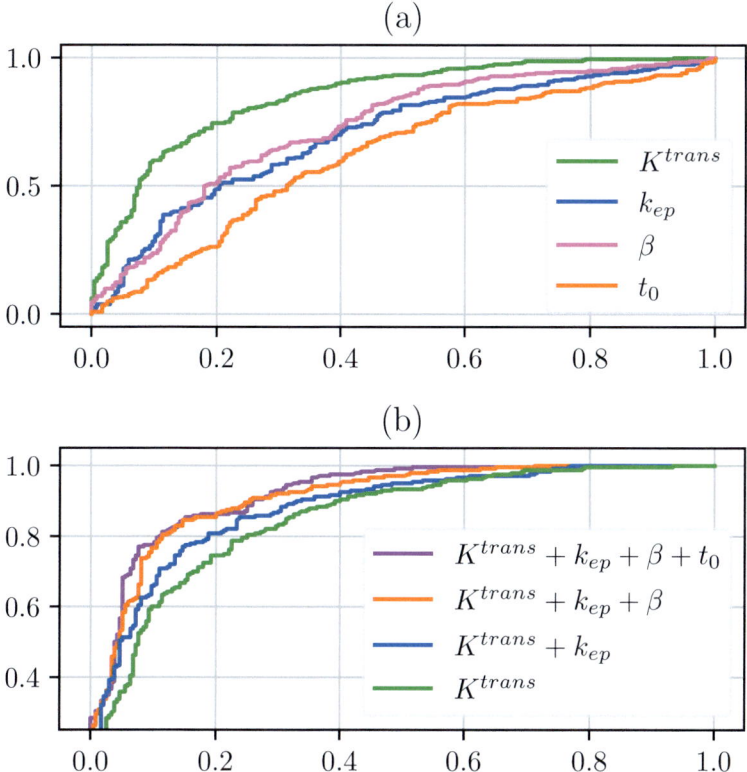

Figure 15. ROC curves from LDA analysis were generated for the entire prostate (PZ + TZ) using various combinations of PK parameters. (**a**) When analyzed individually, K^{trans} exhibited the highest performance, followed by λ and then k_{ep}. Conversely, t_0 demonstrated the lowest performance and could only differentiate lesions from normal tissue to a limited extent. (**b**) When analyzed collectively, excluding t_0 barely impacted the performance, and the inclusion of λ moderately improved the performance.

3.3. Validation with Digital Reference Objects

Our two-phase inference pipeline is more resilient to noise because the neural network provides a stable initial state for subsequent iterative refinement. In this experiment, we tested the robustness of different methods against data noise using digital reference objects (DROs). The DROs are synthetical input data that are generated similarly to our training data using Equation (7) with two exceptions: (1) we used the plain Tofts model without λ for DRO synthesis for a fair comparison; (2) the parameters K^{trans} and k_{ep} were sampled from uniform distributions $U(0, 0.4)$ and $U(0, 2)$ to cover a wider range of possible inputs. The noise level of DROs was controlled via γ in Equation (7), whereas a larger γ indicates a higher level of noise. We synthesized 100K DROs that are grouped into $100 = 10 \times 10$ discrete bins according to their K^{trans} and k_{ep} values. Let $\hat{P} \in \mathbb{R}^2 = \{\hat{K^{trans}}, \hat{k_{ep}}\}$ be the estimated parameter and P be the 'ground-truth', which was used to synthesize the corresponding DRO; the estimation error is calculated as follows: $error = \frac{|\hat{P}-P|^2}{|P|^2}$. We compared the fitting error of NLLS and our method under different noise levels in Figure 16. For example, the first bin comprises 1000 DROs with K^{trans} ranging from 0 to 0.1 and k_{ep} ranging from 0 to 0.2.

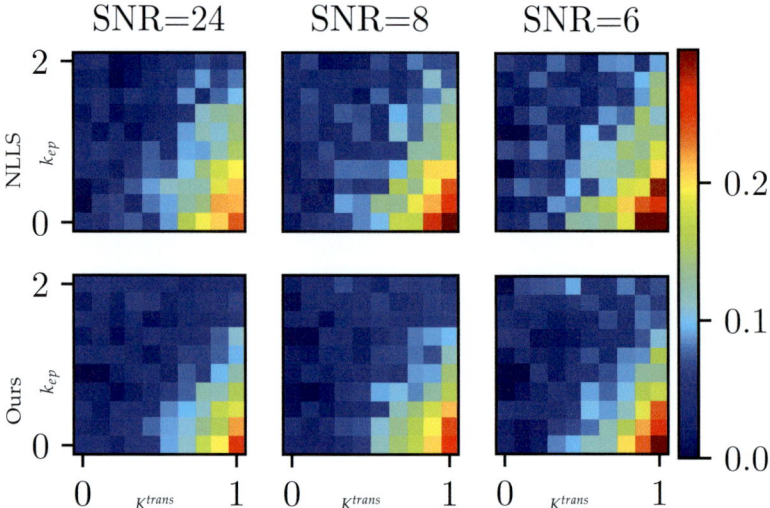

Figure 16. The fitting error of different methods under different noise levels using DROs. The heat maps show fitting errors at different K^{trans} and k_{ep} bins. The table summarizes the average errors at different noise levels.

In the heat maps of Figure 16, we calculated the average estimation error within each bin. We conducted the paired sample t-test to verify that our method achieves lower fitting errors. And the p-values ($p < 0.001$) confirmed the significance of our hypothesis. In general, the fitting errors surge with a higher level of noise. Under the same noise level, the fitting errors increase with the raising of K^{trans} and k_{ep}. Our approach consistently provides more accurate results by reducing estimation errors, especially when dealing with higher levels of noise. This showcases the robustness and superiority of our method in handling noisy data.

4. Discussion

This study introduced the fast MRDI model and a deep learning-based, two-stage framework for efficient prostate DCE-MRI analysis. Existing quantitative DCE-MRI analysis methods rely on the time-consuming, iterative optimization of a pharmacokinetic (PK) model, e.g., the Tofts model [10]. PK modeling requires the characterization of arterial input functions (AIFs), and a population-based AIF is often assumed across patients. MR dispersion imaging (MRDI) [24] characterizes the intravascular dispersion of the contrast agent, yielding voxel-specific AIFs with various dispersion levels. The mMRDI [25] approximates the dispersion-applied AIFs with fewer dispersion-related parameters. The formulation of these models is highly nonlinear and poses difficulty in optimization.

In this study, we first introduced the fast MR dispersion imaging (fMRDI) model that simulates the dispersion-applied AIFs using a weighted sum of a slow and a fast AIF and that effectively forms location-specific AIFs with various dispersion levels, yielding estimates of the intravascular dispersion-related parameter λ. fMRDI is much simpler and easier to optimize compared to MRDI and mMRDI. Additionally, we proposed a deep-learning-based, two-stage framework for PK parameter estimation. We used a transformer-based neural network (NN) to perform a coarse estimation of the PK parameters, and then we used iterative NLLS to further refine the coarse estimation. The

NN estimation essentially serves as an initialization for the subsequent NLLS, and our two-stage framework significantly speeds up and enhances the accuracy of PK modeling. A data-synthesis module was designed to generate synthetic data for neural network training. Two data-preprocessing modules were proposed to enhance the stability of the neural network.

Experimental results on our in-house clinical prostate MRI dataset demonstrated that the fMRDI model improves the fitting accuracy, and the dispersion parameter λ is able to improve the differentiation of csPCa from normal tissue. Our two-stage, deep learning-based method significantly accelerates the quantitative DCE-MRI analysis with more stable estimation.

There were several limitations in the current study. In the quantitative contrast analysis, the regions of interest (ROIs) were annotated on pharmacokinetic (PK) maps instead of being propagated from T2, potentially introducing bias in ROI annotation. Our data acquisition protocol did not include the first pass of the bolus, and the acquisition time was relatively short, which may not have been enough to measure the extra-vascular extracellular space, v_e. This poses challenges in extending our method to other organs, e.g., the liver. Future work will include employing advanced techniques such as neural differentiation equations for continuous-time DCE analysis, as well as extending and applying the proposed computational method to other DCE applications.

5. Conclusions

In conclusion, this study has made two contributions to improve prostate MR dispersion imaging: (i) Introducing the fMRDI model, which efficiently represents AIFs of different dispersion levels using a weighted-sum AIF. (ii) Developing a deep learning-based, two-stage method for estimating PK parameters. We believe the proposed techniques will improve the practical utility of DCE-MRI in oncological applications.

Author Contributions: K.Z.: conceptualization, methodology, software, validation, formal analysis, investigation, data curation, writing—original draft preparation, and visualization. K.P. and A.L.H.: validation, formal analysis, data curation, writing—review and editing, and visualization. H.Z. and R.Y.: formal analysis, data curation, and writing—review and editing. K.S.: resources, supervision, and writing—review and editing. All authors have read and agreed to the published version of the manuscript.

Funding: This research was supported in part by the National Institutes of Health R01-CA248506 and R01-CA272702, and by the Integrated Diagnostics Program, Departments of Radiological Sciences and Pathology, David Geffen School of Medicine, University of California, Los Angeles (UCLA).

Institutional Review Board Statement: Our retrospective study was conducted in compliance with the 1996 Health Insurance Portability and Accountability Act (HIPAA) and approved by the Institutional Review Board (IRB) of the University of California, Los Angeles, with a waiver of the requirement for informed consent due to the study not involving the release of patient privacy or personal identifying information.

Informed Consent Statement: Patient consent was waived by the Institutional Review Board (IRB) of the University of California, Los Angeles, due to the study not involving the release of patient privacy or personal identifying information.

Data Availability Statement: The dataset collected from our institution is currently not publicly available since the IRB only approves its employment for internal usage. The data might be available for research purposes upon reasonable request or for institutional collaborations. Please contact Kyunghyun Sung (ksung@mednet.ucla.edu) for any dataset-specific requests.

Conflicts of Interest: The authors declare no competing interests.

References

Carmeliet, P.; Jain, R.K. Angiogenesis in cancer and other diseases. *Nature* **2000**, *407*, 249–257. [CrossRef] [PubMed]

Russo, G.; Mischi, M.; Scheepens, W.; De la Rosette, J.J.; Wijkstra, H. Angiogenesis in prostate cancer: Onset, progression and imaging. *BJU Int.* **2012**, *110*, E794–E808. [CrossRef] [PubMed]

3. Folkman, J. Tumor angiogenesis. *Adv. Cancer Res.* **1985**, *43*, 175–203. [PubMed]
4. Weidner, N. Tumoural vascularity as a prognostic factor in cancer patients: The evidence continues to grow. *J. Pathol.* **1998**, *184*, 119–122. [CrossRef]
5. Weidner, N.; Carroll, P.; Flax, J.; Blumenfeld, W.; Folkman, J. Tumor angiogenesis correlates with metastasis in invasive prostate carcinoma. *Am. J. Pathol.* **1993**, *143*, 401.
6. Brawer, M.K. Quantitative microvessel density: A staging and prognostic marker for human prostatic carcinoma. *Cancer Interdiscip. Int. J. Am. Cancer Soc.* **1996**, *78*, 345–349. [CrossRef]
7. Rosenkrantz, A.B.; Oto, A.; Turkbey, B.; Westphalen, A.C. Prostate imaging reporting and data system (PI-RADS), version 2: A critical look. *Am. J. Roentgenol.* **2016**, *206*, 1179–1183. [CrossRef]
8. Turco, S.; Lavini, C.; Heijmink, S.; Barentsz, J.; Wijkstra, H.; Mischi, M. Evaluation of dispersion MRI for improved prostate cancer diagnosis in a multicenter study. *Am. J. Roentgenol.* **2018**, *211*, W242–W251. [CrossRef]
9. Fedorov, A.; Fluckiger, J.; Ayers, G.D.; Li, X.; Gupta, S.N.; Tempany, C.; Mulkern, R.; Yankeelov, T.E.; Fennessy, F.M. A comparison of two methods for estimating DCE-MRI parameters via individual and cohort based AIFs in prostate cancer: A step toward practical implementation. *Magn. Reson. Imaging* **2014**, *32*, 321–329. [CrossRef]
10. Tofts, P.S.; Brix, G.; Buckley, D.L.; Evelhoch, J.L.; Henderson, E.; Knopp, M.V.; Larsson, H.B.; Lee, T.Y.; Mayr, N.A.; Parker, G.J.; et al. Estimating kinetic parameters from dynamic contrast-enhanced T1-weighted MRI of a diffusable tracer: Standardized quantities and symbols. *J. Magn. Reson. Imaging Off. J. Int. Soc. Magn. Reson. Med.* **1999**, *10*, 223–232. [CrossRef]
11. Jackson, A.; Buckley, D.L.; Parker, G.J. *Dynamic Contrast-Enhanced Magnetic Resonance Imaging in Oncology*; Springer: Berlin/Heidelberg, Germany, 2005; Volume 12.
12. Folkman, J. The role of angiogenesis in tumor growth. *Semin. Cancer Biol.* **1992**, *3*, 65–71. [PubMed]
13. Parker, G.; Tanner, S.; Leach, M. Pitfalls in the measurement of tissue permeability over short time-scales using a low temporal resolution blood input function. In Proceedings of the 4th Annual Meeting of International Society of Magnetic Resonance in Medicine, New York, NY, USA, 27 April–3 May 1996; Volume 1582.
14. Orton, M.R.; d'Arcy, J.A.; Walker-Samuel, S.; Hawkes, D.J.; Atkinson, D.; Collins, D.J.; Leach, M.O. Computationally efficient vascular input function models for quantitative kinetic modelling using DCE-MRI. *Phys. Med. Biol.* **2008**, *53*, 1225. [CrossRef]
15. Fluckiger, J.U.; Schabel, M.C.; DiBella, E.V. Toward local arterial input functions in dynamic contrast-enhanced MRI. *J. Magn. Reson. Imaging* **2010**, *32*, 924–934. [CrossRef]
16. Huang, W.; Chen, Y.; Fedorov, A.; Li, X.; Jajamovich, G.H.; Malyarenko, D.I.; Aryal, M.P.; LaViolette, P.S.; Oborski, M.J.; O'Sullivan, F.; et al. The impact of arterial input function determination variations on prostate dynamic contrast-enhanced magnetic resonance imaging pharmacokinetic modeling: A multicenter data analysis challenge, part II. *Tomography* **2019**, *5*, 99–109. [CrossRef] [PubMed]
17. Weinmann, H.J.; Laniado, M.; Mützel, W. Pharmacokinetics of GdDTPA/dimeglumine after intravenous injection into healthy volunteers. *Physiol. Chem. Phys. Med. NMR* **1984**, *16*, 167–172.
18. Parker, G.J.; Roberts, C.; Macdonald, A.; Buonaccorsi, G.A.; Cheung, S.; Buckley, D.L.; Jackson, A.; Watson, Y.; Davies, K.; Jayson, G.C. Experimentally-derived functional form for a population-averaged high-temporal-resolution arterial input function for dynamic contrast-enhanced MRI. *Magn. Reson. Med. Off. J. Int. Soc. Magn. Reson. Med.* **2006**, *56*, 993–1000. [CrossRef] [PubMed]
19. Henderson, E.; Rutt, B.K.; Lee, T.Y. Temporal sampling requirements for the tracer kinetics modeling of breast disease. *Magn. Reson. Imaging* **1998**, *16*, 1057–1073. [CrossRef]
20. Fritz-Hansen, T.; Rostrup, E.; Larsson, H.B.; Søndergaard, L.; Ring, P.; Henriksen, O. Measurement of the arterial concentration of Gd-DTPA using MRI: A step toward quantitative perfusion imaging. *Magn. Reson. Med.* **1996**, *36*, 225–231. [CrossRef]
21. Lewis, D.; Zhu, X.; Coope, D.J.; Zhao, S.; King, A.T.; Cootes, T.; Jackson, A.; Li, K.L. Surrogate vascular input function measurements from the superior sagittal sinus are repeatable and provide tissue-validated kinetic parameters in brain DCE-MRI. *Sci. Rep.* **2022**, *12*, 8737. [CrossRef]
22. Miyazaki, K.; Jerome, N.P.; Collins, D.J.; Orton, M.R.; d'Arcy, J.A.; Wallace, T.; Moreno, L.; Pearson, A.D.; Marshall, L.V.; Carceller, F.; et al. Demonstration of the reproducibility of free-breathing diffusion-weighted MRI and dynamic contrast enhanced MRI in children with solid tumours: A pilot study. *Eur. Radiol.* **2015**, *25*, 2641–2650. [CrossRef]
23. Rata, M.; Collins, D.J.; Darcy, J.; Messiou, C.; Tunariu, N.; Desouza, N.; Young, H.; Leach, M.O.; Orton, M.R. Assessment of repeatability and treatment response in early phase clinical trials using DCE-MRI: Comparison of parametric analysis using MR-and CT-derived arterial input functions. *Eur. Radiol.* **2016**, *26*, 1991–1998. [CrossRef]
24. Kuenen, M.; Saidov, T.; Wijkstra, H.; Mischi, M. Contrast-ultrasound dispersion imaging for prostate cancer localization by improved spatiotemporal similarity analysis. *Ultrasound Med. Biol.* **2013**, *39*, 1631–1641. [CrossRef]
25. Sung, K. Modified MR dispersion imaging in prostate dynamic contrast-enhanced MRI. *J. Magn. Reson. Imaging* **2019**, *50*, 1307–1317. [CrossRef]
26. Mischi, M.; Turco, S.; Lavini, C.; Kompatsiari, K.; de la Rosette, J.J.; Breeuwer, M.; Wijkstra, H. Magnetic resonance dispersion imaging for localization of angiogenesis and cancer growth. *Investig. Radiol.* **2014**, *49*, 561–569. [CrossRef] [PubMed]
27. Sourbron, S.; Buckley, D.L. Tracer kinetic modelling in MRI: Estimating perfusion and capillary permeability. *Phys. Med. Biol.* **2011**, *57*, R1. [CrossRef] [PubMed]

28. Jager, A.; Oddens, J.R.; Postema, A.W.; Miclea, R.L.; Schoots, I.G.; Nooijen, P.G.; van der Linden, H.; Barentsz, J.O.; Heijmink, S.W.; Wijkstra, H.; et al. Is There an Added Value of Quantitative DCE-MRI by Magnetic Resonance Dispersion Imaging for Prostate Cancer Diagnosis? *Cancers* **2024**, *16*, 2431. [CrossRef] [PubMed]
29. Kuenen, M.P.; Mischi, M.; Wijkstra, H. Contrast-ultrasound diffusion imaging for localization of prostate cancer. *IEEE Trans. Med. Imaging* **2011**, *30*, 1493–1502. [CrossRef]
30. Yankeelov, T.E.; Gore, J.C. Dynamic contrast enhanced magnetic resonance imaging in oncology: theory, data acquisition, analysis, and examples. *Curr. Med. Imaging* **2007**, *3*, 91–107. [CrossRef]
31. Hsu, Y.H.H.; Ferl, G.Z.; Ng, C.M. GPU-accelerated nonparametric kinetic analysis of DCE-MRI data from glioblastoma patients treated with bevacizumab. *Magn. Reson. Imaging* **2013**, *31*, 618–623. [CrossRef]
32. Vajuvalli, N.N.; Nayak, K.N.; Geethanath, S. Accelerated pharmacokinetic map determination for dynamic contrast enhanced MRI using frequency-domain based Tofts model. In Proceedings of the 2014 36th Annual International Conference of the IEEE Engineering in Medicine and Biology Society, Chicago, IL, USA, 26–30 August 2014; pp. 2404–2407.
33. Murase, K. Efficient method for calculating kinetic parameters using T1-weighted dynamic contrast-enhanced magnetic resonance imaging. *Magn. Reson. Med. Off. J. Int. Soc. Magn. Reson. Med.* **2004**, *51*, 858–862. [CrossRef]
34. Kelm, B.M.; Menze, B.H.; Nix, O.; Zechmann, C.M.; Hamprecht, F.A. Estimating kinetic parameter maps from dynamic contrast-enhanced MRI using spatial prior knowledge. *IEEE Trans. Med. Imaging* **2009**, *28*, 1534–1547. [CrossRef]
35. Dikaios, N.; Arridge, S.; Hamy, V.; Punwani, S.; Atkinson, D. Direct parametric reconstruction from undersampled (k, t)-space data in dynamic contrast enhanced MRI. *Med. Image Anal.* **2014**, *18*, 989–1001. [CrossRef] [PubMed]
36. You, D.; Aryal, M.; Samuels, S.E.; Eisbruch, A.; Cao, Y. Temporal feature extraction from DCE-MRI to identify poorly perfused subvolumes of tumors related to outcomes of radiation therapy in head and neck cancer. *Tomography* **2016**, *2*, 341–352. [CrossRef] [PubMed]
37. Bliesener, Y.; Acharya, J.; Nayak, K.S. Efficient DCE-MRI parameter and uncertainty estimation using a neural network. *IEEE Trans. Med. Imaging* **2019**, *39*, 1712–1723. [CrossRef] [PubMed]
38. Ottens, T.; Barbieri, S.; Orton, M.R.; Klaassen, R.; van Laarhoven, H.W.; Crezee, H.; Nederveen, A.J.; Zhen, X.; Gurney-Champion, O.J. Deep learning DCE-MRI parameter estimation: Application in pancreatic cancer. *Med. Image Anal.* **2022**, *80*, 102512. [CrossRef] [PubMed]
39. Witowski, J.; Heacock, L.; Reig, B.; Kang, S.K.; Lewin, A.; Pysarenko, K.; Patel, S.; Samreen, N.; Rudnicki, W.; Łuczyńska, E.; et al. Improving breast cancer diagnostics with deep learning for MRI. *Sci. Transl. Med.* **2022**, *14*, eabo4802. [CrossRef]
40. Vaswani, A.; Shazeer, N.; Parmar, N.; Uszkoreit, J.; Jones, L.; Gomez, A.N.; Kaiser, Ł.; Polosukhin, I. Attention is all you need. *Adv. Neural Inf. Process. Syst.* **2017**, *30*, 5998–6008.
41. Futterer, J.J.; Engelbrecht, M.R.; Huisman, H.J.; Jager, G.J.; Hulsbergen-van De Kaa, C.A.; Witjes, J.A.; Barentsz, J.O. Staging prostate cancer with dynamic contrast-enhanced endorectal MR imaging prior to radical prostatectomy: Experienced versus less experienced readers. *Radiology* **2005**, *237*, 541–549. [CrossRef]
42. Klaassen, R.; Gurney-Champion, O.J.; Wilmink, J.W.; Besselink, M.G.; Engelbrecht, M.R.; Stoker, J.; Nederveen, A.J.; van Laarhoven, H.W. Repeatability and correlations of dynamic contrast enhanced and T2* MRI in patients with advanced pancreatic ductal adenocarcinoma. *Magn. Reson. Imaging* **2018**, *50*, 1–9. [CrossRef]
43. Wright, S.J. *Numerical Optimization*; Springer: New York, NY, USA, 2006.
44. Ulas, C.; Das, D.; Thrippleton, M.J.; Valdes Hernandez, M.d.C.; Armitage, P.A.; Makin, S.D.; Wardlaw, J.M.; Menze, B.H. Convolutional neural networks for direct inference of pharmacokinetic parameters: Application to stroke dynamic contrast-enhanced MRI. *Front. Neurol.* **2019**, *9*, 1147. [CrossRef]
45. Dosovitskiy, A.; Beyer, L.; Kolesnikov, A.; Weissenborn, D.; Zhai, X.; Unterthiner, T.; Dehghani, M.; Minderer, M.; Heigold, G.; Gelly, S.; et al. An Image is Worth 16x16 Words: Transformers for Image Recognition at Scale. In Proceedings of the International Conference on Learning Representations, Vienna, Austria, 4 May 2021.
46. Adelson, E.H.; Anderson, C.H.; Bergen, J.R.; Burt, P.J.; Ogden, J.M. Pyramid methods in image processing. *RCA Eng.* **1984**, *29*, 33–41.
47. Krizhevsky, A.; Sutskever, I.; Hinton, G.E. ImageNet Classification with Deep Convolutional Neural Networks. In *Advances in Neural Information Processing Systems*; Pereira, F., Burges, C., Bottou, L., Weinberger, K., Eds.; Curran Associates, Inc.: Lake Tahoe, NV, USA 2012; Volume 25.
48. Ioffe, S.; Szegedy, C. Batch normalization: Accelerating deep network training by reducing internal covariate shift. In Proceedings of the International Conference on Machine Learning, PMLR, Lille, France, 7–9 July 2015; pp. 448–456.
49. Wang, H.Z.; Riederer, S.J.; Lee, J.N. Optimizing the precision in T1 relaxation estimation using limited flip angles. *Magn. Reson. Med.* **1987**, *5*, 399–416. [CrossRef] [PubMed]
50. Sun, C.; Chatterjee, A.; Yousuf, A.; Antic, T.; Eggener, S.; Karczmar, G.S.; Oto, A. Comparison of T2-weighted imaging, DWI, and dynamic contrast-enhanced MRI for calculation of prostate cancer index lesion volume: Correlation with whole-mount pathology. *Am. J. Roentgenol.* **2019**, *212*, 351–356. [CrossRef] [PubMed]

Disclaimer/Publisher's Note: The statements, opinions and data contained in all publications are solely those of the individual author(s) and contributor(s) and not of MDPI and/or the editor(s). MDPI and/or the editor(s) disclaim responsibility for any injury to people or property resulting from any ideas, methods, instructions or products referred to in the content.

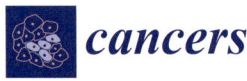

Article

Is There an Added Value of Quantitative DCE-MRI by Magnetic Resonance Dispersion Imaging for Prostate Cancer Diagnosis?

Auke Jager [1], Jorg R. Oddens [1,2], Arnoud W. Postema [3], Razvan L. Miclea [4], Ivo G. Schoots [5,6], Peet G. T. A. Nooijen [7], Hans van der Linden [7], Jelle O. Barentsz [8], Stijn W. T. P. J. Heijmink [6], Hessel Wijkstra [2], Massimo Mischi [2] and Simona Turco [2,*]

[1] Department of Urology, Amsterdam UMC, University of Amsterdam, De Boelelaan 1117, 1081 HV Amsterdam, The Netherlands
[2] Department of Electrical Engineering, Eindhoven University of Technology, 5612 AP Eindhoven, The Netherlands
[3] Leiden University Medical Center, Department of Urology, 2333 ZA Leiden, The Netherlands
[4] Department of Radiology and Nuclear Imaging, Maastricht University Medical Centre+, 6229 HX Maastricht, The Netherlands
[5] Department of Radiology and Nuclear Medicine, Erasmus University Medical Center, 3015 GD Rotterdam, The Netherlands
[6] Department of Radiology, Netherlands Cancer Institute, 1066 CX Amsterdam, The Netherlands
[7] Department of Pathology, Jeroen Bosch Hospital, 5223 GZ 's-Hertogenbosch, The Netherlands
[8] Department of Radiology, Radboud University Nijmegen Medical Center, 6525 GA Nijmegenfi, The Netherlands
* Correspondence: s.turco@tue.nl

Simple Summary: This multicenter, retrospective study assessed the added value of magnetic resonance dispersion imaging (MRDI), a quantitative analysis of dynamic contrast-enhanced MRI (DCE-MRI), alongside standard multiparametric MRI (mpMRI) for detecting clinically significant prostate cancer (csPCa). Seventy-six patients, including fifty-one with csPCa, who underwent mpMRI and radical prostatectomy, were included. Two radiologists evaluated mpMRI, MRDI and a combination of both, with histopathology serving as the reference standard. The study found that MRDI improved inter-observer agreement and enhanced csPCa detection when combined with mpMRI. MRDI enabled the detection of up to 20% more cases compared to mpMRI alone. With the role of DCE-MRI in the context of mpMRI being debated, this study suggests that quantitative analysis of DCE-MRI by MRDI could enhance csPCa detection and reduce variability between observers.

Abstract: In this multicenter, retrospective study, we evaluated the added value of magnetic resonance dispersion imaging (MRDI) to standard multiparametric MRI (mpMRI) for PCa detection. The study included 76 patients, including 51 with clinically significant prostate cancer (csPCa), who underwent radical prostatectomy and had an mpMRI including dynamic contrast-enhanced MRI. Two radiologists performed three separate randomized scorings based on mpMRI, MRDI and mpMRI+MRDI. Radical prostatectomy histopathology was used as the reference standard. Imaging and histopathology were both scored according to the Prostate Imaging-Reporting and Data System V2.0 sector map. Sensitivity and specificity for PCa detection were evaluated for mpMRI, MRDI and mpMRI+MRDI. Inter- and intra-observer variability for both radiologists was evaluated using Cohen's Kappa. On a per-patient level, sensitivity for csPCa for radiologist 1 (R1) for mpMRI, MRDI and mpMRI+MRDI was 0.94, 0.82 and 0.94, respectively. For the second radiologist (R2), these were 0.78, 0.94 and 0.96. R1 detected 4% additional csPCa cases using MRDI compared to mpMRI, and R2 detected 20% extra csPCa cases using MRDI. Inter-observer agreement was significant only for MRDI (Cohen's Kappa = 0.4250, p = 0.004). The results of this study show the potential of MRDI to improve inter-observer variability and the detection of csPCa.

Keywords: prostate cancer; pharmacokinetic analysis; dynamic constrast-enhanced MRI; multiparametric MRI

1. Introduction

Prostate cancer (PCa) is the most commonly diagnosed cancer in males, accounting for nearly one in three new cancer diagnoses in the United States in 2024 [1]. In recent years, multiparametric magnetic resonance imaging (mpMRI) has established itself as a reliable diagnostic tool for PCa detection. There is strong evidence (level 1a) supporting the accuracy of mpMRI in detecting clinically significant PCa (csPCa), with sensitivities reaching up to 91% when compared to template biopsy [2]. Several large-scale clinical trials have further confirmed the benefits of incorporating mpMRI into the prostate cancer evaluation process, with MRI-targeted biopsy (MRI-TBx) finding an additional 6.3% to 7.6% csPCa compared to conventional systematic biopsy (SBx) [2–4]. As a result, the use of pre-biopsy mpMRI has become a standard practice in many institutions for evaluating patients suspected of having PCa.

Traditionally, the prostate MRI protocol consists of T2-weighted imaging (T2W), diffusion-weighted imaging (DWI) and dynamic contrast-enhanced imaging (DCE). While the role of T2W and DWI sequences is well established, the added value of DCE for PCa detection is currently debated [5]. Biparametric MRI (bpMRI), an alternative to mpMRI that does not include DCE, is gaining popularity due to its reduced imaging time and cost. Currently published data on the diagnostic accuracy of bpMRI show mixed results. Multiple recent meta-analyses comparing bpMRI and mpMRI show no difference in diagnostic accuracy [6–8]. However, caution is warranted considering that these data originate from single-center studies, and there are no large, prospective, randomized controlled trials available. Other studies show that DCE MRI does improve sensitivity for csPCa detection [9–11]. DCE can play an especially important role in further characterizing PI-RADS 3 lesions located in the peripheral zone (PZ), with Greer et al. finding an odds ratio of 2.0 ($p = 0.27$) for csPCa detection. In the Prostate Imaging—Reporting and Data System (PI-RADS) V2, DCE is considered to be of secondary importance to T2W and DWI [5]. However, the updated PI-RADS V2.1 protocol states that DCE can still be of value for csPCa detection, especially when either the T2W or DWI sequence is of suboptimal quality (e.g., artifacts or inadequate signal-to-noise ratio) [12]. Additionally, the PI-RADS Steering Committee voices their concerns that widespread implementation of bpMRI can lead to missed csPCa cases [12].

In DCE-MRI, a bolus of gadolinium-based contrast agent is administered intravenously during rapid T1-weighted imaging. The contrast flows through the microvasculature, where it is temporarily confined, after which it diffuses into the extracellular space, or "leakage space" [13]. The rate at which inflow and diffusion take place depends on multiple factors related to the microvascular structure [13]. In PCa, angiogenesis causes alternations to this microvascular structure, leading to abnormalities in perfusion and permeability [14]. These abnormalities can be observed on DCE-MRI as early focal contrast enhancement and fast contrast washout [13]. While visual or qualitative assessment is the most commonly performed method for DCE-MRI assessment, it is subjective and susceptible to inter-observer variability [11]. To increase the reproducibility of DCE-MRI, semi-quantitative and quantitative analysis methods have been proposed. Semi-quantitative analysis of the extracted time–intensity curves provides parameters describing tissue enhancement (e.g., peak enhancement, wash-in, wash-out) as a predictor of malignancy [15]. However, these parameters are subject to high interpatient variability and are difficult to generalize due to variations in acquisition protocols and sequences [16,17].

Quantitative analysis of DCE-MRI is based on the quantification of intravascular contrast leakage to the extracellular space. This can be accomplished using compartmental pharmacokinetic modeling devised by Tofts et al. [18]. The Tofts model (TM) describes two main pharmacokinetics (PK) parameters. These parameters can quantify contrast leakage from plasma to tissue and have shown to be significantly increased in cancerous prostate tissue [19]. The major advantage of quantitative DCE-MRI over qualitative and semi-quantitative analysis is that it does not depend on the MRI scanner brand or model, pulse sequence, observer experience or contrast administration protocol [20]. However, the reliability of the parameters is limited by other factors. TM relies on the Arterial Impulse Function (AIF) for PK parameter estimation. The AIF represents the concentration of the contrast agent in the plasma [21]. When evaluating the AIF determination in a multicenter setting, significant variations are found [22,23]. These variations have a considerable impact on PK parameter estimation and therefore limit the reliability of TM [20]. Studies comparing TM for quantitative DCE-MRI to the semi-quantitative and qualitative methods have thus far not shown an improvement in PCa detection [24].

In an effort to overcome the current limitations of TM, novel methods for quantitative analysis for DCE-MRI are being developed [25,26]. One of these methods is magnetic resonance dispersion imaging (MRDI) [27–29]. This method quantifies the dispersion of an extravascular contrast agent by the local dispersion parameter κ at each voxel in the prostate. The dispersion parameter κ is highly dependent on the microvascular changes caused by angiogenesis and can therefore be used to construct parametric maps that are suitable for PCa detection [28,29]. Contrary to TM, MRDI does not require AIF determination, thus preventing variation in the parameter estimates caused by AIF inaccuracies [20].

Two previous studies comparing MRDI to whole-gland prostate histopathology have proven the potential of MRDI for PCa detection and localization [28,29], with MRDI outperforming all TM parameters and reaching a sensitivity of 91% [28]. To prove the clinical utility of MRDI, further validation is necessary. The aim of this study is to evaluate the diagnostic potential of quantitative DCE-MRI analysis by MRDI for the detection and localization of csPCa as a separate imaging modality and as an addition to mpMRI, using histopathology from radical prostatectomy specimens as the reference standard.

2. Materials and Methods

2.1. Patient Population and Data Acquisition

Participants in this study were recruited from three tertiary healthcare centers in the Netherlands within the framework of the Prostate Cancer Molecular Medicine (PCMM) project. Ethical approval for data utilization was granted by the medical ethics review committee of Erasmus MC (Rotterdam, The Netherlands) under the reference number NL32105.078.10. The PCMM project systematically gathered mpMRI and pathology data from men diagnosed with localized PCa, who were scheduled for prostatectomy. Data collection was performed prospectively from 7 February 2011 to 30 June 2015. All study participants provided written informed consent to have data from their medical records used in research.

The adopted pre-biopsy prostate MRI protocol depended on the center of acquisition. Table 1 gives an overview of the MRI acquisition details for each participating center.

Table 1. mpMRI acquisition details per center of inclusion. TR = repetition time, TE = echo time.

Parameter	T2W			DWI			DCE		
	Center 1	Center 2	Center 3	Center 1	Center 2	Center 3	Center 1	Center 2	Center 3
TR (ms)	3500–7220	5321–10,233	4000–6050	4000–4800	3429–4498	2500–4200	50	4–5.5	3.85–36
TE (ms)	108	120	99–104	87	67–69	60–90	4	1–2	1.40
Thickness (cm)	3	3	3–4	3–3.6	3	3–4	4–5	6	3–4.5
Width (voxels)	512	512	320–512	136	176	84–160	144	176–256	128–160
Height (voxels)	512	512	320–512	160	176	106–168	192	176–256	128–160
Field strength (Tesla)	1.50	3.00	3.00	1.50	3.00	3.00	1.50	3.00	3.00
Flip angle (degrees)	150	90	117–160	90	90	90	70	8–15	12–14
Endorectal coil (Yes/No)	Yes	Yes	No	Yes	Yes	No	Yes	Yes	No
MRI scanner model	SIEMENS Avanto	Philips Achieva	SIEMENS Skyra/TrioTim	SIEMENS Avanto	Philips Achieva	SIEMENS Skyra/TrioTim	SIEMENS Avanto	Philips Achieva	SIEMENS Skyra/TrioTim
Voxel size (mm)	0.31	0.27	0.31–0.80	1.63	1.03	1.40–2.00	1.67	1.02–2.05	1.50–1.63
MRI sequence	Turbo Spin Echo (TSE)	Turbo Spin Echo (TSE)	Turbo Spin Echo (TSE)	Spin Echo—Echo Planar Imaging (EPI SE)	Spin Echo—Echo Planar Imaging (SE-EPI)	Spin Echo—Echo Planar Imaging (EPI SE)	Spoiled Gradient Echo (FLASH)	Spoiled Gradient Echo (T1-FFE)	Spoiled Gradient Echo (FLASH)
Temporal resolution (s)	-	-	-	-	-	-	3.09–3.12	2.90–3.67	3.31–4.24
Contrast agent	-	-	-	-	-	-	Gadobutrol (0.1 mmol/kg)	Gadoterate meglumine (0.1 mmol/kg)	Gadobutrol (0.1 mmol/kg)

2.2. MRDI Analysis

Time–intensity curves were obtained from DCE-MRI images for each pixel and converted to concentration–time curves as explained in [28]. Quantitative analysis was performed by fitting each concentration–time curve by the reduced dispersion model, according to a previously described method known as MRDI [27–29]. Parametric maps of the local dispersion parameter κ were obtained and visualized as color-coded maps using a custom-made software tool (Figure 1a).

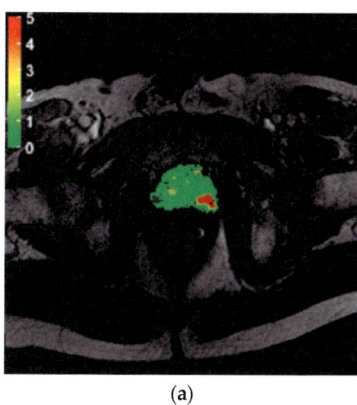
(a)

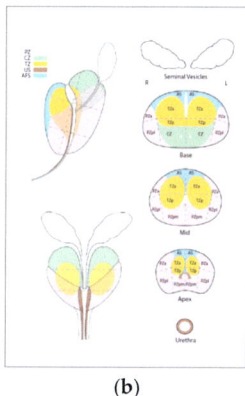
(b)

Figure 1. (a) Example of MRDI map; (b) sector map of PIRADS 2.0 used for scoring.

2.3. MRI and MRDI Scoring

Assessment was performed by two radiologists, R1 and R2, with 9 and 5 years of experience in PIRADS scoring, respectively, who were blinded to the histopathology results. Scoring was performed according to the PIRADS V2.0 prostate sector map (Figure 1b). PIRDS V2.0 was adopted because the development of the protocols and the start of the study occurred before the publication of the updated PIRADS V2.1 [12]. Each radiologist performed three randomized scorings by evaluating mpMRI alone, MRDI maps alone and mpMRI and MRDI in conjunction (mpMRI+MRDI). To reduce the risk of bias, the study protocol dictated a pause of at least 2 weeks between performing the different scoring methods. Moreover, patient numbers and order were randomized for each scoring:

- **mpMRI**: The scoring was performed according to the PIRADS V2.0 guidelines [5].
- **MRDI**: MRDI maps were scored from 0 (no lesion) to 5 according to custom guidelines summarized in Table 2. No size criterium is given for scoring MRDI, as it is based on the assessment of angiogenic vascularization within and surrounding the tumor [28,29].
- **mpMRI+MRDI**: The scoring was performed by integrating the information provided by mpMRI and MRDI, according to the separate scoring models for each modality. In the case of a discrepancy between mpMRI and MRDI scores, the final score was at the radiologist's discretion.

Table 2. MRDI map scoring guidelines.

Score	Assessment Category	MRDI Map Features
0	None (benign)	Continuous area with values below 1
1	Very low (clinically significant cancer is highly unlikely to be present)	Continuous area with values between 1 and 2. Non-continuous area with values mostly below 2
2	Low (clinically significant cancer is unlikely to be present)	Continuous area with values between 2 and 3. Non-continuous area with values mostly below 3
3	Intermediate (the presence of clinically significant cancer is equivocal)	Non-continuous area with values between 2 and 4

Table 2. Cont.

Score	Assessment Category	MRDI Map Features
4	High (clinically significant cancer is likely to be present)	Continuous area with values between 3 and 4. Non-continuous area with values mostly above 4
5	Very high (clinically significant cancer is highly likely to be present)	Continuous area with values above 4

For all scoring methods, a score ≥3 was considered positive (e.g., suspicious for csPCa), while a score <3 was considered to be not suspicious for the presence of csPCa.

2.4. Prostate Histopathology

All patients underwent radical prostatectomy (RP) at their respective institutions, and histopathologic analysis was performed on each prostate specimen after resection. After fixation in formalin, the prostate specimens were cut into slices with a thickness of approximately 4 mm by a pathologist who marked cancer areas on the basis of the microscopic analysis of cellular differentiation (Figure 2). For each patient, at least the index lesion was graded by the pathologist according to the 2005 International Society of Urological Pathology (ISUP) Gleason grading system [30], and the corresponding Gleason score (GS) was noted. Based on the histopathological analysis, each sector in the PIRADS sector map (Figure 1b) was scored in consensus by two uropathologists, who were blinded for MRI and MRDI results, according to the criteria summarized in Table 3.

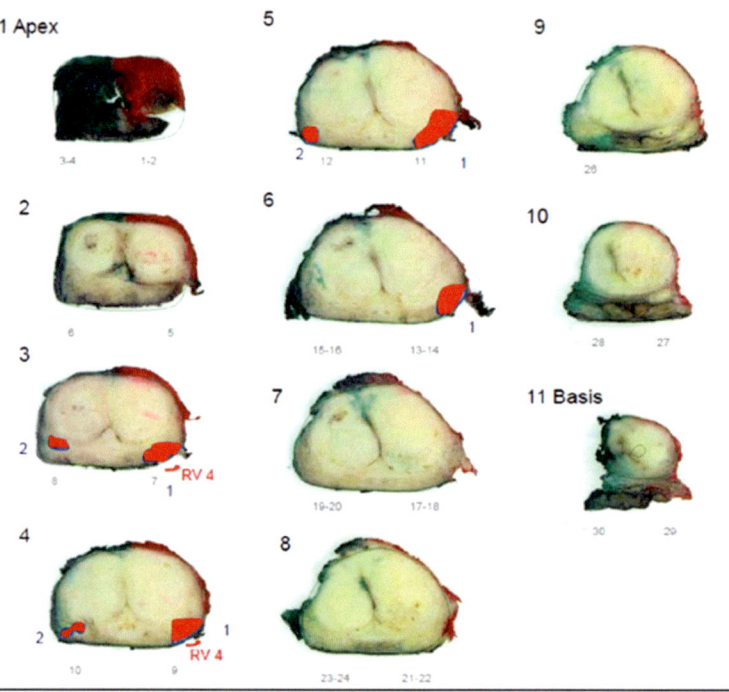

1) GS 3+4=7 Ø 16x10x8 mm Intracapsulaire incisie RV 8 mm, EPE-, VS- pT2cR1
2) GS 3=3=6 Ø 12x4x4 mm

Figure 2. Example of histopathology result.

Table 3. Guidelines for scoring radical prostatectomy histopathology. Size (%) = tumor volume in the corresponding sector. GS = Gleason score.

Score	Histology	
1	• GS ≤ 3 + 3 = 6 • Size ≤ 25%	
2	• GS ≤ 3 + 3 = 6 • Size > 25% & <50&	
3	• GS ≤ 3 + 3 = 6 • Size ≥ 50%	• GS = 3 + 4 = 7 • Size ≤ 50%
4	• GS > 3 + 4 = 7 • Size < 50%	• GS = 3 + 4 = 7 • Size ≥ 50%
5	• GS > 3 + 4 = 7 • Size ≥ 50%	

2.5. Evaluation of Diagnostic Performance

The added value of quantitative DCE-MRI analysis by MRDI to the standard mpMRI protocol for csPCa detection was evaluated on a per-patient level, using RP specimen histopathology as the reference standard. A positive mpMRI, MRDI or mpMRI+MRDI (e.g., suspicious for csPCa) was defined as at least one sector scored as 3 or higher. This was considered a true positive when csPCa, defined as any GS ≥ 3 + 4 = 7, was present in the RP histopathology.

Performance of mpMRI and MRDI was also separately evaluated to determine the number of csPCa prostates missed by mpMRI and detected by MRDI and vice versa.

2.6. Prostate Cancer Localization

The ability to localize csPCa was assessed on a per-sextant level. Sextants were created by dividing each prostate slice from the PIRADS V2.0 prostate sector map (apex, mid, base) into left and right, thereby creating six areas (sextants). The diagnostic performance of mpMRI and MRDI was evaluated using the RP specimen pathology scoring as the reference standard for the corresponding sextants. For mpMRI and MRDI, a sextant was considered to contain csPCa if at least one sector in the sextant was scored ≥3; for the pathology scoring, this was ≥4. To reduce the influence of mismatching errors, a correction was applied by looking at each sector with csPCa in the pathology and considering the corresponding MRDI/mpMRI/MRDI+mpMRI sector to contain csPCa also when the sector adjacent to it in the same slice or the same sector in an adjacent slice (apex-mid or mid-base) contained csPCa. The correction was applied before aggregating the results for each sextant.

2.7. Statistical Analysis

Diagnostic performance was expressed as sensitivity and specificity for both the per-patient and per-sextant analysis. Performance was evaluated for mpMRI, MRDI and MRDI+mpMRI. Statistically significant differences in sensitivity and specificity were evaluated using the McNemar Chi-squared test with Yates's correction. Discrepancies between mpMRI and MRDI were evaluated on a per-case basis.

Inter- and intra-observer variability for the radiologists were evaluated for each scoring method using Cohen's Kappa on a per-patient level.

3. Results

3.1. Patient Population

The PCMM database consisted of 90 patients. After exclusion for insufficient temporal resolution of the DCE exam for MRDI analysis, movement artifacts and missing DICOM files, a total of 76 patients were included for analysis. Table 4 gives an overview of patient characteristics and histopathology findings [31]. Table 5 shows PI-RADS scores for both radiologists.

Table 4. Demographics and histopathological characteristics of the dataset. pT-stage and ISUP grading is based on radical prostatectomy histopathology. PSA = prostate-specific antigen, ISUP = International Society of Urological Pathology.

Patient Characteristics	
Number of patients	76
Age at diagnosis (mean ± std years)	62 ± 6
PSA at biopsy (mean ± std ng/mL)	9 ± 6
Prostate volume (mean ± std mL)	44 ± 18
pT-stage, n (%)	
T2ab	19 (25)
T2c	32 (42)
T3	25 (33)
ISUP grade group [31], n (%)	
1	25 (33)
2	27 (36)
3	15 (20)
4	4 (5)
5	5 (6)

Table 5. PI-RADS scores for radiologists R1 and R2 and corresponding histopathology results. PI-RADS = Prostate Imaging-Reporting and Data System, csPCa = clinically significant prostate cancer.

	R1					R2			
PI-RADS	N	%	N csPCa	% csPCa	PI-RADS	N	%	N csPCa	% csPCa
1	2	2.6	1	50.0	1	0	0.0	0	0.0
2	5	6.6	2	40.0	2	22	28.9	11	50.0
3	13	17.1	8	61.5	3	16	21.1	10	62.5
4	27	35.5	19	70.4	4	23	30.3	16	69.6
5	29	38.2	21	72.4	5	15	19.7	14	93.3
Total	76	100.0	51		Total	76	100.0	51	

3.2. Diagnostic Performance

Most csPCa lesions were found by both mpMRI and MRDI; however, each technique showed additional value above the other. For R1, 16% (8 out of 51) of csPCa was detected on mpMRI only, and 4% (2 out of 51) of csPCa was detected on MRDI only. For R2, this was 4% (2 out of 51) and 20% (10 out of 51), respectively. These results are also described in Figure 3. Two example cases of mpMRI imaging, MRDI maps and corresponding histopathology are shown in Figure 4. The selected histopathology slice was visually matched to the mpMRI. For the case in (a), both R1 and R2 missed the clinically significant lesion (GS = 3 + 4) on MRDI but found it on mpMRI. For the case in (b), both R1 and R2 missed the clinically significant lesion (GS = 3 + 4) on mpMRI but found it on MRDI.

Tables 6 and 7 show the sensitivity, specificity, and accuracy for the csPCa detection of each imaging technique on a per-patient and a per-sextant level, respectively. The per-sextant analysis provides an indication of the localization performance. No significant differences were found in the performance of mpMRI, MRDI and mpMRI+MRDI for either of the radiologists.

Table 6. Diagnostic performance in terms of sensitivity, specificity and accuracy on a patient level. TP = true positive, TN = true negative, FN = false negative, FP = false positive, N = ground-truth negative (TN + FP), P = ground-truth positive (TP + FN).

	Sensitivity (TP/P)			Specificity (TN/N)			Accuracy (TN + TP/N + P)		
Radiologist	mpMRI	MRDI	mpMRI+MRDI	mpMRI	MRDI	mpMRI+MRDI	mpMRI	MRDI	mpMRI+MRDI
R1	0.94 (48/51)	0.82 (42/51)	0.94 (48/51)	0.16 (4/25)	0.32 (8/25)	0.16 (4/25)	0.68 (52/76)	0.66 (50/76)	0.68 (52/76)
R2	0.78 (40/51)	0.94 (48/51)	0.96 (49/51)	0.68 (17/25)	0.16 (4/25)	0.04 (1/25)	0.67 (51/76)	0.68 (52/76)	0.66 (50/76)

Table 7. Diagnostic performance in terms of sensitivity, specificity and accuracy on a sextant level. TP = true positive, TN = true negative, FN = false negative, FP = false positive, N = ground-truth negative (TN + FP), P = ground-truth positive (TP + FN).

Radiologist	Sensitivity (TP/P)			Specificity (TN/N)			Accuracy (TN + TP/N + P)		
	mpMRI	MRDI	mpMRI+ MRDI	mpMRI	MRDI	mpMRI+ MRDI	mpMRI	MRDI	mpMRI+ MRDI
R1	0.81 (103/127)	0.56 (71/127)	0.81 (103/127)	0.85 (279/329)	0.83 (273/329)	0.85 (279/329)	0.84 (382/456)	0.75 (344/456)	0.84 (382/456)
R2	0.51 (65/127)	0.54 (69/127)	0.61 (77/127)	0.92 (302/329)	0.84 (276/329)	0.85 (281/329)	0.80 (367/456)	0.76 (345/456)	0.79 (359/456)

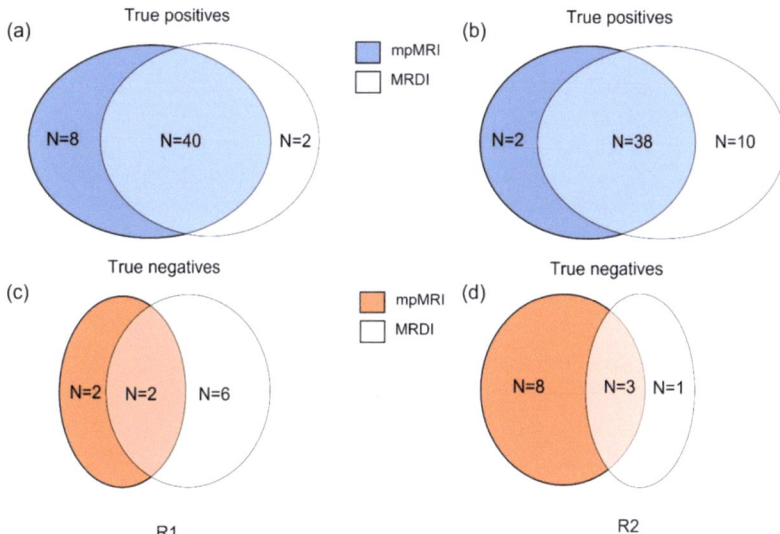

Figure 3. Schematic representation comparing the performance of mpMRI and MRDI. (**a**,**b**) represents the true positives found by mpMRI alone (dark blue), MRDI alone (light blue) and both MRDI and mpMRI (MRDI ∩ mpMRI, mid-tone blue) for radiologists 1 and 2, respectively; (**c**,**d**) represents the true negatives found by mpMRI alone (dark orange), MRDI alone (light orange) and both MRDI and mpMRI (MRDI ∩ mpMRI, mid-tone orange) for radiologists 1 and 2, respectively.

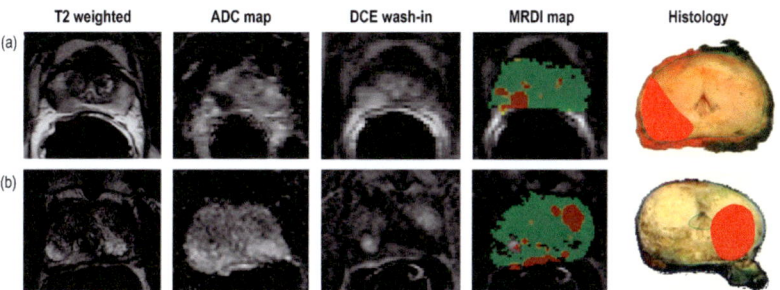

Figure 4. Example cases for two patients showing mpMRI images, MRDI maps and the corresponding visually matched histopathology slice. For both cases, the lesion was diagnosed as Gleason score 4 + 3. For (**a**), both R1 and R2 missed csPCa on MRDI but found it on mpMRI, while for (**b**), both R1 and R2 missed csPCa on mpMRI but found it on MRDI.

3.3. Per-Patient Discrepancies between Imaging and Pathology

For R1, two (3.9%) csPCa cases were missed by mpMRI only, eight (15.6%) on MRDI only and one (2.0%) on both. R2 missed 10 (19.6%) cases of csPCa on mpMRI only, 2 (3.9%) on MRDI only and 1 (2.0%) on both. Table 8 gives an overview of the missed cases per scoring method and corresponding pathology results. Note that the ISUP > 1 is considered csPCa.

Table 8. Diagnostic performance in terms of sensitivity and specificity on a patient level. TP = true positive, TN = true negative, FN = false negative, FP = false positive, N = ground-truth negative (TN + FP), P = ground-truth positive (TP + FN).

	Number of Missed csPCa					
	R1			R2		
ISUP	mpMRI Only	MRDI Only	Missed by Both	mpMRI Only	MRDI Only	Missed by Both
2	1/27	5/27	1/27	5/27	0/27	1/27
3	1/15	2/15	0/15	4/15	2/15	0/15
4	0/4	0/4	0/4	1/4	0/4	0/4
5	0/5	1/5	0/5	0/5	0/5	0/5
Total	2/51	8/51	1/51	10/51	2/51	1/51

3.4. Per-Patient Inter-Observer Variability

Inter-observer agreement between R1 and R2 was fair for mpMRI ($\kappa = 0.1456$, $p = 0.054$), moderate for MRDI ($\kappa = 0.4250$, $p = 0.004$) and poor for mpMRI+MRDI ($\kappa = -0.0585$, $p = 0.681$). Significant inter-observer agreement was only found for MRDI.

Intra-observer agreement for R1 was slight for mpMRI vs. MRDI ($\kappa = 0.1375$, $p = 0.365$), perfect for mpMRI vs. mpMRI+MRDI ($\kappa = 1$, $p = 0.000$) and slight for MRDI vs. mpMRI+MRDI ($\kappa = 0.1375$, $p = 0.365$). For R2, intra-observer agreement was slight for mpMRI vs. MRDI ($\kappa = 0.1582$, $p = 0.340$), poor for mpMRI vs. mpMRI+MRDI ($\kappa = -0.0747$, $p = 0.707$) and poor for MRDI vs. mpMRI+MRDI ($\kappa = -0.0585$, $p = 0.681$). Significant intra-observer agreement was only found for mpMRI vs. mpMRI+MRDI for R1.

4. Discussion

This study presents the first assessment of radiologists' experience with interpreting MRDI in combination with mpMRI in patients undergoing radical prostatectomy (RP). The aim was to determine the additional value of MRDI for the detection of clinically significant prostate cancer (csPCa) compared to the current standard of care, mpMRI. The results of the study suggest that MRDI can be of additional value for PCa diagnosis as there were cases where the radiologist correctly identified csPCa on MRDI, which were not detected on mpMRI.

The sensitivity for csPCa detection varied between the two radiologists, with R1 detecting more csPCa using mpMRI and R2 detecting more csPCa using MRDI. However, for R2, the combined reading of mpMRI and MRDI led to a substantial improvement in csPCa detection compared to mpMRI alone, while R1 did not show any improvement. The differences in added value between the radiologists could be attributed to the challenges of interpreting a new imaging modality, and more extensive training is necessary to fully utilize the potential of MRDI. This is demonstrated by Figure 4a, where both radiologists missed a clear lesion on MRDI. To achieve optimal results, it is important to continuously improve the interpretation and integration of MRDI and mpMRI information.

The low specificity of both imaging modalities on a per-patient level can be attributed to the highly selected patient population in this study. The 25 patients who were deemed negative for csPCa were all treated by RP due to ISUP 1 PCa. ISUP 1 PCa lesions can be visible on mpMRI and are often interpreted as significant lesions, especially in the case of larger ISUP 1 tumors [32]. Bratan et al. evaluated PCa detection by mpMRI using full-mount histopathology as the reference and found that 70% of ISUP 1 tumors larger than 2cc were detected on mpMRI [32]. Therefore, the patient-level specificity in the current study is not representative of the accuracy of the imaging modalities used. This is substantiated by the higher sextant-based specificities.

In this study, we found fair agreement between R1 and R2 for mpMRI ($\kappa = 0.146$, $p = 0.054$). The agreement between R1 and R2 for MRDI was substantially higher, reaching significant moderate agreement ($\kappa = 0.425$, $p = 0.004$). A possible explanation is the relatively easily (compared to mpMRI) interpretable visualization used in quantitative imaging methods, such as MRDI (see Figure 1a). Furthermore, the accessibility of MRDI could also positively impact the steep learning curve generally associated with mpMRI. This is particularly relevant considering the growing need for skilled radiologists due to the increasing adoption of mpMRI for PCa detection and the increasing incidence of PCa [1,33].

This study has several limitations. First, there is an increased risk for selection bias due to the inclusion of RP patients only, with a larger prevalence of aggressive prostate cancer expected in this population. Based on the current guidelines [34,35], with mpMRI being recommended for pre-biopsy risk stratification of intermediate and high-risk patients, future prospective studies are warranted to validate the proposed approach in biopsy-naive patients, e.g., for biopsy targeting. Second, due to the deformation of the prostate after RP and because of the difference in the slicing angle of pathology and MRI, mismatching errors can occur when correlating imaging to pathology. By dividing the prostate into sextants, we attempted to minimize this error. Lastly, due to its retrospective design and limited sample size, the results cannot yet be extrapolated to general practice. However, this is the first study reporting on a cohort evaluated with MRDI; future prospective studies will need to prove the utility of MRDI in clinical practice. Given the recent advances in other imaging modalities, such as multiparametric ultrasound and micro-ultrasound [36,37], the investigation of multimodal imaging approaches, leveraging mpMRI image fusion with these emerging techniques, is also warranted.

5. Conclusions

In this study, we reported the results of the first experience with using MRDI for csPCa detection in patients undergoing RP. The results showed that MRDI has the potential to further increase the diagnostic accuracy of mpMRI, with sensitivity of up to 0.96 achieved with the combination of MRDI and mpMRI. Notably, MRDI could potentially lead to an improvement in detection rate of up to 20% and a reduction in missed csPCa of up to 17% when combined with mpMRI. The quantitative MRDI maps could prove to be especially useful for less-experienced radiologists and for improving inter-observer agreement. However, further validation in a larger, pre-biopsy cohort is necessary before clinical implementation.

Author Contributions: Conceptualization, H.W., M.M. and S.T.; Data curation, A.W.P. and S.T.; Formal analysis, A.J. and S.T.; Investigation, R.L.M., I.G.S., P.G.T.A.N. and H.v.d.L.; Methodology, H.W., M.M. and S.T.; Resources, A.W.P., J.O.B., S.W.T.P.J.H. and H.W.; Software, S.T.; Supervision, H.W. and M.M.; Validation, A.W.P. and S.T.; Writing—original draft, A.J. and S.T.; Writing—review and editing, A.J., A.W.P., J.R.O., R.L.M., I.G.S., J.O.B., S.W.T.P.J.H., H.W., M.M. and S.T. All authors have read and agreed to the published version of the manuscript.

Funding: This study was performed within the framework of CTMM, the Center for Translational Molecular Medicine, PCMM project (grant 03O-203).

Institutional Review Board Statement: This retrospective study was approved by institutional review boards at each participating institution. Ethical approval for data utilization was granted by the medical ethics review committee of Erasmus MC (Rotterdam, The Netherlands) under the reference number NL32105.078.10.

Informed Consent Statement: Informed consent was obtained from all subjects involved in the study.

Data Availability Statement: The original contributions presented in the study are included in the article; further inquiries can be directed to the corresponding author.

Acknowledgments: We acknowledge Chris H. Bangma for approving the use of data.

Conflicts of Interest: The authors declare no conflicts of interest.

References

1. Siegel, R.L.; Giaquinto, A.N.; Jemal, A. Cancer Statistics, 2024. *CA Cancer J. Clin.* **2024**, *74*, 12–49. [CrossRef] [PubMed]
2. Drost, F.-J.H.; Osses, D.; Nieboer, D.; Bangma, C.H.; Steyerberg, E.W.; Roobol, M.J.; Schoots, I.G. Prostate Magnetic Resonance Imaging, with or without Magnetic Resonance Imaging-Targeted Biopsy, and Systematic Biopsy for Detecting Prostate Cancer: Cochrane Systematic Review and Meta-Analysis. *Eur. Urol.* **2020**, *77*, 78–94. [CrossRef] [PubMed]
3. Rouvière, O.; Puech, P.; Renard-Penna, R.; Claudon, M.; Roy, C.; Mège-Lechevallier, F.; Decaussin-Petrucci, M.; Dubreuil-Chambardel, M.; Magaud, L.; Remontet, L.; et al. Use of Prostate Systematic and Targeted Biopsy on the Basis of Multiparametric MRI in Biopsy-Naive Patients (MRI-FIRST): A Prospective, Multicentre, Paired Diagnostic Study. *Lancet Oncol.* **2019**, *20*, 100–10. [CrossRef] [PubMed]
4. van der Leest, M.; Cornel, E.; Israël, B.; Hendriks, R.; Padhani, A.R.; Hoogenboom, M.; Zamecnik, P.; Bakker, D.; Setiasti, A.; Veltman, J.; et al. Head-to-Head Comparison of Transrectal Ultrasound-Guided Prostate Biopsy versus Multiparametric Prostate Resonance Imaging with Subsequent Magnetic Resonance-Guided Biopsy in Biopsy-Naïve Men with Elevated Prostate-Specific Antigen: A Large Prospective Multicenter Clinical Study. *Eur. Urol.* **2019**, *75*, 570–578. [CrossRef] [PubMed]
5. Weinreb, J.C.; Barentsz, J.O.; Choyke, P.L.; Cornud, F.; Haider, M.A.; Macura, K.J.; Margolis, D.; Schnall, M.D.; Shtern, F.; Tempany, C.M.; et al. PI-RADS Prostate Imaging—Reporting and Data System: 2015, Version 2. *Eur. Urol.* **2016**, *69*, 16–40. [CrossRef] [PubMed]
6. Alabousi, M.; Salameh, J.-P.; Gusenbauer, K.; Samoilov, L.; Jafri, A.; Yu, H.; Alabousi, A. Biparametric vs Multiparametric Prostate Magnetic Resonance Imaging for the Detection of Prostate Cancer in Treatment-Naïve Patients: A Diagnostic Test Accuracy Systematic Review and Meta-Analysis. *BJU Int.* **2019**, *124*, 209–220. [CrossRef] [PubMed]
7. Bass, E.J.; Pantovic, A.; Connor, M.; Gabe, R.; Padhani, A.R.; Rockall, A.; Sokhi, H.; Tam, H.; Winkler, M.; Ahmed, H.U. Systematic Review and Meta-Analysis of the Diagnostic Accuracy of Biparametric Prostate MRI for Prostate Cancer in Men at Risk. *Prostate Cancer Prostatic Dis.* **2021**, *24*, 596–611. [CrossRef] [PubMed]
8. Woo, S.; Suh, C.H.; Kim, S.Y.; Cho, J.Y.; Kim, S.H.; Moon, M.H. Head-to-Head Comparison between Biparametric and Multiparametric MRI for the Diagnosis of Prostate Cancer: A Systematic Review and Meta-Analysis. *AJR Am. J. Roentgenol.* **2018**, *211*, W226–W241. [CrossRef]
9. Greer, M.D.; Shih, J.H.; Lay, N.; Barrett, T.; Kayat Bittencourt, L.; Borofsky, S.; Kabakus, I.M.; Law, Y.M.; Marko, J.; Shebel, H.; et al. Validation of the Dominant Sequence Paradigm and Role of Dynamic Contrast-Enhanced Imaging in PI-RADS Version 2. *Radiology* **2017**, *285*, 859–869. [CrossRef]
10. Rosenkrantz, A.B.; Babb, J.S.; Taneja, S.S.; Ream, J.M. Proposed Adjustments to PI-RADS Version 2 Decision Rules: Impact on Prostate Cancer Detection. *Radiology* **2017**, *283*, 119–129. [CrossRef]
11. Krishna, S.; McInnes, M.; Lim, C.; Lim, R.; Hakim, S.W.; Flood, T.A.; Schieda, N. Comparison of Prostate Imaging Reporting and Data System Versions 1 and 2 for the Detection of Peripheral Zone Gleason Score 3 + 4 = 7 Cancers. *AJR Am. J. Roentgenol.* **2017**, *209*, W365–W373. [CrossRef]
12. Turkbey, B.; Rosenkrantz, A.B.; Haider, M.A.; Padhani, A.R.; Villeirs, G.; Macura, K.J.; Tempany, C.M.; Choyke, P.L.; Cornud, F.; Margolis, D.J.; et al. Prostate Imaging Reporting and Data System Version 2.1: 2019 Update of Prostate Imaging Reporting and Data System Version 2. *Eur. Urol.* **2019**, *76*, 340–351. [CrossRef] [PubMed]
13. Brasch, R.C.; Li, K.C.; Husband, J.E.; Keogan, M.T.; Neeman, M.; Padhani, A.R.; Shames, D.; Turetschek, K. In Vivo Monitoring of Tumor Angiogenesis with MR Imaging. *Acad. Radiol.* **2000**, *7*, 812–823. [CrossRef] [PubMed]
14. Russo, G.; Mischi, M.; Scheepens, W.; De La Rosette, J.J.; Wijkstra, H. Angiogenesis in Prostate Cancer: Onset, Progression and Imaging. *BJU Int.* **2012**, *110*, E794–E808. [CrossRef] [PubMed]
15. Isebaert, S.; De Keyzer, F.; Haustermans, K.; Lerut, E.; Roskams, T.; Roebben, I.; Van Poppel, H.; Joniau, S.; Oyen, R. Evaluation of Semi-Quantitative Dynamic Contrast-Enhanced MRI Parameters for Prostate Cancer in Correlation to Whole-Mount Histopathology. *Eur. J. Radiol.* **2012**, *81*, e217–e222. [CrossRef]
16. Verma, S.; Turkbey, B.; Muradyan, N.; Rajesh, A.; Cornud, F.; Haider, M.A.; Choyke, P.L.; Harisinghani, M. Overview of Dynamic Contrast-Enhanced MRI in Prostate Cancer Diagnosis and Management. *Am. J. Roentgenol.* **2012**, *198*, 1277–1288. [CrossRef] [PubMed]
17. Kim, S.H.; Choi, M.S.; Kim, M.J.; Kim, Y.H.; Cho, S.H. Role of Semi-Quantitative Dynamic Contrast-Enhanced MR Imaging in Characterization and Grading of Prostate Cancer. *Eur. J. Radiol.* **2017**, *94*, 154–159. [CrossRef] [PubMed]
18. Tofts, P.S.; Wicks, D.A.; Barker, G.J. The MRI Measurement of NMR and Physiological Parameters in Tissue to Study Disease Process. *Prog. Clin. Biol. Res.* **1991**, *363*, 313–325.
19. van Dorsten, F.A.; van der Graaf, M.; Engelbrecht, M.R.W.; van Leenders, G.J.L.H.; Verhofstad, A.; Rijpkema, M.; de la Rosette, J.J.M.C.H.; Barentsz, J.O.; Heerschap, A. Combined Quantitative Dynamic Contrast-Enhanced MR Imaging and ^{1}H MR Spectroscopic Imaging of Human Prostate Cancer. *J. Magn. Reson. Imaging JMRI* **2004**, *20*, 279–287. [CrossRef]

30. Huang, W.; Chen, Y.; Fedorov, A.; Li, X.; Jajamovich, G.H.; Malyarenko, D.I.; Aryal, M.P.; LaViolette, P.S.; Oborski, M.J.; O'Sullivan, F.; et al. The Impact of Arterial Input Function Determination Variations on Prostate Dynamic Contrast-Enhanced Magnetic Resonance Imaging Pharmacokinetic Modeling: A Multicenter Data Analysis Challenge. *Tomography* **2016**, *2*, 56–66. [CrossRef]
31. Parker, G.J.M.; Roberts, C.; Macdonald, A.; Buonaccorsi, G.A.; Cheung, S.; Buckley, D.L.; Jackson, A.; Watson, Y.; Davies, K.; Jayson, G.C. Experimentally-Derived Functional Form for a Population-Averaged High-Temporal-Resolution Arterial Input Function for Dynamic Contrast-Enhanced MRI. *Magn. Reson. Med.* **2006**, *56*, 993–1000. [CrossRef] [PubMed]
32. Garpebring, A.; Wirestam, R.; Ostlund, N.; Karlsson, M. Effects of Inflow and Radiofrequency Spoiling on the Arterial Input Function in Dynamic Contrast-Enhanced MRI: A Combined Phantom and Simulation Study. *Magn. Reson. Med.* **2011**, *65*, 1670–1679. [CrossRef] [PubMed]
33. Turco, S.; Wijkstra, H.; Mischi, M. Mathematical Models of Contrast-Agent Transport Kinetics for Imaging of Cancer Angiogenesis: A Review. *IEEE Rev. Biomed. Eng.* **2016**, *9*, 121–147. [CrossRef] [PubMed]
34. Ziayee, F.; Ullrich, T.; Blondin, D.; Irmer, H.; Arsov, C.; Antoch, G.; Quentin, M.; Schimmöller, L. Impact of Qualitative, Semi-Quantitative, and Quantitative Analyses of Dynamic Contrast-Enhanced Magnet Resonance Imaging on Prostate Cancer Detection. *PLoS ONE* **2021**, *16*, e0249532. [CrossRef] [PubMed]
35. Parra, N.A.; Pollack, A.; Chinea, F.M.; Abramowitz, M.C.; Marples, B.; Munera, F.; Castillo, R.; Kryvenko, O.N.; Punnen, S.; Stoyanova, R. Automatic Detection and Quantitative DCE-MRI Scoring of Prostate Cancer Aggressiveness. *Front. Oncol.* **2017**, *7*, 259. [CrossRef] [PubMed]
36. Chatterjee, A.; He, D.; Fan, X.; Antic, T.; Jiang, Y.; Eggener, S.; Karczmar, G.S.; Oto, A. Diagnosis of Prostate Cancer by Use of MRI-Derived Quantitative Risk Maps: A Feasibility Study. *AJR Am. J. Roentgenol.* **2019**, *213*, W66–W75. [CrossRef] [PubMed]
37. Mischi, M.; Saidov, T.; Kompatsiari, K.; Engelbrecht, M.R.W.; Breeuwer, M.; Wijkstra, H. Prostate Cancer Localization by Novel Magnetic Resonance Dispersion Imaging. In Proceedings of the 2013 35th Annual International Conference of the IEEE Engineering in Medicine and Biology Society (EMBC), Osaka, Japan, 3–7 July 2013; pp. 2603–2606. [CrossRef]
38. Turco, S.; Lavini, C.; Heijmink, S.; Barentsz, J.; Wijkstra, H.; Mischi, M. Evaluation of Dispersion MRI for Improved Prostate Cancer Diagnosis in a Multicenter Study. *AJR Am. J. Roentgenol.* **2018**, *211*, W242–W251. [CrossRef] [PubMed]
39. Mischi, M.; Turco, S.; Lavini, C.; Kompatsiari, K.; de la Rosette, J.J.M.C.H.; Breeuwer, M.; Wijkstra, H. Magnetic Resonance Dispersion Imaging for Localization of Angiogenesis and Cancer Growth. *Investig. Radiol.* **2014**, *49*, 561–569. [CrossRef] [PubMed]
40. Epstein, J.I.; Allsbrook, W.C.; Amin, M.B.; Egevad, L.L.; ISUP Grading Committee. The 2005 International Society of Urological Pathology (ISUP) Consensus Conference on Gleason Grading of Prostatic Carcinoma. *Am. J. Surg. Pathol.* **2005**, *29*, 1228–1242. [CrossRef]
41. van Leenders, G.J.L.H.; van der Kwast, T.H.; Grignon, D.J.; Evans, A.J.; Kristiansen, G.; Kweldam, C.F.; Litjens, G.; McKenney, J.K.; Melamed, J.; Mottet, N.; et al. The 2019 International Society of Urological Pathology (ISUP) Consensus Conference on Grading of Prostatic Carcinoma. *Am. J. Surg. Pathol.* **2020**, *44*, e87–e99. [CrossRef]
42. Bratan, F.; Niaf, E.; Melodelima, C.; Chesnais, A.L.; Souchon, R.; Mège-Lechevallier, F.; Colombel, M.; Rouvière, O. Influence of Imaging and Histological Factors on Prostate Cancer Detection and Localisation on Multiparametric MRI: A Prospective Study. *Eur. Radiol.* **2013**, *23*, 2019–2029. [CrossRef]
43. Rawla, P. Epidemiology of Prostate Cancer. *World J. Oncol.* **2019**, *10*, 63–89. [CrossRef]
44. Wei, J.T.; Barocas, D.; Carlsson, S.; Coakley, F.; Eggener, S.; Etzioni, R.; Fine, S.W.; Han, M.; Kim, S.K.; Kirkby, E.; et al. Early Detection of Prostate Cancer: AUA/SUO Guideline Part II: Considerations for a Prostate Biopsy. *J. Urol.* **2023**, *210*, 54–63. [CrossRef]
45. European Association of Urology (EAU). Guidelines on Prostate Cancer—DIAGNOSTIC EVALUATION. Available online: https://uroweb.org/guidelines/prostate-cancer/chapter/diagnostic-evaluation (accessed on 19 June 2024).
46. Basso Dias, A.; Ghai, S. Micro-Ultrasound: Current Role in Prostate Cancer Diagnosis and Future Possibilities. *Cancers* **2023**, *15*, 1280. [CrossRef]
47. Wildeboer, R.R.; Mannaerts, C.K.; van Sloun, R.J.G.; Budäus, L.; Tilki, D.; Wijkstra, H.; Salomon, G.; Mischi, M. Automated Multiparametric Localization of Prostate Cancer Based on B-Mode, Shear-Wave Elastography, and Contrast-Enhanced Ultrasound Radiomics. *Eur. Radiol.* **2020**, *30*, 806–815. [CrossRef]

Disclaimer/Publisher's Note: The statements, opinions and data contained in all publications are solely those of the individual author(s) and contributor(s) and not of MDPI and/or the editor(s). MDPI and/or the editor(s) disclaim responsibility for any injury to people or property resulting from any ideas, methods, instructions or products referred to in the content.

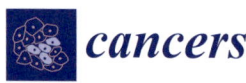

Article

Magnetic Resonance Elastography for the Detection and Classification of Prostate Cancer

Seung Ho Kim [1,*], Joo Yeon Kim [2] and Moon Jung Hwang [3]

[1] Department of Radiology, Inje University College of Medicine, Haeundae Paik Hospital, Busan 48108, Republic of Korea
[2] Department of Pathology, Inje University College of Medicine, Haeundae Paik Hospital, Busan 48108, Republic of Korea; h00311@paik.ac.kr
[3] Advanced Medical Imaging Institute, Korea University Anam Hospital, Seoul 02841, Republic of Korea; mrphd@korea.ac.kr
* Correspondence: radiresi@gmail.com; Tel.: +82-51-797-0382

Simple Summary: Multi-parametric MRI is a first-line imaging modality for prostate cancer detection. Magnetic resonance elastography (MRE) is a useful tool for measuring parenchymal stiffness to diagnose liver fibrosis. A known physical characteristic of prostate cancer is that it is harder than a normal prostate gland. We hypothesized that the quantitative stiffness value derived from MRE could be used to discriminate prostate cancer from benign prostate hyperplasia and normal parenchyma. Until now, the application of MRE to prostate cancer has been sporadic; it has only been used for investigational purposes due to the uncomfortable perineal placement of the acoustic device and inconvenience to patients during preparation. Therefore, we attempted to place an acoustic driver on the lower abdominal wall and determined that detecting and classifying prostate cancer via MRE is feasible. Our observation of 75 consecutive patients revealed that the stiffness value of prostate cancer was significantly different from normal parenchyma, and an accuracy of 87% was estimated at a cutoff value of 4.2 kPa in discriminating prostate cancer from normal parenchyma. In terms of differentiating prostate cancer from benign prostate hyperplasia, an accuracy of 62% was estimated. Additionally, the stiffness values tended to increase as the ISUP grade increased. This observation suggests that the stiffness value derived from pelvic MRE is helpful for detecting and classifying prostate cancer and could be an adjunct to multi-parametric MRI.

Abstract: We investigated the feasibility of magnetic resonance elastography (MRE) using a pelvic acoustic driver for the detection and classification of prostate cancer (PCa). A total of 75 consecutive patients (mean age, 70; range, 56–86) suspected of having PCa and who underwent multi-parametric MRI including MRE and subsequent surgical resection were included. The analyzed regions consisted of cancer (n = 69), benign prostatic hyperplasia (BPH) (n = 70), and normal parenchyma (n = 70). A histopathologic topographic map served as the reference standard for each region. One radiologist and one pathologist performed radiologic–pathologic correlation, and the radiologist measured stiffness values in each region of interest on elastograms automatically generated by dedicated software. Paired t-tests were used to compare stiffness values between two regions. ROC curve analysis was also used to extract a cutoff value between two regions. The stiffness value of PCa (unit, kilopascal (kPa); 4.9 ± 1.1) was significantly different to that of normal parenchyma (3.6 ± 0.3, $p < 0.0001$) and BPH (4.5 ± 1.4, $p = 0.0454$). Under a cutoff value of 4.2 kPa, a maximum accuracy of 87% was estimated, with a sensitivity of 73%, a specificity of 99%, and an AUC of 0.839 for discriminating PCa from normal parenchyma. Between PCa and BPH, a maximum accuracy of 62%, a sensitivity of 70%, a specificity of 56%, and an AUC of 0.598 were estimated at a 4.5 kPa cutoff. The stiffness values tended to increase as the ISUP grade increased. In conclusion, it is feasible to detect and classify PCa using pelvic MRE. Our observations suggest that MRE could be a supplement to multi-parametric MRI for PCa detection.

Keywords: magnetic resonance imaging (MRI); magnetic resonance elastography (MRE); prostate gland; prostate cancer

1. Introduction

Multi-parametric magnetic resonance imaging (MRI), including T2-weighted imaging (T2WI) and diffusion-weighted imaging (DWI), is a first-line imaging modality in the detection and local staging of prostate cancer (PCa) [1–3]. Management of PCa is individually tailored by several factors such as the patient's age, prostate specific antigen (PSA) level, and Gleason score (GS). In particular, GS is a PCa classification system based on the structure of PCa and is related to tumor aggressiveness. Combining of Gleason scores into a three-tiered grouping (6, 7, 8–10) is used most frequently for prognostic and therapeutic purposes [4].

Recent advances in MRI include techniques such as diffusion, perfusion, and texture for acquisition of the physical properties of specific tissues [5–7]. Magnetic resonance elastography (MRE) is an emerging technique for measuring liver stiffness and has shown promising results for staging liver fibrosis [8–10]. Moreover, the prostate gland is one of the organs other than the liver in which MRE could be implemented, considering the previous observation that PCa causes the prostate to have a higher stiffness value than the normal prostate gland [11–13].

MRE is a non-invasive method that can evaluate the mechanical properties of tissues, making it useful for diagnosing and monitoring various diseases. The basic principle of MRE is to transmit external mechanical vibrations to the tissue and measure the resulting displacements to calculate tissue stiffness. As tissue stiffness varies, the phase values of the magnetic resonance (MR) signal change accordingly—stiffer tissues result in greater phase shifts. These phase changes are then inverted to calculate stiffness values. Accurate calculation of these values relies heavily on high signal-to-noise ratios in the base images and phase-contrast imaging. Effective transmission of vibrations and visualization of these small changes are crucial for evaluating the mechanical properties of tissues non-invasively.

Previous studies on prostate gland MRE have used a passive acoustic driver placed in the patient's urethra, rectum, or perineum [14–16]. However, the uncomfortable placement of the acoustic device and inconvenience to patients during preparation is an issue. Therefore, we attempted to place an acoustic driver on the lower abdominal wall and investigated whether this could detect and classify PCa. To our knowledge, this has rarely been attempted for PCa [17–19]; moreover, studies have used relatively small populations and systematic biopsy as the gold standard rather than pathologic whole mount after radical prostatectomy. Our hypothesis was that the quantitative stiffness value derived from MRE could be used to discriminate PCa from benign prostatic hyperplasia (BPH) and normal parenchyma. Thus, the aim of this study was to investigate the feasibility of MRE combined with a pelvic acoustic driver for the detection and classification of PCa with topographic maps as the reference standard.

2. Materials and Methods

Our institutional review board approved this study (IRB 2024-03-016-002), and informed consent was waived due to the extremely low risk to patients associated with this retrospective study.

2.1. Patient Selection Criteria

A total of 151 patients who had suspected PCa and underwent prostate MRI between August 2023 and May 2024 were initially eligible for this study. Patients who satisfied the following inclusion criteria were selected: (1) patients who underwent MRE; (2) patients who underwent subsequent robot-assisted laparoscopic radical prostatectomy; (3) patients who had histopathologic whole mount and relevant full pathologic information including GS. From this population, 56 patients who had undergone systematic biopsy only were excluded. In addition, 19 patients whose tumor size was less than 1 cm were excluded due to the inherent limitations of MRE in detecting small tumors. One patient was excluded due to technical errors during MRE. Finally, 75 patients (mean age, 70; range, 56–86) were included and analyzed. The patient accrual process is presented in Figure 1.

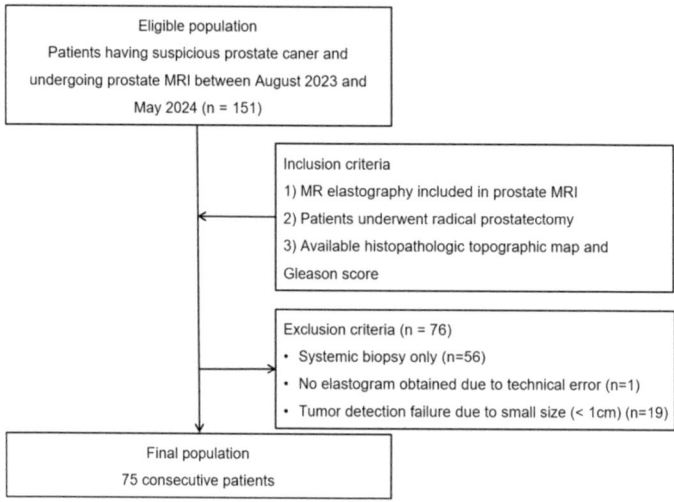

Figure 1. Flowchart of the case-accrual process.

2.2. Magnetic Resonance Imaging

All MRI scans were performed using a 3.0-T MR machine (Signa Architect, GE HealthCare, Chicago, IL, USA) with a torso coil (AIRTM Anterior Array, GE HealthCare Coils, Aurora, OH, USA). The scan protocol comprised bi-parametric MRI including T2WI in the axial, sagittal, and coronal planes, axial DWI sequences (b-values of 0, 100, 1000, and 2000 s/mm^2), and corresponding apparent diffusion coefficient (ADC) maps.

2.3. Magnetic Resonance Elastography

The MRE system consisted of active and passive drivers. The active driver (RESOUNDANT, benchmark electronics Inc. Rochester MN, USA) generates continuous acoustic vibrations at a 60 to 120 Hz frequency, transmitted via a flexible vinyl tube to the passive driver positioned on the patient's lower abdomen. The passive driver converts these vibrations into mechanical waves that propagate through the tissues. These waves are synchronized with a modified two-dimensional (D) spin-echo (SE) echo planar imaging (EPI) pulse sequence, allowing phase-contrast imaging to measure tissue displacements. Since these displacements are proportional to tissue stiffness, this method provides valuable relative stiffness information.

A 2D SE EPI-based phase-contrast sequence was employed to capture the phase displacements correlated with tissue stiffness. The pulse sequence was modified with an oscillating motion-encoding gradient (MEG), applied in the slice direction at 90 Hz. The MEG duration matched the mechanical vibration period, leading to phase shifts in the MR signal corresponding to mechanical excursions. These phase shifts were inverted voxel by voxel to calculate stiffness values using the multi-model direct inversion (MMDI) algorithm. Given that the prostate is a small structure, and to differentiate the lesions within it, relatively shorter wavelengths are required. However, using higher frequencies to achieve shorter wavelengths results in reduced penetration depth, making it challenging for the vibrations to effectively reach the prostate. Therefore, under the current imaging conditions and available MR hardware, a 90 Hz frequency was determined to be optimal for clinical application to the prostate. Future improvements in MR hardware or pulse sequences could allow for effective imaging with even shorter wavelengths.

The MRE acquisition parameters were a TR/TE of 2000/70.5 ms, FOV of 240 mm, matrix size of 80 × 80, and slice thickness of 3.0 mm, with a reconstructed voxel size of 1.5 × 1.5 × 3.0 mm. The imaging sequence utilized chemical fat saturation, a number of excitations (NEX) of 8, a bandwidth of 250 kHz, a temporal phase of 4, an MEG and driver frequency of 90 Hz in the slice direction, and a free-breathing scan time of 2 min and 16 s. The scan parameters are presented in detail in Table 1.

Table 1. MRI sequence parameters.

Parameter	T2WI (Axial, Sagittal, and Coronal)	DWI (b = 0, 100, 1000 and 2000 s/mm^2)	MR Elastography
TR	4680~4930	5260	2000
TE	75~100	88.5	70.5
ETL	15	2	2
Slice thickness	3.0 mm	3.0 mm	3.0 mm
Slice gap	0.3 mm	0.3 mm	0.3 mm
Matrix size (axial)	400 × 320	120 × 120	80 × 80
NEX	1	2, 2, 4, 8	8
FOV (mm)	220 × 220	240 × 240	240 × 240
Acquisition time	1 min 28 s~1 min 51 s	7 min 53 s	2 min 16 s

Repetition time (TR); Echo time (TE); Echo train length (ETL); Field of view (FOV); Number of excitations (NEX); Diffusion-weighted imaging (DWI); MR elastography was performed by utilizing 2-dimensional spin-echo echo planar imaging pulse sequence.

2.4. Image Analysis

Data processing was performed using MR-touch in ReadyView, which is installed within the AW system (AW server 3.2 Ext. 4.9, GE HealthCare). Region-of-interest (ROI) measurements were taken from color-coded elastograms (maximum 8 kilopascals) fused with T2WI using rigid registration, as the elastogram images alone were not sufficient for viewing small anatomical structures. Using the fused images of T2WI and stiffness maps, along with wave images for reference, a freehand ROI was employed to measure the whole tumor volume by tracing the tumor margin across all visible slices.

2.5. Reference Standard

All patients underwent robot-assisted radical prostatectomy. Resected specimens were evaluated by a dedicated pathologist. Histopathologic topographic maps served as the reference standard for the radiologic–pathologic correlation of PCa.

2.6. Statistical Analysis

All the statistical analyses were performed with MedCalc software for Windows (MedCalc Software version 22.032, Mariakerke, Belgium). When the calculated *p*-value was less than 0.05, it was considered a statistically significant difference. Paired t-tests were used to compare stiffness values between two regions. Receiver operating characteristic (ROC) curve analysis was also used to extract an optimal cutoff value between two regions. The area under the ROC curve (AUC) was calculated and represented diagnostic performances.

3. Results

3.1. Patient Demographics

The analyzed regions consisted of cancer (n = 69), benign prostatic hyperplasia (BPH) (n = 70), and normal parenchyma (n = 70). Six patients had high grade prostatic intraepithelial neoplasia, which is considered as the precursor of PCa. The mean interval from preoperative prostate MRI and radical prostatectomy was 58 days (range: 7–137 days), and the mean PSA level was 21.0 ng/mL (range: 0.25–527). Patients were grouped according to International Society of Urologic Pathologists (ISUP) grades and GSs as follows: ISUP grade 1 (GS6, n = 18), ISUP grade 2 (GS3 + 4, n = 24), ISUP grade 3 (GS4 + 3, n = 19), ISUP grade 4 (GS8, n = 4), and ISUP grade 5 (GS9, n = 4). PCa was not found in six patients.

The tumor locations included the peripheral zone (PZ, n = 35), transition zone (TZ, n = 22), diffuse involvement (n = 10), and anterior fibrous stroma (n = 2). The detailed demographic data are summarized in Table 2.

Table 2. Demographic data of the study population.

Parameter	Study Population (n = 75)
Mean age, years [range]	70 (56–86)
Mean PSA, ng/mL [range]	21.0 (0.25–527)
Mean interval from MRI to radical prostatectomy, days [range]	58 (7–137)
Gleason score of prostate cancer	
6	18
7	43
3 + 4	24
4 + 3	19
8	4
9	4
High grade prostatic intraepithelial neoplasia	6
Tumor location	
Peripheral zone	35
Transition zone	22
Anterior fibromuscular stroma	2
Diffuse	10

Prostate-specific antigen (PSA).

3.2. Comparison of Stiffness Values among Three Groups

The stiffness value for PCa (unit, kilopascal; 4.9 ± 1.1) was significantly higher than that for normal parenchyma (3.6 ± 0.3, $p < 0.0001$) and BPH (4.5 ± 1.4, $p = 0.0454$) (Figure 2). At a 4.2 kPa cutoff, a maximum accuracy of 87% was estimated, with a sensitivity of 73%, a specificity of 99%, and an AUC of 0.839 for discriminating PCa from normal parenchyma. Between PCa and BPH, a maximum accuracy of 62%, a sensitivity of 70%, a specificity of 56%, and an AUC of 0.598 were estimated at a 4.5 kPa cutoff.

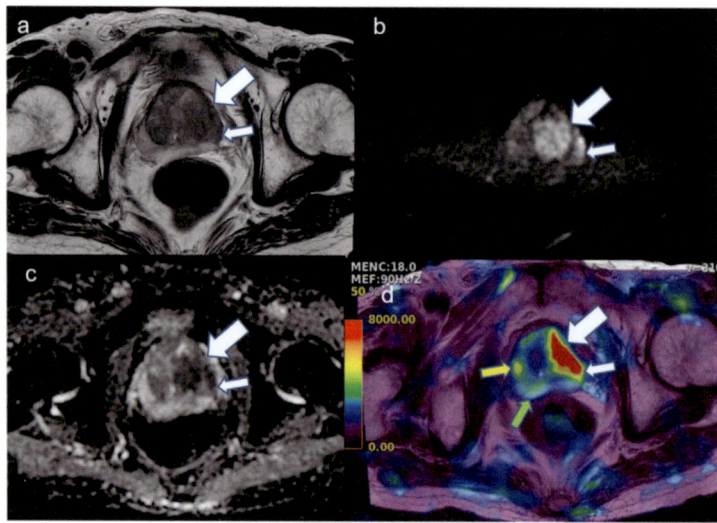

Figure 2. A representative case of a 72-year-old man with prostate cancer with a Gleason score of 7 (4 + 3) in the transition zone. (**a**) T2-weighted image shows a 3 cm low-signal-intensity (SI) lesion (large arrow) in the left transition zone (TZ) with an extension (small arrow) to the neighboring

peripheral zone (PZ). It is difficult to demarcate low SI in the benign prostatic hyperplasia (BPH) nodule in the right TZ. (**b**) Diffusion-weighted image (b value, 2000 s/mm^2) showing a heterogeneous high SI. (**c**) Corresponding apparent diffusion coefficient map also showing a reciprocal low SI in the tumor. Some diffusion-restricted areas are also seen in the BPH nodule in the right TZ. (**d**) Elastogram fused with T2-weighted image showing a high stiffness value (red area, white arrow) in the tumor. Compared with the stiffness value of 7.3 kilopascals in the tumor, the BPH nodule (yellow arrow) was measured at 4.1 kilopascals and normal parenchyma in the PZ (green arrow) indicated 3.2 kilopascals.

3.3. Comparison of Stiffness Values According to Tumor Location

In PZ cancer, the stiffness value for PCa (4.6 ± 1.1) was higher than that for normal parenchyma (3.6 ± 0.3, p = 0.0001) but was not significantly different to that for BPH (4.4 ± 1.2, p = 0.3350). A similar trend was observed for TZ cancer between PCa (5.2 ± 1.0) and normal parenchyma (3.7 ± 0.3, p < 0.0001) as well as BPH (4.5 ± 1.6, p = 0.1400). Box and whisker plots are presented in Figure 3, and the detailed results are summarized in Table 3.

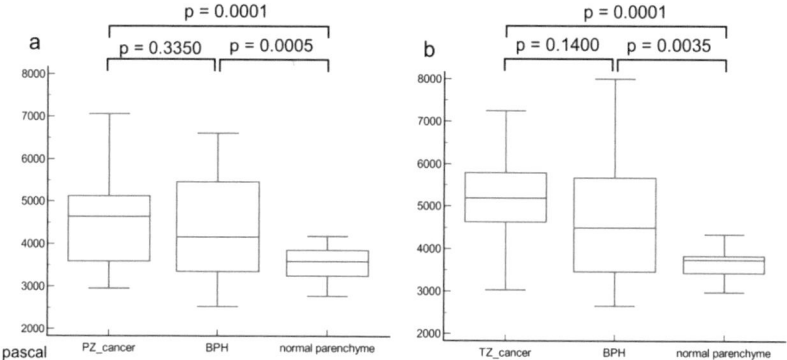

Figure 3. Box and whisker plots comparing the stiffness values of prostate cancer, benign prostatic hyperplasia (BPH), and normal parenchyma according to tumor location. For both peripheral-zone (**a**) and transition-zone cancers (**b**), the stiffness value of prostate cancer was higher than normal parenchyma; however, it did not show a significant difference compared to BPH. The middle line in each box represents the median. The lower and upper boundaries of the boxes represent the lower and upper quartiles (25th and 75th percentiles, respectively). The whiskers indicate the range from the maximum to the minimum calculated stiffness values in pascals.

Table 3. Comparison of stiffness values of three groups according to cancer location.

Location	PZ Cancer		TZ Cancer	
	Stiffness Value	p Value	Stiffness Value	p Value
Prostate cancer	4.6 ± 1.1	0.3350 *	5.2 ± 1.0	0.1400 *
BPH	4.4 ± 1.2	0.0005 †	4.5 ± 1.6	0.0035 †
Normal parenchyma	3.6 ± 0.3	0.0001 ‡	0.7 ± 0.3	0.0001 ‡

* comparison between prostate cancer and BPH; † comparison between BPH and normal parenchyma; ‡ comparison between prostate cancer and normal parenchyma; PZ cancer, peripheral zone cancer; TZ cancer, transition zone cancer; BPH, benign prostatic hyperplasia.

3.4. Comparison of Stiffness Values According to ISUP Grade Group

Stiffness values tended to increase as the ISUP grade increased. The mean stiffness values between grade 1 (4.5 ± 0.8) and grades 4 and 5 (5.1 ± 1.0) were not significantly different (p = 0.2243). This was also true between grade 1 and grade 2 (4.7 ± 1.0, p = 0.5821) and between grade 2 and grade 3 (5.2 ± 1.4, $p = 0.2574$). A box and whisker plot is presented in Figure 4, and the detailed results are described in Table 4.

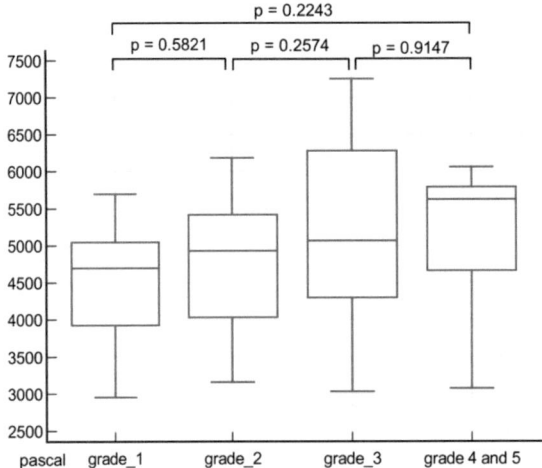

Figure 4. A box and whisker plot comparing the stiffness values of prostate cancer according to International Society of Urologic Pathologists (ISUP) grade group. The mean stiffness value of prostate cancer shows an increasing tendency as ISUP grade increases. The middle line in each box represents the median. The lower and upper boundaries of the boxes represent the lower and upper quartiles (25th and 75th percentiles, respectively). The whiskers indicate the range from the maximum to the minimum calculated stiffness values in pascals.

Table 4. Comparison of stiffness values according to ISUP grade group.

ISUP Grade	Stiffness Value (unit, kilopascal)	p Value
Grade 1 (GS 6)	4.5 ± 0.8	0.5821 *
Grade 2 (GS 3 + 4)	4.7 ± 1.0	0.2574 †
Grade 3 (GS 4 + 3)	5.2 ± 1.4	0.9147 ‡
Gr.4 (GS8) & Gr.5(GS9)	5.1 ± 1.0	0.2243 §

* comparison between Gr. 1 and Gr. 2; † comparison between Gr. 2 and Gr. 3; ‡ comparison between Gr. 3 and Gr. 4 and 5; § comparison between Gr. 1 and Gr. 4 and 5; Data are presented as mean ± standard deviations; ISUP, international society of urologic pathologists; GS, Gleason score.

4. Discussion

Our study found that the stiffness value for PCa was higher than that for normal parenchyma, regardless of location. Our observation corresponds well with previous studies [13,18,19]. Previous studies have reported that the stiffness of PCa was higher than that of normal parenchyma. Li et al. reported that the shear wave velocity that corresponds to the tissue stiffness value for PCa was higher than that for normal parenchyma (unit, m/sec, 3.4 ± 06, 2.2 ± 0.1, $p < 0.001$) according to multi-frequency MRE [19]. In addition, this finding has also been observed with sonoelastography [11,12]. The stiffness of PCa was also found to be higher than that of normal parenchyma (unit, kPa, 8.7 ± 3.4, 3.6 ± 1.3) in a small study population (less than 10 patients in each group).

The difference between PCa and normal parenchyma can be explained from a histologic perspective [20–23]. The epithelium–stroma interaction has a major role in maintaining the structure and function of normal tissue. In carcinomas, this balance is disrupted, leading to the generation of an abnormal tumor microenvironment consisting of fibroblasts, immune cells, and extracellular matrix proteins [20]. Cancer cells interact with these stromal components through many signaling factors [21]. In particular, cancer-associated fibroblasts (CAFs) play an essential role in PCa by overproducing various extracellular matrix components such as collagens, consequently increasing matrix stiffening and thereby promoting tumor growth and invasion [22–24].

Although the overall results comparing PCa and BPH showed a difference in the stiffness values, our subgroup analyses found that the stiffness values for PCa were not different from those for BPH in both PZ and TZ. These results differ from those of previous studies [18,19,25], which observed that the stiffness of PCa was higher than that of BPH. Li et al. observed that TZ cancers had a higher shear wave velocity (stiffness value) than did BPH (unit, m/s; 3.1 ± 0.4, 2.6 ± 0.3, $p < 0.001$) [19]. Lee et al. also reported stiffness values for PCa and BPH nodules (unit, kPa; 5.99 ± 1.46, 4.67 ± 1.54, $p = 0.045$) based on systematic biopsy rather than radical prostatectomy specimens [25]. However, these studies have limited generalizability due either to their small study population (19 PCa and 10 BPH nodules) [25] or their gold standard being based on cognitive fusion biopsy rather than histologic topographic maps of the excised specimens [19].

Therefore, the substantial overlap of stiffness values between PCa and BPH might have been overlooked in previous studies. In our opinion, the discrepancy with previous studies could be explained by two factors: the measurement method for ROIs and the heterogeneity of PCa and BPH. In terms of measuring the stiffness values of focal prostate lesions including PCa and BPH, the previous studies have used either one single slice covering the focal lesion [25] or three consecutive slices [19]. However, this method could not represent the whole BPH nodule volume. To overcome this drawback, we used the whole volume measurement method instead, which is known to be robust and the most reproducible among the various quantitative measurement methods in the field of oncology [26]. Based on our observation, we suggest that the wide range of stiffness values for BPH could be attributed to some overlap with PCa. Our observation is supported by a recent study [27] by Reiter et al., who also reported that PCa is characterized by a homogeneous stiff biomechanical signature, possibly due to the unique nondestructive growth pattern of PCa with intervening stroma. Increased heterogeneity in neighboring BPH was also observed [27]. The larger the BPH nodule, the wider the range of heterogeneity of the BPH nodule. In this regard, we suggest that the stiffness value measured by MRE has an inherent limitation in discriminating PCa from BPH, particularly in the TZ (Figure 5). Our opinion can be supported by the histopathologic explanation of BPH. Histological BPH can be defined as epithelial and stromal proliferation in the prostate TZ, with a predominance of stromal cells. Compared with normal prostatic tissue, the balance between the growth and apoptosis of stromal cells in hyperplastic nodules is lost, resulting in an increase in stromal volume, which leads to the increased stiffness of BPH [28].

In terms of differentiating ISUP grade groups, the diagnostic performance of the imaging technique is important in treatment planning and risk stratification in patients with PCa. Various MRI techniques have been used to discriminate clinically significant cancer (CSC, GS $\geq$ 7) from non-CSC (GS6) [5–7]. Our study revealed that the stiffness value tended to increase as the ISUP grade increased. Similar results were reported in a previous study [13]. Reiter et al. also observed a similar increasing tendency for stiffness as the GS increased from GS6 to GS8/9. However, the diagnostic task of discriminating CSC from non-CSC is challenging when using other imaging modalities, in light of the inherent limitations in analyzing the tumor microenvironment. This is the case with MRE. Based on our observation, the potential use of MRE to discriminate ISUP grade 2 (GS 3 + 4) from grade 3 (GS 4 + 3) is also limited.

In this study, we validated the technical feasibility of MRE with a pelvic acoustic driver. In contrast to the other acoustic drivers used in previous studies that may cause discomfort associated with their endo-rectal, perineal, or transurethral placement and inconvenience to patients during preparation [14–16], the placement of the acoustic driver on the low abdominal wall can be easily adopted and incorporated into clinical practice, with good compliance of patients.

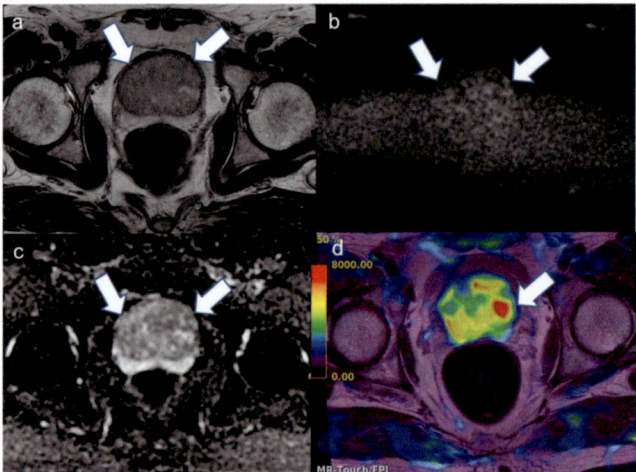

Figure 5. A representative case of a 73-year-old man with a benign prostatic hyperplasia (BPH) nodule (arrows) showing the internal heterogeneity of the stiffness value. (**a**) T2-weighted image shows a large BPH nodule with heterogeneous signal intensity (SI) in the transition zone. (**b**) Diffusion-weighted image (b value, 2000 s/mm^2) showing a heterogeneous high SI in the BPH nodule. (**c**) The corresponding apparent diffusion coefficient map also shows a reciprocal heterogeneous low SI in the BPH nodule. (**d**) Elastogram fused with T2-weighted image shows a wide range of stiffness values in the BPH nodule. Some portions indicate a stiffness value of 8 kilopascals, which is similar to that of prostate cancer.

Several limitations in our study should be acknowledged. First, there could be selection bias associated with the retrospective study design. Patients undergoing systemic biopsy were excluded in this study. However, radical prostatectomy was necessary to obtain a topographic map, which was a ground truth for the segmentation of PCa, BPH, and normal parenchyma. We believe that the histologic whole mount is an ideal guide for radiologic–pathologic correlation. Moreover, measurement was performed based on a relatively large study population compared with previous studies, which is a merit of this study. Another limitation is that we excluded small PCa (less than 1 cm) from further analyses based on our experience and previous observations [25]. In this study, we used a high frequency of 90 Hz for prostate imaging, which provided shorter wavelengths and better resolution, which is crucial for assessing smaller structures. However, it was challenging to measure tumors smaller than 1 cm with MRE. This limitation suggests that using frequencies higher than 90 Hz to produce shorter wavelengths could improve resolution and potentially solve this issue. However, higher frequencies result in reduced penetration depth, making it difficult for the vibrations to effectively reach the prostate gland. Lastly, we did not compare the diagnostic performance of MRE with that of other techniques, including DWI and corresponding ADC maps, for specific tasks such as discriminating CSC from non-CSC. It would be intriguing to compare the diagnostic efficacy of MRE with that of DWI and corresponding ADC for incorporation into clinical practice. However, this task is beyond the scope of this study; thus, we focused on the feasibility of MRE with a pelvic acoustic driver. Further efficacy studies are warranted.

5. Conclusions

In conclusion, it is feasible to detect PCa via MRE with a pelvic acoustic driver. Our observations suggest that MRE could be a supplement to multi-parametric MRI for PCa detection. In addition, the wide range of stiffness values for BPH could be attributed to the substantial overlap between PCa and BPH.

Author Contributions: Conceptualization, S.H.K.; Methodology, S.H.K.; Software, S.H.K.; Validation, S.H.K., J.Y.K. and M.J.H.; Formal analysis S.H.K., J.Y.K. and M.J.H.; Investigation, S.H.K., J.Y.K. and M.J.H.; Resources, S.H.K., J.Y.K. and M.J.H.; Data curation, S.H.K., J.Y.K. and M.J.H.; Writing—original draft preparation, S.H.K., J.Y.K. and M.J.H.; Writing—review and editing, all authors; Visualization, S.H.K.; Supervision, S.H.K.; Project administration, S.H.K.; Funding acquisition, S.H.K. All authors have read and agreed to the published version of the manuscript.

Funding: This work was supported by the 2023 Inje University research grant.

Institutional Review Board Statement: The study was conducted in accordance with the Declaration of Helsinki, and approved by the Institutional Review Board (IRB 2024-03-016-002).

Informed Consent Statement: Patient consent was waived due to extremely low risk to patients associated with this retrospective study.

Data Availability Statement: The data presented in this study are available on request from the corresponding author. The data are not publicly available due to patients' privacy.

Conflicts of Interest: The authors declare no conflicts of interest.

References

1. Turkbey, B.; Rosenkrantz, A.B.; Haider, M.A.; Padhani, A.R.; Villeirs, G.; Macura, K.J.; Tempany, C.M.; Choyke, P.L.; Cornud, F.; Margolis, D.J.; et al. Prostate Imaging Reporting and Data System Version 2.1: 2019 Update of Prostate Imaging Reporting and Data System Version 2. *Eur. Urol.* **2019**, *76*, 340–351. [CrossRef] [PubMed]
2. Weinreb, J.C.; Barentsz, J.O.; Choyke, P.L.; Cornud, F.; Haider, M.A.; Macura, K.J.; Margolis, D.; Schnall, M.D.; Shtern, F.; Tempany, C.M.; et al. PI-RADS Prostate Imaging—Reporting and Data System: 2015, Version 2. *Eur. Urol.* **2016**, *69*, 16–40. [CrossRef]
3. Gupta, R.T.; Spilseth, B.; Patel, N.; Brown, A.F.; Yu, J. Multiparametric prostate MRI: Focus on T2-weighted imaging and role in staging of prostate cancer. *Abdom. Radiol.* **2016**, *41*, 831–843. [CrossRef]
4. Epstein, J.I.; Zelefsky, M.J.; Sjoberg, D.D.; Nelson, J.B.; Egevad, L.; Magi-Galluzzi, C.; Vickers, A.J.; Parwani, A.V.; Reuter, V.E.; Fine, S.W.; et al. A contemporary prostate cancer grading system: A validated alternative to the Gleason Score. *Eur. Urol.* **2016**, *69*, 428–435. [CrossRef]
5. Park, H.; Kim, S.H.; Lee, Y.; Son, J.H. Comparison of diagnostic performance between diffusion kurtosis imaging parameters and mono-exponential ADC for determination of clinically significant cancer in patients with prostate cancer. *Abdom. Radiol.* **2020**, *45*, 4235–4243. [CrossRef]
6. Park, H.; Kim, S.H.; Kim, J.Y. Dynamic contrast-enhanced magnetic resonance imaging for risk stratification in patients with prostate cancer. *Quant. Imaging Med. Surg.* **2022**, *12*, 742–751. [CrossRef] [PubMed]
7. Baek, T.W.; Kim, S.H.; Park, S.J.; Park, E.J. Texture analysis on bi-parametric MRI for evaluation of aggressiveness in patients with prostate cancer. *Abdom. Radiol.* **2020**, *45*, 4214–4222. [CrossRef] [PubMed]
8. Lee, D.H.; Lee, J.M.; Han, J.K.; Choi, B.I. MR elastography of healthy liver parenchyma: Normal value and reliability of the liver stiffness value measurement. *J. Magn. Reson. Imaging* **2013**, *38*, 1215–1223. [CrossRef] [PubMed]
9. Chang, W.; Lee, J.M.; Yoon, J.H.; Han, J.K.; Choi, B.I.; Yoon, J.H.; Lee, K.B.; Lee, K.W.; Yi, N.J.; Suh, K.S. Liver fibrosis staging with MR elastography: Comparison of diagnostic performance between patients with chronic hepatitis B and those with other etiologic causes. *Radiology* **2016**, *280*, 88–97. [CrossRef]
10. Kim, S.W.; Lee, J.M.; Park, S.; Joo, I.; Yoon, J.H.; Chang, W.; Kim, H. Diagnostic Performance of Spin-Echo Echo-Planar Imaging Magnetic Resonance Elastography in 3T System for Noninvasive Assessment of Hepatic Fibrosis. *Korean J. Radiol.* **2022**, *23*, 180–188. [CrossRef]
11. Hoyt, K.; Castaneda, B.; Zhang, M.; Nigwekar, P.; di Sant'agnese, P.A.; Joseph, J.V.; Strang, J.; Rubens, D.J.; Parker, K.J. Tissue elasticity properties as biomarkers for prostate cancer. *Cancer Biomark.* **2008**, *4*, 213–225. [CrossRef] [PubMed]
12. Zhang, M.; Nigwekar, P.; Castaneda, B.; Hoyt, K.; Joseph, J.V.; di Sant'Agnese, A.; Messing, E.M.; Strang, J.G.; Rubens, D.J.; Parker, K.J. Quantitative characterization of viscoelastic properties of human prostate correlated with histology. *Ultrasound Med. Biol.* **2005**, *34*, 1033–1042. [CrossRef] [PubMed]
13. Reiter, R.; Majumdar, S.; Kearney, S.; Kajdacsy-Balla, A.; Macias, V.; Crivellaro, S.; Caldwell, B.; Abern, M.; Royston, T.J.; Klatt, D. Prostate cancer assessment using MR elastography of fresh prostatectomy specimens at 9.4 T. *Magn. Reson. Med.* **2020**, *84*, 396–404. [CrossRef] [PubMed]
14. Chopra, R.; Arani, A.; Huang, Y.; Musquera, M.; Wachsmuth, J.; Bronskill, M.; Plewes, D. In vivo MR elastography of the prostate gland using a transurethral actuator. *Magn. Reson. Med.* **2009**, *62*, 665–671. [CrossRef] [PubMed]
15. Arani, A.; Plewes, D.; Krieger, A.; Chopra, R. The feasibility of endorectal MR elastography for prostate cancer localization. *Magn. Reson. Med.* **2011**, *66*, 1649–1657. [CrossRef]
16. Sahebjavaher, R.S.; Baghani, A.; Honarvar, M.; Sinkus, R.; Salcudean, S.E. Transperineal prostate MR elastography: Initial in vivo results. *Magn. Reson. Med.* **2013**, *69*, 411–420. [CrossRef]

17. Dittmann, F.; Reiter, R.; Guo, J.; Haas, M.; Asbach, P.; Fischer, T.; Braun, J.; Sack, I. Tomoelastography of the prostate using multifrequency MR elastography and externally placed pressurized-air drivers. *Magn. Reson. Med.* **2018**, *79*, 1325–1333. [CrossRef]
18. Asbach, P.; Ro, S.R.; Aldoj, N.; Snellings, J.; Reiter, R.; Lenk, J.; Köhlitz, T.; Haas, M.; Guo, J.; Hamm, B.; et al. In Vivo Quantification of Water Diffusion, Stiffness, and Tissue Fluidity in Benign Prostatic Hyperplasia and Prostate Cancer. *Investig. Radiol.* **2020**, *55*, 524–530. [CrossRef]
19. Li, M.; Guo, J.; Hu, P.; Jiang, H.; Chen, J.; Hu, J.; Asbach, P.; Sack, I.; Li, W. Tomoelastography Based on Multifrequency MR Elastography for Prostate Cancer Detection: Comparison with Multiparametric MRI. *Radiology* **2021**, *299*, 362–370. [CrossRef]
20. Silva, M.M., Jr.; Matheus, W.E.; Garcia, P.V.; Stopiglia, R.M.; Billis, A.; Ferreira, U.; Favaro, W.J. Characterization of reactive stroma in prostate cancer: Involvement of growth factors, metalloproteinase matrix, sexual hormones receptors and prostatic stem cell. *Int. Braz. J. Urol.* **2015**, *41*, 849–858. [CrossRef]
21. Hinshaw, D.C.; Shevde, L.A. The Tumor Microenvironment Innately Modulates Cancer Progression. *Cancer Res.* **2019**, *79*, 4557–4566. [CrossRef] [PubMed]
22. Bonollo, F.; Thalmann, G.N.; Kruithof-de Julio, M.; Karkampouna, S. The Role of Cancer-Associated Fibroblasts in Prostate Cancer Tumorigenesis. *Cancers* **2020**, *12*, 1887. [CrossRef] [PubMed]
23. Luthold, C.; Hallal, T.; Labbé, D.P.; Bordeleau, F. The extracellular matrix stiffening: A trigger of prostate cancer progression and castration resistance? *Cancers* **2022**, *14*, 2887. [CrossRef]
24. Heidegger, I.; Frantzi, M.; Salcher, S.; Tymoszuk, P.; Martowicz, A.; Gomez-Gomez, E.; Blanca, A.; Cano, G.L.; Latosinska, A.; Mischak, H.; et al. Prediction of Clinically Significant Prostate Cancer by a Specific Collagen-related Transcriptome, Proteome and Urinome Signature. *Eur. Urol. Oncol.* **2024**, *7*, 969–1158. [CrossRef] [PubMed]
25. Lee, H.J.; Cho, S.B.; Lee, J.K.; Kim, J.S.; Oh, C.H.; Kim, H.J.; Yoon, H.; Ahn, H.K.; Kim, M.; Hwang, Y.G.; et al. The feasibility of MR elastography with transpelvic vibration for localization of focal prostate lesion. *Sci. Rep.* **2024**, *14*, 3864. [CrossRef] [PubMed]
26. Lambregts, D.M.; Beets, G.L.; Maas, M.; Curvo-Semedo, L.; Kessels, A.G.; Thywissen, T.; Beets-Tan, R.G. Tumour ADC measurements in rectal cancer: Effect of ROI methods on ADC values and interobserver variability. *Eur. Radiol.* **2011**, *21*, 2567–2574. [CrossRef]
27. Reiter, R.; Majumdar, S.; Kearney, S.; Kajdacsy-Balla, A.; Macias, V.; Crivellaro, S.; Abern, M.; Royston, T.J.; Klatt, D. Investigating the heterogeneity of viscoelastic properties in prostate cancer using MR elastography at 9.4T in fresh prostatectomy specimens. *Magn. Reson. Imaging* **2022**, *87*, 113–118. [CrossRef]
28. Peng, Y.C.; Joyner, A.L. Hedgehog signaling in prostate epithelial-mesenchymal growth regulation. *Dev. Biol.* **2015**, *400*, 94–104. [CrossRef]

Disclaimer/Publisher's Note: The statements, opinions and data contained in all publications are solely those of the individual author(s) and contributor(s) and not of MDPI and/or the editor(s). MDPI and/or the editor(s) disclaim responsibility for any injury to people or property resulting from any ideas, methods, instructions or products referred to in the content.

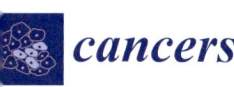

Article

Prostate Cancers Invisible on Multiparametric MRI: Pathologic Features in Correlation with Whole-Mount Prostatectomy

Aritrick Chatterjee [1,2,*], Alexander Gallan [3], Xiaobing Fan [1,2], Milica Medved [1,2], Pranadeep Akurati [4], Roger M. Bourne [5], Tatjana Antic [6], Gregory S. Karczmar [1,2] and Aytekin Oto [1,2]

1. Department of Radiology, University of Chicago, Chicago, IL 60637, USA; xfan@uchicago.edu (X.F.); mmedved@uchicago.edu (M.M.); gskarczm@uchicago.edu (G.S.K.); aoto@uchicagomedicine.org (A.O.)
2. Sanford J. Grossman Center of Excellence in Prostate Imaging and Image Guided Therapy, University of Chicago, Chicago, IL 60637, USA
3. Department of Pathology, Medical College of Wisconsin, Milwaukee, WI 53226, USA; agallan@mcw.edu
4. Department of Biology, Loyola University, Chicago, IL 60611, USA
5. Discipline of Medical Imaging Science, Sydney School of Health Sciences, Faculty of Medicine and Health, The University of Sydney, Sydney, NSW 2006, Australia; roger.bourne@sydney.edu.au
6. Department of Pathology, University of Chicago, Chicago, IL 60637, USA; tatjana.antic@uchospitals.edu
* Correspondence: aritrick@uchicago.edu; Tel.: +1-773-702-4467

Simple Summary: We investigated why some prostate cancers (PCas) are not identified on multiparametric MRI (mpMRI) by using ground truth reference from whole-mount prostatectomy specimens. A total of 61 patients with PCa underwent 3T mpMRI followed by prostatectomy. Lesions visible on MRI prospectively or retrospectively identified after correlating with histology were considered "identified cancers" (ICs). Lesions that could not be identified on mpMRI were considered "unidentified cancers" (UCs). Pathologists marked the Gleason score, stage, size, and density of cancer glands and performed quantitative histology to calculate the tissue composition. The UCs were significantly smaller, had lower Gleason scores and clinical stage lesions, with a lower density of cancer glands, compared with the ICs. Independent from size and Gleason score, tissue composition differences, specifically, the higher lumen and lower epithelium in UCs (associated with higher T2 and ADC), can explain why some of the prostate cancers cannot be identified on mpMRI.

Abstract: We investigated why some prostate cancers (PCas) are not identified on multiparametric MRI (mpMRI) by using ground truth reference from whole-mount prostatectomy specimens. A total of 61 patients with biopsy-confirmed PCa underwent 3T mpMRI followed by prostatectomy. Lesions visible on MRI prospectively or retrospectively identified after correlating with histology were considered "identified cancers" (ICs). Lesions that could not be identified on mpMRI were considered "unidentified cancers" (UCs). Pathologists marked the Gleason score, stage, size, and density of the cancer glands and performed quantitative histology to calculate the tissue composition. Out of 115 cancers, 19 were unidentified on MRI. The UCs were significantly smaller and had lower Gleason scores and clinical stage lesions compared with the ICs. The UCs had significantly ($p < 0.05$) higher ADC (1.34 ± 0.38 vs. 1.02 ± 0.30 $\mu m^2/ms$) and T2 (117.0 ± 31.1 vs. 97.1 ± 25.1 ms) compared with the ICs. The density of the cancer glands was significantly ($p = 0.04$) lower in the UCs. The percentage of the Gleason 4 component in Gleason 3 + 4 lesions was nominally ($p = 0.15$) higher in the ICs ($20 \pm 12\%$) compared with the UCs ($15 \pm 8\%$). The UCs had a significantly lower epithelium (32.9 ± 21.5 vs. $47.6 \pm 13.1\%$, $p = 0.034$) and higher lumen volume (20.4 ± 10.0 vs. $13.3 \pm 4.1\%$, $p = 0.021$) compared with the ICs. Independent from size and Gleason score, the tissue composition differences, specifically, the higher lumen and lower epithelium in UCs, can explain why some of the prostate cancers cannot be identified on mpMRI.

Keywords: prostate cancer; MRI; invisible lesion; tissue composition

1. Introduction

Prostate cancer (PCa) is the most common non-cutaneous cancer in men in the United States, with one out of nine men affected by it [1]. Magnetic resonance imaging (MRI) is increasingly being used for prostate cancer diagnosis and for guiding biopsies due to its advantages over traditional prostate-specific antigen (PSA) screening and transrectal ultrasound (TRUS)-guided biopsies in its ability to reliably visualize the whole prostate noninvasively [2–4]. MRI not only provides information about the presence of PCa, but also about the location and size of PCa lesions [5,6]. Despite MRI's good soft tissue contrast, higher sensitivity, and negative predictive value for PCa detection, a large number of prostate cancers still go undetected [3,7–9]. It has been noted that up to 30% of clinically significant cancers can be missed even by expert radiologists on multiparametric MRI (mpMRI) using the PIRADS guidelines [9–12], with a large variation seen between radiologists and imaging centers [13,14].

An improved understanding of why some lesions are missed by mpMRI may be critical to improving prostate MR imaging protocol and may lead to increased diagnostic accuracy. The few studies that have looked into the characteristics of these missed cancers suggest that missed cancers tend to be of smaller size or volume, have a lower Gleason score and PSA density, and are located in a specific location (apical or anterior) compared with cancer lesions that were identified on mpMRI [9,10,12,15–18]. However, only a handful of studies have investigated histologic differences between identified and unidentified cancer lesions [19,20]. A significant fraction of missed cancers cannot be explained by their small size or low Gleason score, and some biophysical explanation as to why some cancers are missed is needed. In addition, mpMRI is also known to underestimate the true index lesion pathological volume [21,22] and represents the foundation to further investigate invisible vs. visible tumors. Because the contrast on prostate MRI scans heavily depends on the tissue's microstructures and their distinct MR properties [23], we hypothesize that histological features (such as tissue composition and cancer cell density) may impact the MR visibility of certain cancers. Therefore, this study aims to investigate why some prostate cancers are not identified on mpMRI using ground truth reference from whole-mount prostatectomy specimens.

2. Materials and Methods

2.1. Study Patients

This institutional-review-board-approved study involved a retrospective analysis of prospectively acquired data. It was conducted with prior informed patient consent and was HIPAA compliant. Inclusion criteria for this study included patients with prior biopsy-proven prostate cancer that underwent prostate mpMRI on a 3T scanner, followed by subsequent radical prostatectomy with whole-mount processing and digitization of histology slides. Exclusion criteria included the receipt of radiation or hormonal therapy prior to MRI that could have led to alterations in prostatic signal on MRI and impaired renal function (glomerular filtration rate or GFR less than 60 mL/min). Of the 108 patients that had initially consented and were imaged at our research center between March 2014 and June 2017, only 61 patients that fit the criteria were recruited for this study. There is an overlap between some of the research subjects used in this study and some of our previously published works [24,25], but none of the previous papers investigated why some prostate cancers are not identified on mpMRI.

2.2. MR Imaging

Patients underwent preoperative multiparametric MRI using a 3T Philips Achieva MR scanner along with an endorectal coil (Medrad, Warrendale, PA, USA) and a 16-channel phased array coil (Philips, Eindhoven, Netherlands) placed around the pelvis. The prostate mpMRI protocol included axial and coronal T2-weighted, axial multi-echo T2-weighted, axial diffusion-weighted, and axial dynamic contrast-enhanced images. Typical MR imaging parameters that were used are described in further detail in Table 1.

Table 1. MR imaging parameters.

Imaging Sequence	Pulse Sequence	FOV (mm)	Scan Matrix Size	In Plane Resolution (mm)	TE (ms)	TR (ms)	Slice Thickness (mm)	Flip Angle (°)
Axial T2W	SE-TSE	160 × 160	400 × 400	0.4 × 0.4	115	8230	3	90
Multi-echo T2W (T2 mapping)	SE-TSE	160 × 160	212 × 212	0.75 × 0.75	30, 60, 90, 120, 150, 180, 210, 240, 270	7850	3	90
DWI [a]	SE-EPI	180 × 180	120 × 120	1.5 × 1.5	80	6093	3	90
DCE-MRI [b]	T1-FFE	250 × 385	200 × 308	1.25 × 1.25	3.3	4.8	3.5	10

SE—spin echo; TSE—turbo spin echo; EPI—echo planar imaging; FFE—fast field echo. [a] b-values used: 0, 50, 150, 990, 1500 s/mm^2, δ/Δ = ms. [b] Contrast agent: gadobenate dimeglumine (MultiHance, Bracco, Minneapolis, MI, USA) was injected at a rate of 2.0 mL/s followed by a 20-mL saline flush. Contrast dose amount was based on patient's weight (0.1 mmol/kg). DCE-MRI T1-weigthed images were taken with temporal resolution of ~8.3 s at 60 dynamic scan points over 8.2 min.

2.3. Histology Processing

The subjects underwent radical prostatectomy. The excised prostate specimens were fixed overnight in 10% buffered formalin. The fixed organ was then serially sectioned transversely (4 mm slice thickness), approximately in the same plane as the axial MR images. Sectioned tissue was embedded in paraffin and microtomed into 5 µm sections, and whole-mount hematoxylin and eosin (H&E) stained slides were made. The slides were evaluated for prostate cancer by expert pathologists (T.A. and A.G., 15 and 5 years' experience, respectively) and all PCas were marked on the histologic slides for correlation with MR images. However, only cancer lesions meeting the minimum size criteria of 5 mm × 5 mm were included in the analysis. The whole-mount sections were scanned and digitized using a brightfield Olympus VS120 whole-mount digital microscope (Olympus Corporation, Waltham, MA, USA) at 20× magnification.

2.4. MR Image Analysis

MRI and histology sections were matched by the consensus of an experienced radiologist (18 years' experience with prostate MRI), pathologist (15 years' experience), and medical physicist (8 years' experience). The lesions that were visible on conventional multi-parametric MRI (T2-weighted, diffusion-weighted images along with apparent diffusion coefficient maps and dynamic contrast-enhanced images) and were prospectively (blinded to pathology results) or retrospectively identified after correlating with histology were considered "identified cancers". Lesions that could not be identified (invisible) on mpMRI even after radiological–pathological correlation were considered "unidentified cancers".

Using the axial T2-weighted images as the reference image, other mpMRI sequences—diffusion-weighted and contrast-enhanced MRI—were co-registered using rigid registration in 3D Slicer (https://github.com/rcc-uchicago/PCampReview, accessed on 1 November 2016) and matched with corresponding histological sections. Subsequently, MR images were analyzed by an expert radiologist (A.O., 15 years' experience with prostate MRI), and regions of interest (ROIs) were marked on axial T2-weighted images on regions of known PCa verified on whole prostatectomy sections. The ROIs for the cancer lesions were drawn by the radiologist based on outlines by pathologists on whole-mount histologic sections. These ROIs drawn on T2W images were then transferred to other mpMRI sequences, keeping the same shape and size as on the T2W images using 3D Slicer, similar to previous studies [24–26].

Quantitative analysis of MRI data was performed using in-house programs in MATLAB v2019a (Mathworks, Natick, MA, USA) and Interactive Data Language (IDL, Harris Geospatial Solutions, Boulder, CO, USA). Apparent diffusion coefficient (ADC) and quantitative T2 maps were calculated from diffusion-weighted and multi-echo T2-weighted images, respectively, using a mono-exponential signal decay model using custom written code in MATLAB on a voxel-by-voxel basis, and mean values (ADC and T2) for the ROIs were calculated. For DCE-MRI, the percent signal enhancement (PSE) curve (relative to unenhanced image intensity) is calculated using the formula

$$\text{PSE}(t) = \frac{S(t) - S_0}{S_0} \times 100$$

where S_0 is the baseline signal intensity and $S(t)$ is the DCE signal at each time point (t). Subsequently, PSE vs. time curves were analyzed in IDL using the empirical mathematical model (EMM) described in Fan et al. [27] with the following equation:

$$\text{PSE}(t) = A\left(1 - e^{-\alpha t}\right)e^{-\beta t}$$

where A (%) is the amplitude of the relative percent signal enhancement curve or PSE, α describes the signal enhancement due to contrast agent uptake, and β is the washout rate.

2.5. Pathology Image Analysis

Two experienced, board-certified genitourinary pathologists (T.A. and A.G., with 15 and 5 years of experience with prostate pathology, respectively), working in consensus, marked the Gleason score, pathologic stage, and size (dimensions at the section of largest extent) for all cancers.

We further investigated all cancers that were undetected, along with identified cancers with matching size and grade (Gleason 3 + 3 and 3 + 4). The relative density, which is defined as the density of cancer glands with respect to surrounding tissue (category or scale 1–5, with 5 being highly dense compared with surrounding tissue), and the absolute density scale, which is defined as how sparse or dense the cancer glands are in the lesion [28] (category 1–4, with 4 being highly dense cancer), were determined visually by the experienced pathologists. In cancers with Gleason score 3 + 4, the percentage of Gleason pattern 4 was also determined.

The cancer regions of interest (rectangular area) were extracted from digitized whole-mount images using the BIOP VSI reader plugin on ImageJ v1.51(National Institutes of Health, Bethesda, MD, USA). The software was used to crop the intended area and convert the digitized pathology slides from the proprietary virtual slide image (.vsi) file format (Olympus proprietary format) to the commonly used tagged image file format (TIFF). To avoid errors during tissue segmentation, luminal secretions were removed from the glandular space using Microsoft Paint (https://mspaint.humanhead.com/, accessed on 1 November 2016) (Microsoft Corporation, Redmond, WA, USA). Quantitative histology was then performed to calculate fractional volumes of tissue components using image segmentation of H&E-stained prostate tissue to separate the stroma, epithelium, and lumen using Image Pro Premier v9.2. This was performed on the basis of color, intensity, morphology, and background using the "Smart Segment" functionality, which was described in a previous study [23]. Like in the previous study, segmentation performed with the software was visually inspected by the consensus of a pathologist and medical physicist and rectified iteratively until the final segmented image was determined to have fewer than 5% errors. The tissue fractional volumes were calculated using the "Count" functionality and defined as the percentage of image pixels that were segmented as that tissue type. The segmentation function of this tool has been validated to estimate prostate tissue composition and used in previous studies with reported correlation greater than 0.9 with manual segmentation [23,29,30].

2.6. Statistical Analysis

Statistical analysis was performed using SPSS v28 (IBM Corporation, Armonk, NY, USA). A one-sided *t*-test (parametric test for scalar data: lesion size, ADC, T2, DCE parameters, proportion of Gleason 4 pattern, and tissue volumes) or Mann–Whitney U test (nonparametric test for categorical/ordinal data: Gleason score, stage, and relative and absolute density of lesions) was performed to determine whether any significant differences between the identified and unidentified cancers were present. The significance level was set as $p < 0.05$.

3. Results

3.1. Participant and Tumor Characteristics

A total of 61 patients who fit the criteria (imaged at our research center, followed by subsequent prostatectomy and digitized pathology) were recruited for this study. The mean age (± standard deviation) of all included men was 59 ± 8 years (range 40–76 years), and mean PSA was 8.2 ± 7.9 ng/mL (range 0.8–66.1 ng/mL). A total of 115 confirmed cancers met the minimum size criteria and were included in the study.

Only 19 of 115 (17%) confirmed cancerous lesions were unidentified on mpMRI. These unidentified cancers came from 17 subjects, while the identified lesions came from 57 subjects. Of the 96 identified lesions, 83 lesions were found prospectively on mpMRI (blinded to pathology results) and 13 were retrospectively identified after correlating with histology. However, no difference in quantitative mpMRI parameters was found for the identified cancer lesions. Representative images of identified and unidentified cancers are shown in Figures 1 and 2.

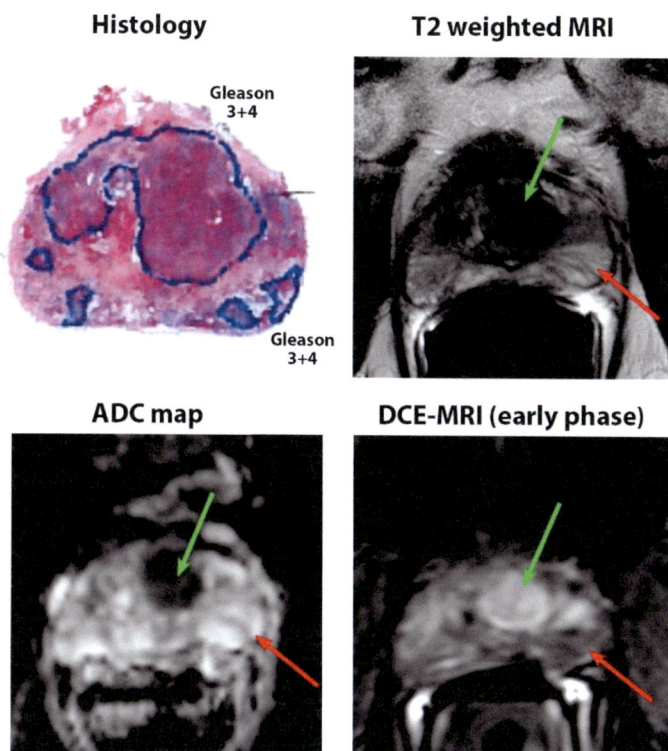

Figure 1. A 67-year-old patient with PSA of 9.5 ng/mL with a Gleason 3 + 4 anterior lesion (green arrow) that was clearly identified on mpMRI. The lesion was highly hypointense on T2W (T2 = 61 ± 8 ms) and ADC (0.58 ± 0.09 µm^2/ms) and showed focal enhancement on early-phase DCE-MRI. However, another Gleason 3 + 4 lesion in the left peripheral zone (red arrow) was unidentified on MRI. The lesion was isointense on T2W (T2 = 194 ± 34 ms) and ADC (1.51 ± 0.25 µm^2/ms) and showed no focal enhancement on early-phase DCE-MRI. It was found to have lower glandular density than the surrounding benign tissue and was interspersed between atrophic benign glands.

Of the identified lesions, 78 lesions (81%) were primarily in the peripheral zone, while 18 lesions (19%) were in the transition zone. A similar zonal distribution was found for the unidentified lesions, with 15 (79%) peripheral zone lesions and 4 (21%) transition zone lesions. The unidentified cancers (1.4 ± 1.0 cm × 0.7 ± 0.4 cm) were significantly smaller ($p < 0.001$) in size compared with the identified cancers (2.1 ± 1.2 cm × 1.0 ± 0.5 cm). The unidentified cancers were predominantly low grade ($p < 0.001$) (11 Gleason 3 + 3, 8 Gleason 3 + 4) and stage ($p < 0.01$) (all 19 were stage T2) compared with the identified cancers (Grade: 20 Gleason 3 + 3, 59 Gleason 3 + 4, 13 Gleason 4 + 3, 4 Gleason 4 + 5; Stage: 68 Stage T2, 27 Stage T3). Additional details can be found in Table 2.

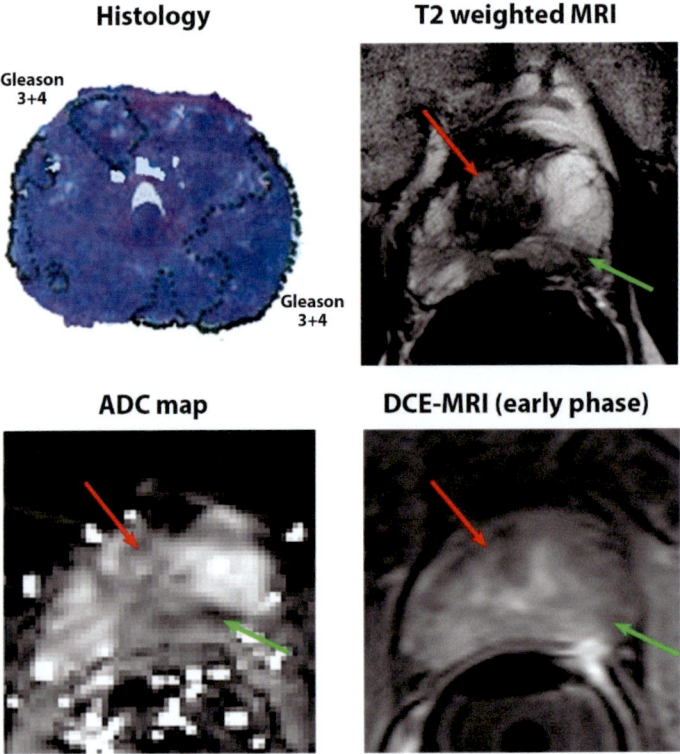

Figure 2. A 53-year-old patient with PSA of 5.1 ng/mL with a Gleason 3 + 4 lesion (green arrow) in the left peripheral zone that was identified on mpMRI. The lesion was focally hypointense on T2W (T2 = 94 ± 34 ms) and ADC (1.13 ± 0.26 μm^2/ms) but showed no focal enhancement on early-phase DCE-MRI. However, another Gleason 3 + 4 lesion in the right transition zone (red arrows) was unidentified on MRI (no focal area of abnormal MR signal that correlates with cancer presence). The lesion was isointense on T2W (T2 = 138 ± 52 ms) and ADC (1.45 ± 0.41 μm^2/ms) and showed no focal enhancement on early-phase DCE-MRI, making it indistinguishable from the surrounding benign tissue. Even though it was found to have high glandular density, it was adjacent to very dense benign glands.

Table 2. Cancer lesion properties.

Gleason Score	Identified Cancers	Unidentified Cancers	All Cancers
3 + 3	20	11	31
3 + 4	59	8	67
4 + 3	13	-	13
4 + 5	4	-	4
Overall	96	19	115
	Relative density		
Relative density category	Identified Cancers [+]	Unidentified Cancers	All Cancers
Significantly less glandular density than surrounding benign tissue (Category 1)	0	1	1
Somewhat less glandular density than surrounding benign tissue (Category 2)	0	3	3
Similar glandular density to surrounding benign tissue (Category 3)	4	3	7
Somewhat higher glandular density than surrounding benign tissue (Category 4)	12	9	21
Significantly higher glandular density than surrounding benign tissue (Category 5)	9	3	12
Overall	25	19	44
	Absolute density		
Absolute density category (% of cancer tissue)	Identified Cancers [+]	Unidentified Cancers	All Cancers
Highly sparse (0–25%) (Category 1)	0	1	1
Sparse (25–50%) (Category 2)	2	7	9
Dense (50–75%) (Category 3)	16	7	23
Highly dense (75–100%) (Category 4)	7	4	11
Overall	25	19	44

[+] Only size and Gleason score matched identified cancers used in this analysis.

3.2. Quantitative MRI Characteristics

Unidentified cancers had significantly higher ADC (1.34 ± 0.38 vs. 1.02 ± 0.30 μm^2/ms, $p < 0.001$) and T2 (117.0 ± 31.1 vs. 97.1 ± 25.1 ms, $p = 0.005$) compared with cancers identified on MRI (Figure 3). However, the DCE-MRI parameters from EMM analysis, A or amplitude (110.7 ± 45.3 vs. $129.2 \pm 51.1\%$, $p = 0.206$), α or enhancement rate (5.24 ± 2.84 vs. $6.79 \pm 5.08\%$ per s, $p = 0.263$), and β or washout rate (0.031 ± 0.083 vs. $0.081 \pm 0.072\%$ per s, $p = 0.222$), were not significantly different between the unidentified and identified cancers.

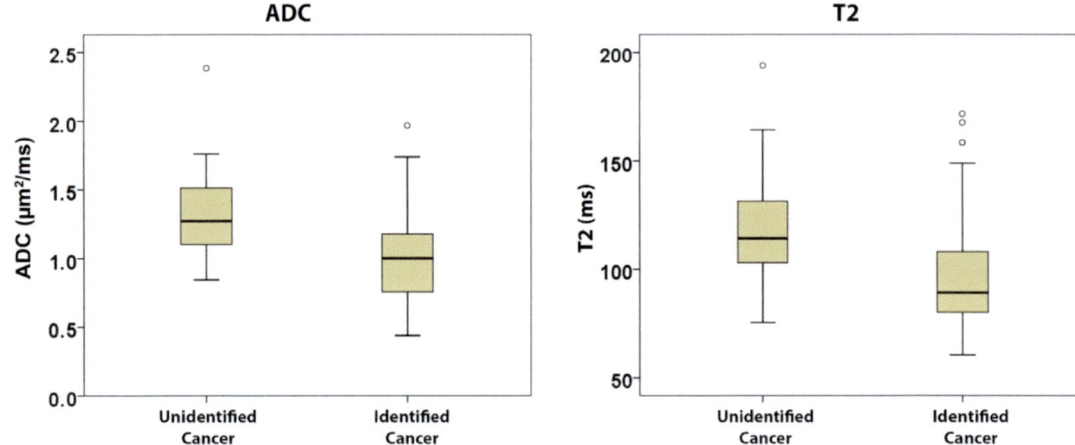

Figure 3. Unidentified cancers had significantly higher ADC (1.34 ± 0.38 vs. 1.02 ± 0.30 μm^2/ms, $p < 0.001$) and T2 (117.0 ± 31.1 vs. 97.1 ± 25.1 ms, $p = 0.005$) compared with cancers identified on MRI.

3.3. Pathologic Characteristics

Nineteen unidentified cancers and twenty-five identified cancers with similar sizes and grades were selected for analysis. While investigating all undetected cancers along with size and grade (Gleason 3 + 3 and 3 + 4) matched identified cancers, the relative density and absolute density of cancer glands were found to be significantly ($p = 0.04$) higher in the cancers identified on MRI compared with the unidentified cancers. A large percentage of the unidentified cancers tended to have lower relative density compared with the surrounding tissue (4/19 = 21% vs. 0/25 = 0%) and to be categorized as sparse cancers (8/19 = 42% vs. 2/25 = 8%) compared with the MR-visible cancers. Detailed results can be found in Table 2. However, the percentage of the Gleason 4 component in Gleason 3 + 4 lesions was only nominally ($p = 0.15$) higher in the identified cancers (20 ± 12%) compared with the unidentified cancers on MRI (15 ± 8%).

An investigation into the tissue composition of these cancers using matching lesion size and grade showed that nonvisible cancers on MRI had significantly lower epithelium volume, 32.9 ± 21.5 vs. 47.6 ± 13.1% ($p = 0.034$), and higher lumen volume, 20.4 ± 10.0 vs. 13.3 ± 4.1% ($p = 0.021$), compared with identified cancers. However, no difference in stroma volume was found between the unidentified and identified cancers (46.6 ± 19.9 vs. 39.1 ± 13.3%, $p = 0.154$). Representative examples of histologic images and corresponding segmented images for a cancer identified on MRI and a cancer undefined on MRI can be seen in Figure 4. Box plots showing the differences in tissue composition (fractional volumes of stroma, epithelium, and lumen) between identified and unidentified cancers are shown in Figure 5.

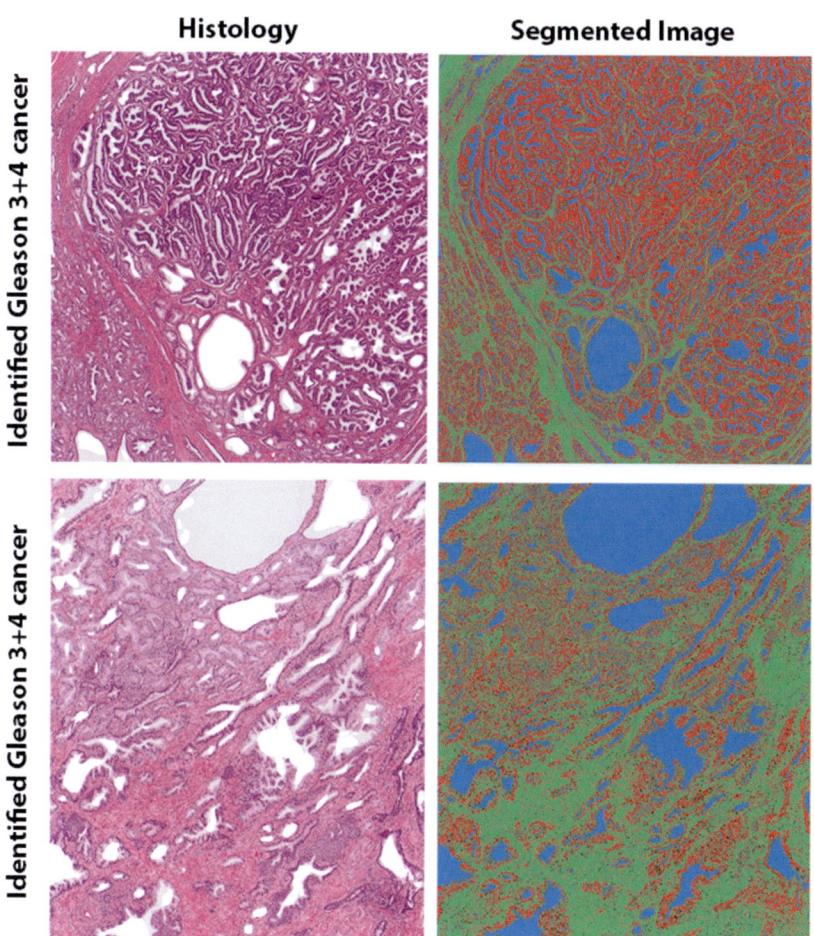

Figure 4. The identified Gleason 3 + 4 cancer from the posterior peripheral zone from the apex midline (**top**) had higher glandular density compared with the MR-unidentified Gleason 3 + 4 cancer from the right peripheral zone (**bottom**) from the same patient (76 years old). Tissue components were segmented into stroma (green), epithelium (red), and lumen (blue). The tissue composition in the identified cancer and the unidentified cancer was different: stroma, 21.5 vs. 45.7%; epithelium, 60.6 vs. 34.0%; and lumen, 17.9 vs. 20.4%. In addition, the identified cancer (40%) had a greater proportion of Gleason pattern 4 than the unidentified cancer (10%).

Some additional observations by pathologists, possibly explaining why some cancers were not identified, were: cystic changes adjacent to the cancer lesions ($n = 2$), small cancer focus ($n = 2$), cancers being interspersed between atrophic ($n = 2$) or benign glands ($n = 4$), and dense glands surrounding the cancer ($n = 1$).

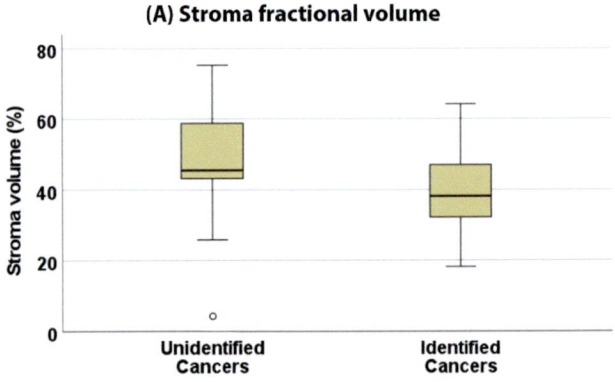
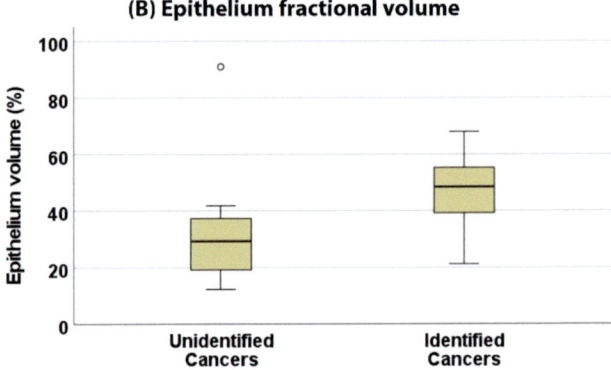
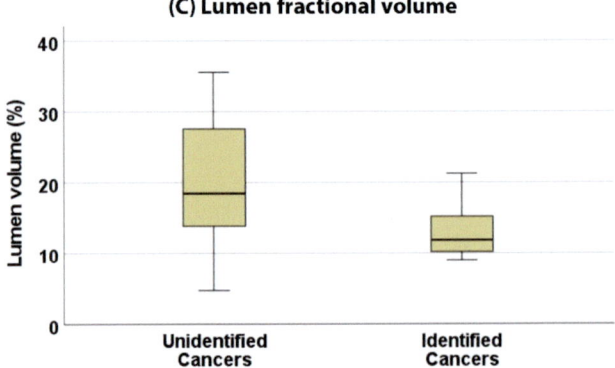

Figure 5. An investigation into the tissue composition of these cancers as presented in these box-plots showed that unidentified cancers had significantly lower epithelium volume (**B**), 32.9 ± 21.5 vs. 47.6 ± 13.1% ($p = 0.034$), and significantly higher lumen volume (**C**), 20.4 ± 10.0 vs. 13.3 ± 4.1% ($p = 0.021$), compared with identified cancers. However, no difference in stroma volume (**A**) was found between the unidentified and identified cancers (46.6 ± 19.9 vs. 39.1 ± 13.3%, $p = 0.154$).

4. Discussion

In this study, we investigated why some prostate cancers are not identified on mpMRI by using ground truth reference from whole-mount prostatectomy specimens. Our results showed that unidentified cancers tend to exhibit a lower Gleason score and pathologic stage, smaller size, and lower density of glands compared with the surrounding tissue (sparse cancer lesions), and they have different tissue compositions compared with cancer lesions identified on MRI. Independent from size and Gleason score, tissue composition differences, specifically, a higher proportion of lumen (associated with high T2 and ADC values) and lower epithelium (associated with lower T2 and ADC) in unidentified cancers compared with identified cancers, can explain why some of the prostate cancers cannot be identified on mpMRI.

The unidentified cancers are smaller in size and have predominantly lower Gleason scores. These results are in agreement with previous studies, including the large multicenter PROMIS study [9,10,12,15–18]. The fact that we see that a higher percentage of the unidentified cancers is non-clinically significant cancer reinforces the role mpMRI plays in risk stratification of men with suspected prostate cancer: detecting clinically significant cancers (Gleason 3 + 4 and above) while missing non-clinically significant cancers (Gleason 3 + 3). Future studies may consider looking at the oncological implications of mpMRI visible versus invisible lesions and whether that may affect decisions on treatment options. A negative correlation between the cancer Gleason score and the ADC [31] and T2 [32] has been noted in the literature. This can also be attributed to tissue composition differences in different Gleason patterns, as shown by a previous study [23], which showed that Gleason pattern 3 is closely similar to normal prostate (preserved glandular morphology), whereas in pattern 4 and higher, there is gradually less lumen and more dense epithelial cells. This leads to a reduction in MR contrast in ADC and T2 maps and T2-weighted images in lower-grade lesions, making detection challenging.

Differences in quantitative mpMRI parameters were also found. The unidentified cancers had significantly higher ADC and T2 compared with the identified cancers, confirming why these lesions were not visualized on mpMRI. Conversely, the DCE-MRI parameters were not significantly different between the identified and nonidentified cancers. Considering DCE-MRI is used as a secondary sequence to T2W and DWI (primary sequences) for prostate cancer diagnosis, and that up to 50% of prostate lesions are not seen on DCE-MRI [33], it is not surprising that a number of lesions remained invisible on DCE as well.

We chose identified cancers with sizes and Gleason scores similar to the unidentified cancers for subsequent analysis. While looking at size- and Gleason score-matched cancers, the relative density and absolute density of cancer glands were higher in the identified cancers compared with the unidentified cancers. A large percentage of the unidentified cancers tended to have lower relative density compared with the surrounding tissue, and were categorized as sparse cancers, compared with the identified cancers. This is consistent with a study by Langer et al. [28] that showed that sparse prostate tumors have similar mpMRI (ADC and T2 values) to those of benign peripheral zone tissue, which may limit their detection and the assessment of tumor volume of these sparse cancer lesions in mpMRI. Another study by van Houdt et. al. also reported lower tumor density and heterogeneous tumor morphology in undetected prostate cancers on MRI [20], while Miyai et. al. reported that cancer cells cover a larger area in detected cancers (60.9%) versus undetected cancers (42.7%) [34]. Other histologic differences, such as loose or desmoplastic stroma and the presence of intermixed benign glands, along with cancer glands that represent sparse cancers, have also been reported [19].

We found that the percentage of the Gleason 4 component in the Gleason 3 + 4 lesions was not significantly higher in the identified cancers (20 ± 12%) compared with the unidentified cancers (15 ± 8%). While this result is similar to another study [34], the percentage of Gleason pattern 4 reported was higher for lesions in that study due to a slightly different definition of unidentified cancers and the cohort containing Gleason 4 + 3 unidentified lesions (which, by definition, are expected to have more than 50% Gleason 4 pattern).

Most importantly, tissue composition differences, specifically, the higher lumen and lower epithelium in unidentified cancers, are likely to be the major contributor to clinically observed variations in different appearances of identified and unidentified cancers on mpMRI and may explain why these lesions were missed on MRI. Most prostate cancers are epithelial in nature and are characterized by rapidly proliferating cancer epithelial cells that concomitantly replace the surrounding stromal cells and luminal space. Epithelial cells are associated with low ADC and T2, while lumen is associated with high ADC and T2. Our results show that identified cancers have similarly higher epithelium and reduced lumen compared with unidentified cancers; therefore, identified cancers have lower ADC and T2, making them easily visible on mpMRI, unlike unidentified cancers. In addition, comparing tissue composition with the previous literature [23,35], the tissue composition of identified cancers in this study (47.6 ± 13.1% epithelium, 13.3 ± 4.1% lumen) matches well with the literature values for Gleason pattern 3 and 4 cancers visualized on MRI and confirmed by pathology (~52–58% epithelium, 11–16% lumen). However, unidentified cancers (32.9 ± 21.5% epithelium, 20.4 ± 10.0% lumen) were found to have tissue compositions closely similar to benign prostatic tissue (~33% epithelium, ~27% lumen), and thus, appear similar to the surrounding benign tissue and remain undetected. Therefore, the biophysical basis of MRI signal changes in prostate tissue can be attributed to tissue composition changes, namely, in differences in the proportions of lumen, epithelium, and stroma. Conventional imaging, measuring ADC and T2 using the mono-exponential signal model, may not be able to isolate signals specific to the cancer cells due to signal averaging when tissue composition changes are not spread out. However, a multicompartment tissue model of the prostate (using the components stroma, epithelium, and lumen) can exploit the distinct biophysical properties of each of these tissue components. This is a basis of some of the newer tissue microstructural imaging models, such as hybrid multidimensional MRI (HM-MRI) [36,37], luminal water imaging [38], VERDICT [39], etc., as well as high b-value non-Gaussian DWI models that have the potential to better identify focal areas of tissue where the tissue composition starts to deviate from the surrounding benign tissue and thus, potentially, to detect lesions that cannot be detected on conventional mpMRI. These results may also suggest the need to develop MRI methods that detect intrinsic properties of cancer cells (i.e., the properties of individual cells) rather than extrinsic properties such as cell density. For example, quadrant analysis of hybrid multidimensional MRI detects signals from enlarged nuclei associated with rapidly growing cancers [40]. Even if cancer cells are dispersed within a voxel, the aggregate signal from these enlarged nuclei may be detectable. However, if cancer cells are dispersed within a voxel, they may not produce a low ADC, but they may have a distinct and detectable signal from cancers cells in quadrant analysis. The use of machine-learning-based or deep-learning-based methods has shown promise in identifying a greater percentage of clinically significant prostate cancers [41,42], and the use of these methods to identify these unidentified lesions may also be considered for future studies.

There are a few limitations to this study. First, this study is a retrospective single-center study, where MRIs were performed using a single MR vendor with a standardized imaging protocol. Additionally, any changes in hardware or imaging parameters may affect image contrast and thus affect whether a lesion is identified on MRI. Therefore, it would be preferable to validate these results for invisible cancers in both a multivendor and multicenter setting using a large sample size (especially that of MR-invisible lesions), including consideration such as the use of independent measures, such that only one lesion is considered for each patient. Third, because whole-mount prostatectomy specimens were needed for the analysis, there is an intrinsic selection bias in the cohort of MR-invisible cancers, as only subjects referred to surgery were enrolled. These may not reflect the population of men with MR-unidentified prostate cancer who did not undergo surgery. Fourth, there may be small uncertainty in the radiology–pathology correlation. The sectioning of the prostate was performed in approximately the same plane as the MRI images, without the use of any patient-specific sectioning mold. In addition, formalin fixation results in tissue shrinkage, which may affect radiology–pathology registration, but this is not unique to our work. Finally, the labeling of unidentified cancers can be subjective as per the visual interpretation of mpMRI, which has been shown to have large inter-reader variation. Combining the prospectively identified lesions and the lesions retrospectively identified after correlating with histology as identified lesions may introduce a bias. The intention was to have a cohort of MR-unidentifiable lesions that are truly MR-invisible lesions, as some of these retrospectively identified lesions could possibly have been identified by other radiologists. While no differences were found for the identified cancer lesions found prospectively on mpMRI or retrospectively identified after correlating with histology, this could be influenced by background signal in the surrounding benign tissue [43].

5. Conclusions

Our study reveals that, independent from size and Gleason score, there are tissue composition differences, specifically, a higher lumen (associated with high T2 and ADC) and a lower epithelium (associated with lower T2 and ADC) in unidentified cancers compared with identified cancers, which might explain why some of the prostate cancers cannot be identified on mpMRI. Some of the newer tissue microstructural imaging models, such as hybrid multidimensional MRI [44], luminal water imaging [38], VERDICT [39], etc., or the development of new MRI methods that detect the intrinsic properties of cancer cells, may have the potential to detect these lesions that cannot be detected on conventional mpMRI.

Author Contributions: Conceptualization, A.C., A.G. and A.O.; methodology, A.C., A.G., X.F., R.M.B., G.S.K. and A.O.; software, A.C., R.M.B. and X.F.; validation, A.C., T.A. and A.O.; formal analysis, A.C., A.G., T.A., P.A., X.F., M.M. and A.O.; investigation, A.C., T.A. and A.O.; resources, T.A., G.S.K. and A.O.; data curation, A.C., A.G., X.F. and P.A.; writing—original draft preparation, A.C.; writing—review and editing, A.C., A.G., X.F., M.M., P.A., R.M.B., T.A., G.S.K. and A.O.; visualization, A.C., A.G., X.F., T.A., G.S.K. and A.O.; supervision, A.C., T.A., G.S.K. and A.O.; project administration, A.C., T.A., G.S.K. and A.O.; funding acquisition, G.S.K. and A.O. All authors have read and agreed to the published version of the manuscript.

Funding: This research was funded by the NIH (R01 CA227036, 1R41CA244056-01A1, R01 CA17280, 1S10OD018448-01) and the Sanford J. Grossman Charitable Trust.

Institutional Review Board Statement: The study was conducted in accordance with the Health Insurance Portability and Accountability Act and approved by the Institutional Review Board of the University of Chicago (IRB13-0756).

Informed Consent Statement: The institutional-review-board-approved study involved retrospective analysis of prospectively acquired data. It was conducted with prior informed patient consent and was HIPAA compliant.

Data Availability Statement: In accordance with the institutional review board, the data acquired in this study contain person-sensitive information, which can be shared only in the context of scientific collaboration.

Conflicts of Interest: The authors state that they have no conflict of interest related to the material discussed in this article. A.C., A.O. and G.S.K. have equity in QMIS, LLC., which is unrelated to this study.

References

1. Siegel, R.L.; Miller, K.D.; Fuchs, H.E.; Jemal, A. Cancer Statistics, 2021. *CA Cancer J. Clin.* **2021**, *71*, 7–33. [CrossRef] [PubMed]
2. Litwin, M.S.; Tan, H. The diagnosis and treatment of prostate cancer: A review. *JAMA* **2017**, *317*, 2532–2542. [CrossRef] [PubMed]
3. Ahmed, H.U.; El-Shater Bosaily, A.; Brown, L.C.; Gabe, R.; Kaplan, R.; Parmar, M.K.; Collaco-Moraes, Y.; Ward, K.; Hindley, R.G.; Freeman, A.; et al. Diagnostic accuracy of multi-parametric MRI and TRUS biopsy in prostate cancer (PROMIS): A paired validating confirmatory study. *Lancet* **2017**, *389*, 815–822. [CrossRef]
4. Panebianco, V.; Barchetti, F.; Sciarra, A.; Ciardi, A.; Indino, E.L.; Papalia, R.; Gallucci, M.; Tombolini, V.; Gentile, V.; Catalano, C. Multiparametric magnetic resonance imaging vs. standard care in men being evaluated for prostate cancer: A randomized study. *Urol. Oncol.* **2015**, *33*, 17.e1–17.e17. [CrossRef]
5. Woo, S.; Suh, C.H.; Kim, S.Y.; Cho, J.Y.; Kim, S.H. Diagnostic Performance of Prostate Imaging Reporting and Data System Version 2 for Detection of Prostate Cancer: A Systematic Review and Diagnostic Meta-analysis. *Eur. Urol.* **2017**, *72*, 177–188. [CrossRef] [PubMed]
6. Isebaert, S.; Van den Bergh, L.; Haustermans, K.; Joniau, S.; Lerut, E.; De Wever, L.; De Keyzer, F.; Budiharto, T.; Slagmolen, P.; Van Poppel, H.; et al. Multiparametric MRI for prostate cancer localization in correlation to whole-mount histopathology. *J. Magn. Reson. Imaging* **2013**, *37*, 1392–1401. [CrossRef]
7. Moldovan, P.C.; Van den Broeck, T.; Sylvester, R.; Marconi, L.; Bellmunt, J.; van den Bergh, R.C.N.; Bolla, M.; Briers, E.; Cumberbatch, M.G.; Fossati, N.; et al. What Is the Negative Predictive Value of Multiparametric Magnetic Resonance Imaging in Excluding Prostate Cancer at Biopsy? A Systematic Review and Meta-analysis from the European Association of Urology Prostate Cancer Guidelines Panel. *Eur. Urol.* **2017**, *72*, 250–266. [CrossRef]
8. Hansen, N.L.; Barrett, T.; Kesch, C.; Pepdjonovic, L.; Bonekamp, D.; O'Sullivan, R.; Distler, F.; Warren, A.; Samel, C.; Hadaschik, B.; et al. Multicentre evaluation of magnetic resonance imaging supported transperineal prostate biopsy in biopsy-naïve men with suspicion of prostate cancer. *BJU Int.* **2018**, *122*, 40–49. [CrossRef]
9. Mohammadian Bajgiran, A.; Afshari Mirak, S.; Shakeri, S.; Felker, E.R.; Ponzini, D.; Ahuja, P.; Sisk, A.E.; Lu, D.S.; Raman, S. Characteristics of missed prostate cancer lesions on 3T multiparametric-MRI in 518 patients: Based on PI-RADSv2 and using whole-mount histopathology reference. *Abdom. Radiol.* **2019**, *44*, 1052–1061. [CrossRef]
10. Borofsky, S.; George, A.K.; Gaur, S.; Bernardo, M.; Greer, M.D.; Mertan, F.V.; Taffel, M.; Moreno, V.; Merino, M.J.; Wood, B.J.; et al. What Are We Missing? False-Negative Cancers at Multiparametric MR Imaging of the Prostate. *Radiology* **2018**, *286*, 186–195. [CrossRef]
11. Fütterer, J.J.; Briganti, A.; De Visschere, P.; Emberton, M.; Giannarini, G.; Kirkham, A.; Taneja, S.S.; Thoeny, H.; Villeirs, G.; Villers, A. Can Clinically Significant Prostate Cancer Be Detected with Multiparametric Magnetic Resonance Imaging? A Systematic Review of the Literature. *Eur. Urol.* **2015**, *68*, 1045–1053. [CrossRef] [PubMed]
12. Schouten, M.G.; van der Leest, M.; Pokorny, M.; Hoogenboom, M.; Barentsz, J.O.; Thompson, L.C.; Futterer, J.J. Why and Where do We Miss Significant Prostate Cancer with Multi-parametric Magnetic Resonance Imaging followed by Magnetic Resonance-guided and Transrectal Ultrasound-guided Biopsy in Biopsy-naive Men? *Eur. Urol.* **2017**, *71*, 896–903. [CrossRef]
13. Stabile, A.; Sorce, G.; Barletta, F.; Brembilla, G.; Mazzone, E.; Pellegrino, F.; Cannoletta, D.; Cirulli, G.O.; Gandaglia, G.; De Cobelli, F.; et al. Impact of prostate MRI central review over the diagnostic performance of MRI-targeted biopsy: Should we routinely ask for an expert second opinion? *World J. Urol.* **2023**, *41*, 3231–3237. [CrossRef] [PubMed]
14. Westphalen, A.C.; McCulloch, C.E.; Anaokar, J.M.; Arora, S.; Barashi, N.S.; Barentsz, J.O.; Bathala, T.K.; Bittencourt, L.K.; Booker, M.T.; Braxton, V.G.; et al. Variability of the Positive Predictive Value of PI-RADS for Prostate MRI across 26 Centers: Experience of the Society of Abdominal Radiology Prostate Cancer Disease-focused Panel. *Radiology* **2020**, *296*, 76–84. [CrossRef] [PubMed]
15. Tan, N.; Margolis, D.J.; Lu, D.Y.; King, K.G.; Huang, J.; Reiter, R.E.; Raman, S.S. Characteristics of Detected and Missed Prostate Cancer Foci on 3-T Multiparametric MRI Using an Endorectal Coil Correlated With Whole-Mount Thin-Section Histopathology. *AJR Am. J. Roentgenol.* **2015**, *205*, W87–W92. [CrossRef]
16. Coker, M.A.; Glaser, Z.A.; Gordetsky, J.B.; Thomas, J.V.; Rais-Bahrami, S. Targets missed: Predictors of MRI-targeted biopsy failing to accurately localize prostate cancer found on systematic biopsy. *Prostate Cancer Prostatic Dis.* **2018**, *21*, 549–555. [CrossRef]
17. Norris, J.M.; Carmona Echeverria, L.M.; Bott, S.R.J.; Brown, L.C.; Burns-Cox, N.; Dudderidge, T.; El-Shater Bosaily, A.; Frangou, E.; Freeman, A.; Ghei, M.; et al. What Type of Prostate Cancer Is Systematically Overlooked by Multiparametric Magnetic Resonance Imaging? An Analysis from the PROMIS Cohort. *Eur. Urol.* **2020**, *78*, 163–170. [CrossRef]
18. Park, K.J.; Kim, M.-h.; Kim, J.K.; Cho, K.-S. Characterization and PI-RADS version 2 assessment of prostate cancers missed by prebiopsy 3-T multiparametric MRI: Correlation with whole-mount thin-section histopathology. *Clin. Imaging* **2019**, *55*, 174–180. [CrossRef]
19. Rosenkrantz, A.B.; Mendrinos, S.; Babb, J.S.; Taneja, S.S. Prostate Cancer Foci Detected on Multiparametric Magnetic Resonance Imaging are Histologically Distinct From Those Not Detected. *J. Urol.* **2012**, *187*, 2032–2038. [CrossRef]
20. van Houdt, P.J.; Ghobadi, G.; Schoots, I.G.; Heijmink, S.W.T.P.J.; de Jong, J.; van der Poel, H.G.; Pos, F.J.; Rylander, S.; Bentzen, L.; Haustermans, K.; et al. Histopathological Features of MRI-Invisible Regions of Prostate Cancer Lesions. *J. Magn. Reson. Imaging* **2020**, *51*, 1235–1246. [CrossRef]
21. Sorce, G.; Stabile, A.; Lucianò, R.; Motterle, G.; Scuderi, S.; Barletta, F.; Pellegrino, F.; Cucchiara, V.; Gandaglia, G.; Fossati, N.; et al. Multiparametric magnetic resonance imaging of the prostate underestimates tumour volume of small visible lesions. *BJU Int.* **2022**, *129*, 201–207. [CrossRef]

2. Sun, C.; Chatterjee, A.; Yousuf, A.; Antic, T.; Eggener, S.; Karczmar, G.S.; Oto, A. Comparison of T2-Weighted Imaging, DWI, and Dynamic Contrast-Enhanced MRI for Calculation of Prostate Cancer Index Lesion Volume: Correlation With Whole-Mount Pathology. *Am. J. Roentgenol.* **2018**, *212*, 351–356. [CrossRef] [PubMed]
3. Chatterjee, A.; Watson, G.; Myint, E.; Sved, P.; McEntee, M.; Bourne, R. Changes in Epithelium, Stroma, and Lumen Space Correlate More Strongly with Gleason Pattern and Are Stronger Predictors of Prostate ADC Changes than Cellularity Metrics. *Radiology* **2015**, *277*, 751–762. [CrossRef] [PubMed]
4. Chatterjee, A.; Gallan, A.J.; He, D.; Fan, X.; Mustafi, D.; Yousuf, A.; Antic, T.; Karczmar, G.S.; Oto, A. Revisiting quantitative multi-parametric MRI of benign prostatic hyperplasia and its differentiation from transition zone cancer. *Abdom. Radiol.* **2019**, *44*, 2233–2243. [CrossRef]
5. Chatterjee, A.; Tokdemir, S.; Gallan, A.J.; Yousuf, A.; Antic, T.; Karczmar, G.S.; Oto, A. Multiparametric MRI Features and Pathologic Outcome of Wedge-Shaped Lesions in the Peripheral Zone on T2-Weighted Images of the Prostate. *Am. J. Roentgenol.* **2019**, *212*, 124–129. [CrossRef] [PubMed]
6. Chatterjee, A.; Turchan, W.T.; Fan, X.; Griffin, A.; Yousuf, A.; Karczmar, G.S.; Liauw, S.L.; Oto, A. Can Pre-treatment Quantitative Multi-parametric MRI Predict the Outcome of Radiotherapy in Patients with Prostate Cancer? *Acad. Radiol.* **2022**, *29*, 977–985. [CrossRef]
7. Fan, X.; Medved, M.; River, J.N.; Zamora, M.; Corot, C.; Robert, P.; Bourrinet, P.; Lipton, M.; Culp, R.M.; Karczmar, G.S. New model for analysis of dynamic contrast-enhanced MRI data distinguishes metastatic from nonmetastatic transplanted rodent prostate tumors. *Magn. Reson. Med.* **2004**, *51*, 487–494. [CrossRef]
8. Langer, D.L.; van der Kwast, T.H.; Evans, A.J.; Sun, L.; Yaffe, M.J.; Trachtenberg, J.; Haider, M.A. Intermixed normal tissue within prostate cancer: Effect on MR imaging measurements of apparent diffusion coefficient and T2—sparse versus dense cancers. *Radiology* **2008**, *249*, 900–908. [CrossRef]
9. Lin, Y.-C.; Lin, G.; Hong, J.-H.; Lin, Y.-P.; Chen, F.-H.; Ng, S.-H.; Wang, C.-C. Diffusion radiomics analysis of intratumoral heterogeneity in a murine prostate cancer model following radiotherapy: Pixelwise correlation with histology. *J. Magn. Reson. Imaging* **2017**, *46*, 483–489. [CrossRef]
10. Chatterjee, A.; Oto, A. Future Perspectives in Multiparametric Prostate MR Imaging. *Magn. Reson. Imaging Clin.* **2019**, *27*, 117–130. [CrossRef]
11. Turkbey, B.; Merino, M.J.; Shih, J.H.; Wood, B.J.; Pinto, P.A.; Choyke, P.L.; Shah, V.P.; Pang, Y.; Bernardo, M.; Xu, S.; et al. Is apparent diffusion coefficient associated with clinical risk scores for prostate cancers that are visible on 3-T MR images? *Radiology* **2011**, *258*, 488–495. [CrossRef]
12. Chatterjee, A.; Devaraj, A.; Matthew, M.; Szasz, T.; Antic, T.; Karczmar, G.; Oto, A. Performance of T2 maps in the detection of prostate cancer. *Acad. Radiol.* **2019**, *26*, 15–21. [CrossRef] [PubMed]
13. He, D.; Chatterjee, A.; Fan, X.; Wang, S.; Eggener, S.; Yousuf, A.; Antic, T.; Oto, A.; Karczmar, G.S. Feasibility of Dynamic Contrast-Enhanced Magnetic Resonance Imaging Using Low-Dose Gadolinium: Comparative Performance With Standard Dose in Prostate Cancer Diagnosis. *Investig. Radiol.* **2018**, *53*, 609–615. [CrossRef] [PubMed]
14. Miyai, K.; Mikoshi, A.; Hamabe, F.; Nakanishi, K.; Ito, K.; Tsuda, H.; Shinmoto, H. Histological differences in cancer cells, stroma, and luminal spaces strongly correlate with in vivo MRI-detectability of prostate cancer. *Mod. Pathol.* **2019**, *32*, 1536–1543. [CrossRef] [PubMed]
15. Langer, D.L.; van der Kwast, T.H.; Evans, A.J.; Plotkin, A.; Trachtenberg, J.; Wilson, B.C.; Haider, M.A. Prostate tissue composition and MR measurements: Investigating the relationships between ADC, T2, K(trans), v(e), and corresponding histologic features. *Radiology* **2010**, *255*, 485–494. [CrossRef]
16. Chatterjee, A.; Mercado, C.; Bourne, R.M.; Yousuf, A.; Hess, B.; Antic, T.; Eggener, S.; Oto, A.; Karczmar, G.S. Validation of Prostate Tissue Composition by Using Hybrid Multidimensional MRI: Correlation with Histologic Findings. *Radiology* **2022**, *302*, 368–377. [CrossRef]
17. Chatterjee, A.; Bourne, R.M.; Wang, S.; Devaraj, A.; Gallan, A.J.; Antic, T.; Karczmar, G.S.; Oto, A. Diagnosis of Prostate Cancer with Noninvasive Estimation of Prostate Tissue Composition by Using Hybrid Multidimensional MR Imaging: A Feasibility Study. *Radiology* **2018**, *287*, 864–873. [CrossRef]
18. Sabouri, S.; Fazli, L.; Chang, S.D.; Savdie, R.; Jones, E.C.; Goldenberg, S.L.; Black, P.C.; Kozlowski, P. MR measurement of luminal water in prostate gland: Quantitative correlation between MRI and histology. *J. Magn. Reson. Imaging* **2017**, *46*, 861–869. [CrossRef]
19. Bailey, C.; Bourne, R.M.; Siow, B.; Johnston, E.W.; Brizmohun Appayya, M.; Pye, H.; Heavey, S.; Mertzanidou, T.; Whitaker, H.; Freeman, A.; et al. VERDICT MRI validation in fresh and fixed prostate specimens using patient-specific moulds for histological and MR alignment. *NMR Biomed.* **2019**, *32*, e4073. [CrossRef]
20. Sadinski, M.; Karczmar, G.; Peng, Y.; Wang, S.; Jiang, Y.; Medved, M.; Yousuf, A.; Antic, T.; Oto, A. Pilot Study of the Use of Hybrid Multidimensional T2-Weighted Imaging–DWI for the Diagnosis of Prostate Cancer and Evaluation of Gleason Score. *Am. J. Roentgenol.* **2016**, *207*, 592–598. [CrossRef]
21. Oerther, B.; Engel, H.; Nedelcu, A.; Schlett, C.L.; Grimm, R.; von Busch, H.; Sigle, A.; Gratzke, C.; Bamberg, F.; Benndorf, M. Prediction of upgrade to clinically significant prostate cancer in patients under active surveillance: Performance of a fully automated AI-algorithm for lesion detection and classification. *Prostate* **2023**, *83*, 871–878. [CrossRef] [PubMed]

42. Giannini, V.; Mazzetti, S.; Defeudis, A.; Stranieri, G.; Calandri, M.; Bollito, E.; Bosco, M.; Porpiglia, F.; Manfredi, M.; De Pascale, A.; et al. A Fully Automatic Artificial Intelligence System Able to Detect and Characterize Prostate Cancer Using Multiparametric MRI: Multicenter and Multi-Scanner Validation. *Front. Oncol.* **2021**, *11*, 718155. [CrossRef] [PubMed]
43. Hötker, A.M.; Mazaheri, Y.; Aras, Ö.; Zheng, J.; Moskowitz, C.S.; Gondo, T.; Matsumoto, K.; Hricak, H.; Akin, O. Assessment of Prostate Cancer Aggressiveness by Use of the Combination of Quantitative DWI and Dynamic Contrast-Enhanced MRI. *AJR Am. J. Roentgenol.* **2016**, *206*, 756–763. [CrossRef]
44. Chatterjee, A.; Antic, T.; Gallan, A.J.; Paner, G.P.; Lin, L.I.K.; Karczmar, G.S.; Oto, A. Histological validation of prostate tissue composition measurement using hybrid multi-dimensional MRI: Agreement with pathologists' measures. *Abdom. Radiol.* **2022**, *47*, 801–813. [CrossRef] [PubMed]

Disclaimer/Publisher's Note: The statements, opinions and data contained in all publications are solely those of the individual author(s) and contributor(s) and not of MDPI and/or the editor(s). MDPI and/or the editor(s) disclaim responsibility for any injury to people or property resulting from any ideas, methods, instructions or products referred to in the content.

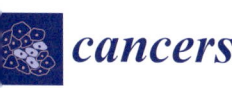

Systematic Review

The Role of Radiomics in the Prediction of Clinically Significant Prostate Cancer in the PI-RADS v2 and v2.1 Era: A Systematic Review

Andreu Antolin [1,2,*], Nuria Roson [1], Richard Mast [3], Javier Arce [1], Ramon Almodovar [3], Roger Cortada [3], Almudena Maceda [4], Manuel Escobar [3], Enrique Trilla [2,5,†] and Juan Morote [2,5,†]

1. Department of Radiology, Institut de Diagnòstic per la Imatge (IDI), Hospital Universitari Vall d'Hebron, 08035 Barcelona, Spain; nuria.roson.idi@gencat.cat (N.R.); javier.arce.idi@gencat.cat (J.A.)
2. Department of Surgery, Universitat Autònoma de Barcelona, 08193 Bellaterra, Spain; enrique.trilla@vallhebron.cat (E.T.); juan.morote@uab.cat (J.M.)
3. Department of Radiology, Hospital Universitari Vall d'Hebron, 08035 Barcelona, Spain; richard.mast@vallhebron.cat (R.M.); ramon.almodovar@vallhebron.cat (R.A.); roger.cortada@vallhebron.cat (R.C.); manel.escobar@vallhebron.cat (M.E.)
4. Vall d'Hebron Research Institute, 08035 Barcelona, Spain; almudena.maceda@vhir.org
5. Department of Urology, Vall d'Hebron University Hospital, 08035 Barcelona, Spain
* Correspondence: antolin.andreu@gmail.com
† These authors contributed equally to this work.

Simple Summary: There is still an overdiagnosis of indolent prostate cancer (iPCa) lesions using the Prostate Imaging-Reporting and Data System (PI-RADS), and radiomics has emerged as a promising tool to improve the diagnosis of clinically significant prostate cancer (csPCa) lesions. However, the current state and applicability of radiomics remains a challenge. This systematic review aims at evaluating the evidence of handcrafted and deep radiomics in differentiating lesions at risk of having csPCa from those with iPCa and benign pathology. The review highlighted a good performance of radiomics but without significant differences with radiologist assessment (PI-RADS), as well as several methodological limitations in the reported studies, which might induce bias. Future studies should improve methodological aspects to ensure the clinical applicability of radiomics, especially the need for clinical prospective studies and the comparison with PI-RADS.

Abstract: Early detection of clinically significant prostate cancer (csPCa) has substantially improved with the latest PI-RADS versions. However, there is still an overdiagnosis of indolent lesions (iPCa), and radiomics has emerged as a potential solution. The aim of this systematic review is to evaluate the role of handcrafted and deep radiomics in differentiating lesions with csPCa from those with iPCa and benign lesions on prostate MRI assessed with PI-RADS v2 and/or 2.1. The literature search was conducted in PubMed, Cochrane, and Web of Science databases to select relevant studies. Quality assessment was carried out with Quality Assessment of Diagnostic Accuracy Studies 2 (QUADAS-2), Radiomic Quality Score (RQS), and Checklist for Artificial Intelligence in Medical Imaging (CLAIM) tools. A total of 14 studies were deemed as relevant from 411 publications. The results highlighted a good performance of handcrafted and deep radiomics methods for csPCa detection, but without significant differences compared to radiologists (PI-RADS) in the few studies in which it was assessed. Moreover, heterogeneity and restrictions were found in the studies and quality analysis, which might induce bias. Future studies should tackle these problems to encourage clinical applicability. Prospective studies and comparison with radiologists (PI-RADS) are needed to better understand its potential.

Keywords: clinically significant prostate cancer; PI-RADS; magnetic resonance imaging; radiomics; deep learning; machine learning; systematic review; prediction

1. Introduction

Prostate cancer (PCa) is the most frequent malignant tumor diagnosed in men, and the second cause of cancer-related death among men [1]. The modified Gleason Score is the recommended PCa grading, and it is based on the microscopic patterns seen in sample tissues obtained from prostate biopsies, ranging from 6 (better prognosis) to 10 (worse prognosis). In 2014, the ISUP Gleason Grading Conference on Gleason Grading of PCa introduced grade groups to better stratify men with PCa, ranging from 1 to 5. ISUP grade 1 (equivalent to Gleason Score of 6) carcinomas have a better prognosis than ISUP grade > 1 (equivalent to Gleason Score of 7 or above) carcinomas [2]. Men with ISUP grade 1 PCa have a better prognosis and can benefit from active surveillance programs in the right conditions, while men with ISUP grade > 1 PCa tend to require curative treatment and follow-up. Consequently, PCa can be further divided into indolent PCa (iPCa), which has an ISUP grade 1, and clinically significant PCa (csPCa), which has an ISUP grade > 1. Risk-stratified PCa screening focuses on improving early detection of csPCa and reducing the overdetection of iPCa, thus avoiding unnecessary prostate biopsies and related side effects [3–5].

Much of the progress in the early detection of csPCa comes from multiparametric or biparametric prostate magnetic resonance imaging (mpMRI or bpMRI) performed before prostate biopsy, which allows the identification of suspicious lesions and the estimation of a semiquantitative risk of csPCa through the Prostate Imaging-Report and Data System (PI-RADS), currently in its version 2.1 [6]. The indication for prostate biopsy is established when the PI-RADS is ≥ 3 since the negative predictive value of MRI when using PI-RADS 2.1 ranges between 96% and 98% for PI-RADS 1 and 2, respectively. The positive predictive value of PI-RADS 3 is 20%, that of PI-RADS 4 is 52%, and that of PI-RADS 5 is 89% [7,8]. Moreover, MRI increases sensitivity for the detection of csPCa by enabling targeted biopsies of suspicious lesions, although it is complemented by the classic systematic biopsy since a small percentage of csPCa is found only in this type of biopsy [9]. Such is the evidence that the European Union recommends PCa screening based on serum prostate-specific antigen (PSA) and MRI [3]. Therefore, the current approach is to perform an MRI in men with a serum PSA > 3.0 ng/mL and/or an abnormal digital rectal examination (DRE), followed by a targeted biopsy of PI-RADS ≥ 3 lesions, complemented with a systematic prostate biopsy [10]. Even though the paradigm of early diagnosis has radically changed thanks to the introduction of MRI, there are still limitations in the application of the latest PI-RADS version [11]. Moreover, there is still important inter-reader variability when assessing prostate lesions using PI-RADS version 2 and 2.1 [12,13], and the overdiagnosis of iPCa in PI-RADS 3 lesions remains a challenge [8]. Consequently, there is a need for new biomarkers and csPCa predictive models to reduce the number of false positives [14].

Radiomics is the extraction of quantitative imaging features from radiological images that are imperceptible to radiologists with the use of specific artificial intelligence (AI) software. These mineable high-dimensional data maximize the information that can be extracted from medical images, as a diagnostic tool or even as prognostic one to improve clinical decisions in the context of personalized precision medicine [15]. Traditional defined and well-known quantitative features known as handcrafted radiomics have been widely used in medical imaging [15]. However, the inception of deep learning algorithms has allowed the automatic extraction of new unknown quantitative features, known as deep radiomics, which might overcome the classical approach [16].

Radiomics has shown promising results in computed tomography (CT) and MRI for improving PCa detection, PCa risk-group classification, risk of biochemical recurrence, and risk of metastatic disease, as well as the identification of extra-prostatic extension or even the evaluation of treatment toxicity, among others [17]. The discrimination between csPCa and iPCa is the main field of research in radiomics applied to PCa [17,18] due to the current diagnostic limitations previously highlighted. A radiomic or multivariable model capable of improving the prediction of PI-RADS in detecting csPCa might help in reducing the number of false positives and unnecessary biopsies in men with iPCa.

Due to this, the European Society of Urogenital Radiology (ESUR) and European Association of Urology (EAU) have advocated for developing robust AI models to overcome these limitations [19]. However, there is still limited evidence of the role of radiomics in real clinical scenarios, as well as its role in predictive models using other clinical variables and the comparison with the PI-RADS.

The main aim of this systematic review is to evaluate the current evidence of the role of handcrafted and deep radiomics in differentiating lesions with csPCa from those with iPCa and benign lesions on prostate MRI assessed with PI-RADS v2 and/or 2.1. Secondary objectives include the comparison between radiomic models and radiologists reporting through the latest PI-RADS versions, as well as the performance in predictive models when combined with other clinical variables.

2. Evidence Acquisition

2.1. Literature Search

The search was conducted in PubMed, Cochrane, and Web of Science databases to select relevant studies for assessing the aims of this review which were published before 30 April 2024. The Boolean strings and keywords used in the search were (Radiomic OR Machine Learning OR Deep Learning) AND Clinically Significant Prostate Cancer AND (Magnetic Resonance Imaging OR PI-RADS). Two independent reviewers, A.A. and J.M., double-blind-reviewed the retrieved reports according to the eligibility criteria. In case of disagreement, consensus was achieved by mutual accordance between both reviewers. References of selected articles were also manually reviewed for additional citations. The Preferred Reporting Items for Systematic Reviews and Meta-analyses (PRISMA) criteria were followed for conducting this systematic review [20]. This systematic review was registered in PROSPERO (International Prospective Register of Systematic Reviews), with the ID number CRD42024527768. A narrative synthesis was chosen for this systematic review due to the heterogeneity of the selected studies.

2.2. Eligibility Criteria

The eligible studies were selected according to inclusion criteria based on the Population, Intervention, Comparator, Outcome (PICO) framework [21], with the detailed breakdown depicted in Supplementary Table S1. The inclusion criteria derived from PICO were (i) men with suspected PCa with consequent evaluation with prostatic mpMRI or bpMRI; (ii) retrospective or prospective assignment of prostatic lesions with PI-RADS v2 or v2.1; (iii) targeted +/− systematic biopsy or radical prostatectomy performed after the mpMRI or bpMRI; (iv) diagnosis of PCa based on histopathological findings, defining csPCa as International Society of Urogenital Pathology (ISUP) grade group > 1 and iPCa as ISUP grade group 1 [2]; (v) outcome measured as diagnostic performance of a handcrafted or deep radiomics model for differentiating csPCa from iPCa and benign lesions with a measurable metric: area under the curve (AUC), sensitivity, specificity, accuracy, positive predictive value (PPV), and negative predictive value (NPV). Exclusion criteria were (i) men in active surveillance or with prior prostate cancer treatment (if specified in the methodology); (ii) studies derived from public datasets (excluding external validation sets). Men with only systematic biopsies were incorporated if no positive findings were detected in bpMRI or mpMRI.

Observational studies were included in this review due to the current lack of randomized clinical trials using AI in clinical settings. Systematic reviews, meta-analyses, letters, conference abstracts and unpublished manuscripts were excluded. In the case of different studies using the same population or datasets, the best methodological study was selected and the rest were discharged. Studies not written in English were excluded.

2.3. Quality Assessment

Risk of bias assessment was analyzed with the Quality Assessment of Diagnostic Accuracy Studies 2 (QUADAS-2) tool [22]. The risk was evaluated by two independent reviewers (A.A. and J.M.) as unclear, low, or high. In case of disagreement, consensus was achieved by mutual accordance between both reviewers. If all the domains were regarded as low risk, the study was given a low risk of bias. If the study had one or more unclear risk of bias, it was considered as an unclear risk of bias. If the study contained any high-risk domain, it was considered as having a high risk.

2.4. Artificial Intelligence Quality Assessment

In addition to the QUADAS-2 [22] risk of bias assessment, each study was also reviewed with specific AI-quality standards guidelines. For studies using handcrafted radiomics and traditional machine learning (ML) methods, the quality was evaluated using the Radiomics Quality Score (RQS), giving a score out of 36 points for each paper included [15]. The RQS v2.0 was not used since it was still under development at the time of this systematic review. Studies using deep radiomics were assessed using the Checklist for Artificial Intelligence in Medical Imaging (CLAIM) [23]. The 42-item checklist of this guideline was evaluated in each case, regarded as fulfilled or not. The 2024 update was not available at the time of this systematic review.

2.5. Data Collection

The data to be extracted were agreed upon between A.A. and J.M. before the beginning of the extraction, detailed in Supplementary File S2. Both authors were responsible for data collection of the studies included. A tabular structure was used to display the results of individual studies, referenced based on author and year of publication. A comprehensive synthesis of the main findings based on each table was then performed, adding extra information not included in the tables.

3. Evidence Synthesis

3.1. Study Selection

A total of 411 titles were obtained according to the search strategy, and 250 were excluded because of duplicates. The remaining 161 were analyzed based on the title and abstract, and 39 were deemed as relevant. A total of 21 reviews, systematic reviews, and meta-analyses were discarded, as well as three editorials and 10 conference-related papers. Three articles were written in a different language than English and were also discarded. The full texts were finally reviewed for definite inclusion, with a final number of 13 studies fulfilling the required criteria. An extra study was incorporated from the references of the analyzed papers, for a total of 14 selected studies [24–37]. The flow diagram is depicted in Figure 1.

3.2. QUADAS-2 Risk of Bias Assessment

The results of the QUADAS-2 [22] assessment for each paper included are presented in Figure 2. A total of 4 out of 14 (29%) studies [26,29–31] had low risk of bias, while 7 out of 14 (50%) [24,25,27,32–34,36] had high risk of bias. The remaining three studies (21%) [28,35,37] had an unclear risk of bias. All papers had low applicability concerns.

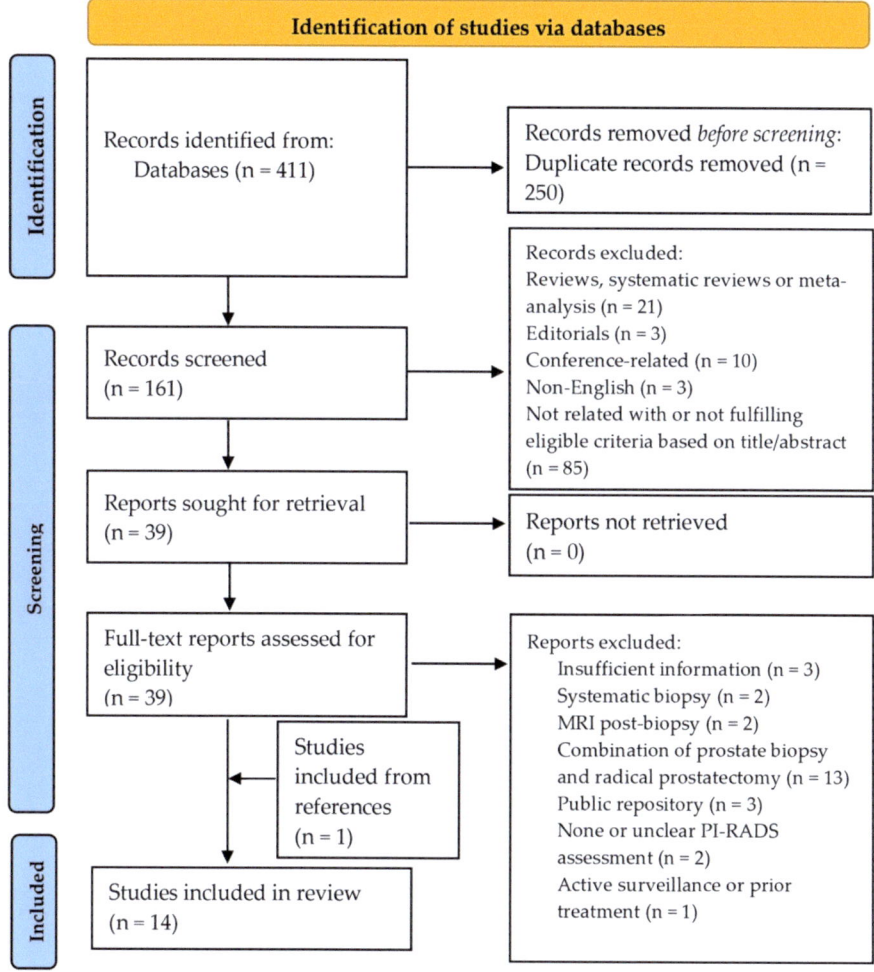

Figure 1. Preferred Reporting Items for Systematic Reviews and Meta-Analysis (PRISMA 2020) flow diagram for the selection of relevant studies based on the search strategy.

Among the seven studies with high risk of bias, four of them had inadequate patient selection [24,25,33,36] because of inappropriate exclusion criteria (exclusion of lesions < 5 mm or advanced stages) [24,25,36] or case–control design [33], which might overestimate the results and conclusions. Moreover, there was also a high risk of bias in the index test in two studies [25,32] because the threshold used was not clearly specified to the best of our knowledge. There was also a high risk of bias in flow and timing in another two studies [27,34] because the period between the MRI and the prostate biopsy or radical prostatectomy exceeded three months in some cases. This might underestimate the risk of csPCa based on MRI interpretation because of a potential tumor progression during the waiting time. Finally, two studies (21%) had an unclear risk of bias in patient selection because the enrollment of the patients and/or exclusion criteria were not clear/reported [32,37].

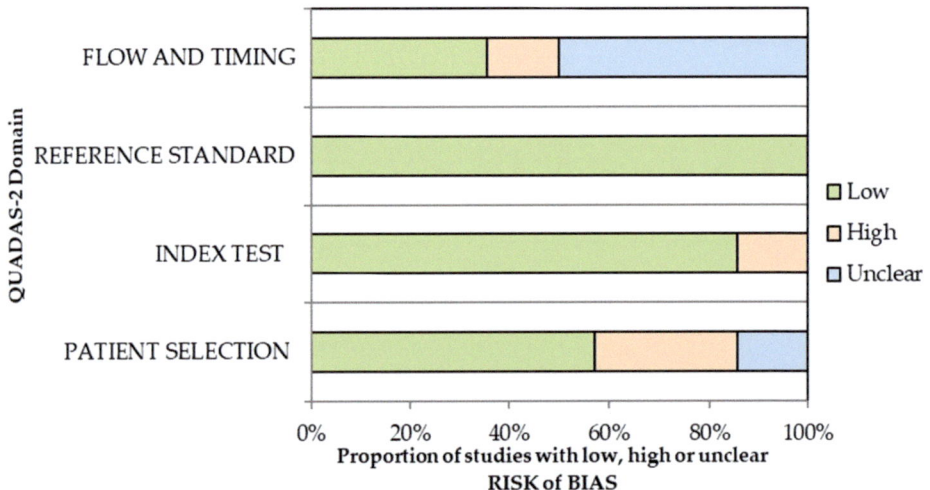

Figure 2. QUADAS-2 risk of bias and applicability concerns of the selected studies (**top**, [24–37]) and its corresponding graphical representation (**bottom**).

3.3. Quality Assessment Based on RQS and CLAIM

The results of AI-specific quality assessment are first presented for the studies based on handcrafted radiomics using RQS [15], detailing the overall score and the specific results for each item in the checklist. Afterwards, the results of the studies based on deep radiomics are presented using CLAIM [23], highlighting the most important or controversial items of the checklist.

Eight studies (57%) used handcrafted radiomics for extracting image features [24–26,29,33–35]. The overall quality based on RQS [15] was low, with a median of 10.5 and interquartile range (IQR) of 2.5, out of a maximum of 36 points. All the studies reported the image quality protocol (item 1) and feature reduction or adjustment for multiple testing (item 4). However, none of them performed phantom studies (item 3), imaging at multiple timepoints (item 4), biological correlation (item 7), prospective studies (item 11), potential clinical applications (item 14), or cost-effectiveness analysis (item 15). Three studies (38%) performed multiple segmentations and/or feature robustness assessments (item 2) [26,29,36]. Multivariable analysis was performed in five studies [24,25,29,34,36], while the rest opted for an exclusive radiomic model [26,33,35]. Interestingly, four studies also made a comparison of the radiomic model or multivariable model with the PI-RADS classification (item 6) [24,25,29,35], albeit in only two was a statistical comparison between both given [24,29]. Moreover, only three studies conducted external validation (item 12) [26,29,35]. Discrimination statistics (item 9) were given in all the studies, although the confidence intervals were not reported in a single study [25]. Cut-off analysis (item 8) and calibration statistics (item 9) were reported in three [24,34,36] and two [26,29] studies, respectively. Lastly, a single study published the code used for creating the model [33].

Six studies (43%) used deep radiomics for extracting image features [27,28,30–32,37], and were assessed with CLAIM [23]. Among the different items in the methods section, none of the studies reported deidentification methods (item 12) nor how missing data were handled (item 13), although no study reported missing data, per se. The intended sample size and how it was determined (item 19) was also not specified in any of the studies, nor was robustness analysis (item 30). Although annotations were generally well explained, measurement of inter- and intrareader variability was not well reported. A detailed description of the model and its training (items 22 to 25) was generally well reported, although the initialization of model parameters (item 24) was only reported in one study [37], which used transfer learning. Metrics of model performance (item 28) were reported in all the studies, with the corresponding statistical measures of significance (item 29) except in a single study [28]. External validation (item 32) was carried out in half of the studies [27,28,31]. Importantly, a single study used explainability or interpretability methods (item 31) [27]. In the results section, two studies did not present the flow of participants in a diagram (item 33) [32,37]. The demographic and clinical characteristics in each partition (item 34) was partially, or not, performed in two studies [30,37]. Failure analysis of incorrectly classified cases was only properly conducted in a single study [31]. Finally, in the discussion and other information section, it is important to note that two studies used open code [27,31].

3.4. Study Characteristics

The characteristics of the selected studies are represented in five consecutive tables (Tables 1–5) following a continuous flow from the main clinical and demographic characteristics to specific details of the radiomic pipeline and, lastly, the metrics of the radiomic, clinical, or combined models developed in each paper.

Table 1. Basic demographics, MRI/PI-RADS characteristics, and reference standard details of the selected studies.

Reference, Year	Data Source, n, Country	Dataset Year/s	csPCa, n (%)	PZ, n (%)	MRI Vendor, Tesla	PI-RADS lesions	Reference Standard, MRI to Procedure	Biopsy Technique
Dominguez et al. 2023 [24]	Single-center, 86, Chile	2017–2021	66 (0.77)	81 (0.94)	Philips, 3	≥3	PB, NR	MRI/US fusion, TRUS
Prata et al. 2023 [25]	Single-center, 91, Italy	2019–2020	39 (0.43)	NR	Siemens, 1.5	≥3	PB, within 4 weeks	MRI/US fusion, TRUS
Jin et al. 2023 [26]	Multicenter, 463, China	2018–2019	100 (0.22)	216 (0.47)	Siemens/Philips, 3	3	PB, within 4 weeks	MRI/US fusion, TRUS
Hamm et al. 2023 [a] [27]	Single-center, 1224, GER	2012–2017	595 (0.49) [b]	1935 (0.59) [b]	Siemens, 3	≥1	PB, within 6 months	NR
Hong et al. 2023 [a] [28]	Single-center, 171, Korea	2018–2022	40 (0.37)	81 (0.47)	Multivendor, 3	≥3	RP, NR	NA
Jing et al. 2022 [29]	Multicenter, 389, China	2016–2021	270 (0.69)	190 (0.49)	GE/UI, 3	≥2	RP, within 12 weeks	NA
Zhu et al. 2022 [30]	Single-center, 347, China	2017–2020	235 (0.68) [c]	212 (0.68) [c]	GE, 3	NR	PB, within 12 weeks	CT, TRUS
Jiang et al. 2022 [a] [31]	Single-center, 1230, China	2012–2019	856 (0.63) [b]	853 (0.63) [b]	Siemens/UI, 3	≥1	PB, within 4 weeks	MRI/US fusion, TRUS
Liu et al. 2021 [32]	Single-center, 402, USA	2010–2018	303 (0.75) [b]	364 (0.78) [b]	NR, 3	≥3	RP, NR	NA
Lim et al. 2021 [33]	Multicenter, 158, Canada	2015–2018	29 (0.18) [b]	79 (0.49) [b]	Siemens/GE, 3	3	PB, NR	CT, TRUS
Hectors et al. 2021 [34]	Single-center, 240, USA	2015–2020	28 (0.12)	NR	Siemens/GE, 3	3	PB, within 12 months	MRI/US fusion, TRUS
Castillo et al. 2021 [35]	Multicenter, 107, NL	2011–2014	112 (0.55) [b]	137 (0.67) [b]	GE/Siemens/Philips, 3/1.5	≥1	RP, NR	NA
Li et al. 2020 [36]	Single-center, 381, China	2014–2017	142 (0.37)	NR	Philips, 3	NR	PB, NR	TRUS
Zhong et al. 2019 [37]	Single-center, 140, USA	2010–2016	105 (0.49) [b]	NR	Siemens, 3	NR	RP, NR	NA

csPCa = clinically significant prostate cancer, CT = cognitive targeting, GE = General Electrics, GER = Germany, MRI = magnetic resonance imaging, NA = not applicable, NL = Netherlands, NR = not reported, PB = prostate biopsy, PZ = peripheral zone, PI-RADS = Prostate Imaging Reporting and Data System, RP = radical prostatectomy, TRUS = trans-rectal ultrasound, UI = United Imaging, US = ultrasound, USA = United States of America. [a] Data from external validation sets are not included in the description (see reference for further details); [b] Data referred to as annotated lesions; [c] Data are for csPCa lesions.

Table 2. Main characteristics of the machine learning process of the selected studies.

Reference, Year	Sequences	Segmentation	Feature Extraction	Image Preprocessing	Data Imbalance techniques, Data Augmentation	Feature Selection	Train/Test (%) [b]	Algorithm
Dominguez et al. 2023 [24]	T2, ADC	Lesion	Shape, FO, HTF	Not performed	NR	RFE	80 (CV)/20	LR
Prata et al. 2023 [25]	T2, ADC	Lesion	FO, HTF, BLP	NR	NR	Wrapper (RF)	CV	RF
Jin et al. 2023 [26]	T2, ADC, DWI (b2000)		FO, HTF, wavelet features	IN, grey-level quantization, resampling, IR	SMOTE, NR	ANOVA	70/30	SVM

Reference, Year	Sequences	Segmentation	Feature Extraction	Image Preprocessing	Data Imbalance techniques, Data Augmentation	Feature Selection	Train/Test (%) [b]	Algorithm
Hamm et al. 2023 [27]	T2, ADC, DWI (high-b value)	Lesion, prostate, PZ, TZ	Deep radiomics	IN, resampling, lesion cropping	NR, Yes	NA	80 (CV)/20	Visual Geometry Group Net-based CNN
Hong et al. 2023 [28]	ADC	Lesion, prostate	Deep radiomics	IN, resizing, prostate cropping, cut-off filtering	Image allocation, NR	NA	80/20	DenseNet 201
Jing et al. 2022 [29]	T2, DWI (b1500)	Lesion, prostate	Shape, FO, HTF, higher-order features	IN, Resampling	NR	Variance threshold algorithm, Select K-best, LASSO	70/30	LR
Zhu et al. 2022 [30]	T2, ADC	Lesion	Deep radiomics	IN, resampling, prostate cropping, IR	NR, Yes	NA	60/40	Res-UNet
Jiang et al. 2022 [31]	T2, DWI (b1500), ADC	Lesion, prostate	Deep radiomics	IN, resampling, prostate cropping, IR	NR, Yes	NA	66.6/33.3	Attention-Gated TrumpetNet
Liu et al. 2021 [32]	T2, ADC	Lesion	Deep radiomics	IN, lesion cropping, IR	NR	NA	70/30	3D GLCM extractor + CNN
Lim et al. 2021 [33]	T2, ADC	Lesion	Shape, FO, HTF	NR	NR	Mann-Whitney U-test	CV	XGBoost
Hectors et al. 2021 [34]	T2	Lesion	Shape, FO, HTF	IN, grey-level quantization, resampling	SMOTE, NR	RF	80 (CV)/20	RF, LR
Castillo et al. 2021 [35]	T2, DWI (highest-b value), ADC	Lesion	Shape, FO, HTF, higher-order features	Resampling	WORC Workflow [a]	WORC Workflow [a]	80 (CV)/20	WORC Workflow [a]
Li et al. 2020 [36]	T2, ADC	Lesion	FO, HTF	IN, grey-level quantization, resampling	NR	mRMR, LASSO	60/40	LR
Zhong et al. 2019 [37]	T2, ADC	Lesion	Deep radiomics	IN, resizing, lesion cropping	Not necessary, Yes	NA	80/20	ResNet with TL

BLP = binary local pattern, CNN = convolutional neural network, CV = cross-validation, FO = first order, GLCM = gray-level co-occurrence matrix, HTF = hand-crafted texture features, IN = image normalization, IR = image registration, LASSO = least absolute shrinkage and selection operator, LR = logistic regression, mRMR = minimum redundancy maximum relevance, NR = not reported, NA = not applicable, PZ = peripheral zone, RFE = recursive feature elimination, RF = random forest, SMOTE = synthetic minority oversampling technique, SVM = support vector machine, TZ = transitional zone. [a] Uses a radiomics workflow called Workflow for Optimal Radiomics Classification (WORC), which includes different workflow processes (see reference for further details). [b] Presented as % of the data selected for the training and test partitions. CV stands for cross-validation performed in the training set.

Table 3. Analysis, validation, and results for csPCa prediction in the selected studies based on handcrafted radiomics as the feature extraction method.

Reference, Year	Analysis	Validation	Sequence for the Best Model	Best Radiomic Model [CI, 95%] [a]			PI-RADS Cut-Off	PI-RADS Model [CI, 95%] [a]		
				AUC	Sensitivity	Specificity		AUC	Sensitivity	Specificity
Dominguez et al. 2023 [24]	Index	CV//Hold-out set	ADC	0.81 [0.56–0.94]//0.71	NR	NR	NR	0.66 [0.57–0.74]//NR	NR	NR
Prata et al. 2023 [25]	Index	CV	ADC	0.77	NR	NR	NR	0.68	NR	NR
Jin et al. 2023 [26]	Index	Hold-out set//External (1 set)	T2 + ADC + DWI (b2000)	0.80//0.80	0.80//0.73	0.65//0.92	NA	NA	NA	NA
Jing et al. 2022 [29]	Index	Hold-out set//External (2 sets)	T2 (prostate) + DWI b1500 (lesion)	0.96 [0.90, 1.00]//0.95 [0.87, 1.00]//0.94 [0.90, 0.99] [b]	0.95//0.98//0.86 [b]	0.94//0.86//0.91 [b]	NR	0.84 [0.74, 0.95]//0.82 [0.72, 0.93]//0.80 [0.71, 0.88]	0.98//0.98//0.50	0.56//0.52//0.94
Lim et al. 2021 [33]	All	CV	ADC	0.68 [0.65–0.72]	NR	NR	NA	NA	NR	NA
Hectors et al. 2021 [34]	Index	Hold-out set	T2	0.76 [0.60–0.92]	0.75	0.8	NA	NA	NA	NA
Castillo et al. 2021 [35]	Index	CV//External	T2 + ADC + DWI (highest-b value)	0.72 [0.64, 0.79]//0.75	0.76 [0.66, 0.89]//0.88	0.55 [0.44, 0.66]//0.63	≥3	0.50//0.44 (2 radiologists, External Validation)	0.76//0.88	0.25//0
Li et al. 2020 [36]	Index	Hold-out set	T2 + ADC	0.98 [0.97–1.00]	0.95	0.87	NA	NA	NA	NA

All = all lesions, AUC = area under the curve, CI = confidence interval, csPCa = clinically significant prostate cancer, CV = cross-validation, Index = index lesion, NA = not applicable, NR = not reported, PI-RADS = Prostate Imaging Reporting and Data System. [a] Data are expressed in the corresponding metric and the CI, 95% for each validation method separated by //. If the CI is not included, it means that it was not reported in the study. [b] The combined model (radiomic model + PI-RADS) is included since there are no data for the radiomic model.

Table 4. Analysis, validation, and results for csPCa prediction in the selected studies based on deep radiomics as the feature extraction method.

Reference, Year	Analysis	Validation	Sequence for the Best Model	Best Radiomic Model [CI, 95%] [a]			PI-RADS Cut-Off	PI-RADS Model [CI, 95%] [a]		
				AUC	Sensitivity	Specificity		AUC	Sensitivity	Specificity
Hamm et al. 2023 [27]	All	Hold-out set//External (PROSTATEx)	T2 + ADC + DWI (high-b value)	0.89 [0.85, 0.93]//0.87 [0.81, 0.93]	0.77 [0.69, 0.85]//0.90 [0.83, 0.97]	0.89 [0.84, 0.95]//0.85 [0.80, 0.90]	NA	NA	NA	NA
	Index			0.78//NR	0.98 [0.95, 1.00] [b]//NR	NR				
Hong et al. 2023 [28]	Index	Hold-out set//External (1 set)	ADC	NR//0.63	0.72//0.84	0.74//0.48	NA	NA	NA	NA
Zhu et al. 2022 [30]	All	Hold-out set	T2 + ADC	NR	0.96 [0.89, 0.99]	NR	≥3	NR	0.94 [0.87, 0.98]	NR
	Sextant			NR	0.96 [0.90, 0.99]	0.92 [0.89, 0.93]		NR	0.93 [0.87, 0.97]	0.92 [0.90, 0.94]
	Index			NR	0.99 [0.92, 0.99]	0.65 [0.53, 0.76]		NR	0.99 [0.92, 0.99]	0.66 [0.54, 0.77]

Table 5. Analysis, validation, and results for csPCa prediction in the selected studies based on clinical and combined models.

Reference, Year	Analysis	Validation	Sequence for the Best Model	Best Radiomic Model [CI, 95%] [a]			PSA-D [CI, 95%] [a]			PI-RADS Cut-Off	PI-RADS Model [CI, 95%] [a]		
				AUC	Sensitivity	Specificity	AUC	Sensitivity	Specificity		AUC	Sensitivity	Specificity
Jiang et al. 2022 [31]	All	Hold-out set//External (PROSTATEx)	T2 + ADC + DWI (b1500)	0.85 [0.81, 0.88]//0.86 [0.81, 0.91]	0.93//0.87	0.5//0.66	0.77 [0.66–0.87]//NR	NR	NR	≥3	0.92 [0.89, 0.95]//0.86 [0.80, 0.90]	0.94//0.77	0.79//0.87
Liu et al. 2021 [32]	All	Hold-out set	T2 + ADC	0.85 [0.79, 0.91]	0.90 [0.83, 0.96]	0.70 [0.59, 0.82]	NA	NA	NA	≥4	0.73 [0.65, 0.80]	0.83 [0.75, 0.92]	0.47 [0.35, 0.59]
	Index			0.73 [0.59, 0.88]	0.90 [0.83, 0.96]	0.47 [0.21, 0.72]	0.71//0.69	0.84//0.77	0.60//0.62		0.65 [0.52, 0.78]	0.83 [0.75, 0.91]	0.27 [0.04, 0.72]
Zhong et al. 2019 [37]	All	Hold-out set	T2 + ADC	0.73 [0.58, 0.88]	0.64	0.8	NA	NA	NA	≥4	0.71 [0.58, 0.87]	0.86	0.48

All = all lesions, AUC = area under the curve, CI = confidence interval, csPCa = clinically significant prostate cancer, CV = cross-validation, Index = index lesion, NA = not applicable, NR = not reported, PI-RADS = Prostate Imaging Reporting and Data System. [a] Data are expressed in the corresponding metric and the CI, 95% for each validation method separated by //. If the CI is not included it means that it was not reported in the study. [b] At 2 false-positive rate.

Table 5. Analysis, validation, and results for csPCa prediction in the selected studies based on clinical and combined models.

Reference, Year	Analysis	Validation	PSA-D [CI, 95%] [a]			Clinical Model [CI, 95%] [a]			Combined Model [CI, 95%] [a]		
			AUC	Sensitivity	Specificity	AUC	Sensitivity	Specificity	AUC	Sensitivity	Specificity
Dominguez et al. 2023 [24]	Index	CV//Hold-out set	0.77 [0.66–0.87]//NR	NR	NR	0.76 [0.62–0.87]//0.80 (PV-MR, PSA, PSA-D)	NR	NR	0.91 [0.76–0.99]//0.80 (Clinical Model and Radiomic Model)	NR	NR
Prata et al. 2023 [25]	Index	Hold-out set	NA	NA	NA	0.69 (DRE, PI-RADS)	NR	NR	0.80 (DRE, PI-RADS and Radiomic Model)	0.915	0.844
Jin et al. 2023 [26]	Index	Hold-out set//External (1 set)	0.71//0.69	0.84//0.77	0.60//0.62	NA	NA	NA	N/A	NA	NA
Jing et al. 2022 [29]	Index	Hold-out set//External (2 sets)	NA	NA	NA	NA	N/A	N/A	0.96 [0.90, 1.00]//0.95 [0.87, 1.00]//0.94 [0.90, 0.99] (Radiomic Model + PI-RADS)	0.952//0.978//0.861	0.944//0.857//0.907
Hectors et al. 2021 [34]	Index	Hold-out set	0.61 [0.41, 0.80]	0.72	0.52	NA	NA	NA	NA	NA	NA
Li et al. 2020 [36]	Index	Hold-out set	NA	NA	NA	0.79 [0.70–0.88] (Age, PSA, PSA-D)	0.76	0.74	0.98 [0.97–1.00] (Age, PSA, PSA-D and Radiomic Model)	0.82	0.97

AUC = area under the curve, CI = confidence intervals, CV = cross-validation, csPCa = clinically significant prostate cancer, DRE = digital rectal examination, Index = index lesion, NA = not applicable, NR = not reported, PI-RADS = Prostate Imaging Reporting and Data System, PSA = prostate-specific antigen, PSA-D = prostate-specific antigen density, PV-MR = prostate volume calculated with magnetic resonance. [a] Data are expressed in the corresponding metric and the CI, 95% for each validation method separated by //. If the CI is not included it means that it was not reported in the study.

Table 1 presents the main clinical, demographic, and radiological characteristics of the different cohorts included in the 14 selected studies [24–37]. The number of participants, origin (i.e., United States of America), and whether it was a unicentric or multicentric study is depicted, as well as the years in which the dataset was obtained. The amount of csPCa included in each paper and the number of lesions in the peripheral zone is also summarized. The MRI manufacturer and the magnetic field strength used for each cohort are represented, as well as the PI-RADS score of the lesions reported. Finally, the reference standard (prostate biopsy or radical prostatectomy) as well as the biopsy technique and the time between the MRI and the procedure are specified.

As seen in this table, most of the selected papers (10 of 14, 71%) used data from single institutions [24,25,27,28,30–32,34,36,37]. The number of men included ranged from 86 to 1230 patients, with a median of 294 and an IQR of 262 [24–37]. Two of the studies had more than 1000 patients [27,31]. All the studies were retrospective, in which eight (57%) had data collected for ≥4 years [24,27–29,31,32,34,37]. There was a general disbalance in the number of csPCa cases of the selected studies. Four studies had between 40 and 60% of csPCa cases [25,27,35,37], while the rest were more disbalanced, with 12% of csPCa cases as the lowest percentage [34] and 77% as the highest [24]. Almost half or more of the lesions were in the peripheral zone [24,26–33,35], with a median of 61% and IQR of 19%. The second most common location was the transitional zone, with a median of 33% and IQR of 7%. Five studies included a few lesions in other locations such as anterior fibromuscular stroma, central zone, or diffuse [27–29,32,35]. Four studies did not report the specific prostate location of the lesions [25,34,36,37].

Half of the selected studies included images from more than one MRI vendor (7 of 13, 54%) [26,28,29,31,33–35]. One study did not report the specific vendor [32] and another reported multiple vendors, but the brand was not specified [28]. Siemens and Philips were the most frequent vendors, present in 10 of the 12 studies (83%) [24–27,31,33–37]. A total of 12 of the 14 studies (86%) used a 3 Tesla as the magnetic field [24,26–34,36,37], and one used a 1.5 Tesla machine [25]. The remaining study used MRIs with both magnitudes [35]. Only two studies included some patients in which an endorectal coil was used [35,37]. A total of 10 of 14 studies specified the PI-RADS of the lesions included [24–29,31–35]. Seven (70%) included PI-RADS 3 and/or higher lesions [24–26,28,32–34], of which three included only PI-RADS 3 lesions [26,34,36].

Most of the studies (9 of 14, 64%) were based on prostate biopsy as the reference standard [24–27,30,31,33,34], and the remaining five (36%) were based on radical prostatectomy [28,29,32,35,37]. All of them had the procedure performed after the MRI, but half of the studies did not report the period between the MRI and the procedure. It ranged from four weeks to 12 months in the studies in which it was reported [25–27,29–31,33]. Transrectal ultrasound (US) was the preferred approach for performing the prostate biopsy in all the studies except in one case, which was not reported [27]. Five studies specified MRI/US fusion technique as the preferred choice [24–26,31,34] while only two preferred cognitive targeting [30,33]. The remaining two studies did not specify [27,36].

Table 2 describes the basic characteristics of the radiomic pipeline. As such, the technique used for extracting the features, either handcrafted radiomics or deep radiomics, is specified. The MRI sequences in which the radiomic features were obtained are given, as well as the origin (i.e., lesion segmentation or other parts of the prostate). Furthermore, several steps in a machine learning process such as image preprocessing, data imbalance or augmentation techniques, feature selection, and train/test split ratio are detailed. Finally, the algorithm used for constructing the model is also depicted.

Eight studies (57%) used handcrafted radiomics for extracting image features [24–26,29,33–36], while the remaining six (43%) relied on deep radiomics [27,28,30–32,37]. All the selected studies extracted the features from MRI T2 and/or ADC sequences, and in five (36%) [26,27,29,31,35], they were also extracted from high b-value DWI sequences. None of the studies extracted features from dynamic contrast-enhanced (DCE) sequences. Imaging features were extracted in all the selected studies from the lesion segmentations. Additional prostate segmentations were performed in four studies (29%) [27–29,31], although in only one study were they used for extracting image biomarkers [29]. The peripheral and transitional zones were also additionally segmented in one study [27]. All the segmentations were manually carried out except in one study, in which a predefined bounding box was created around the annotated lesions, and the prostate and prostate zones were automatically segmented with nn-Unet [27]. OsiriX was the most used software for performing the manual segmentations, which was used in three studies (21%) [25,32,37]. Slicer [24,33] and ITK-SNAP [26,30] were the second most used software tools. One study did not report the tool [34]. The radiologist experience was specified in all but one study [37], ranging from 3 to more than 10 years of experience. In three studies [25,33,34], the segmentations and/or relabeling of the lesions were performed by a single radiologist.

Image preprocessing was reported and performed in 11 studies (79%) [26–32,34–37]. One study reported that image preprocessing was not needed since all the images were acquired with the same protocol and resolution [24]. Intensity normalization and resampling were the most frequently performed. Image registration was reported in four studies (29%) [26,30–32], in which the images were spatially matched using Elastix software in two of them [26,31]. In contrast, data imbalance techniques and data augmentation were barely reported. The former was reported in five studies (36%) [26,28,34,35,37]. The most common method was synthetic minority oversampling technique (SMOTE) [26,34]. In one study it was regarded as not necessary [37]. Data augmentation was performed in five studies [27,29,31,35,37].

Among the eight studies that used handcrafted radiomics [24–26,29,33–36], PyRadiomics was the most used library for extracting the imaging features [24,29,33,34]. Feature robustness was assessed in three of them (38%) [26,29,36]. Feature normalization was also reported in three studies (38%) [24,26,35], with z-Score as the method used. Feature harmonization was reported in one study [35], which used ComBat. Finally, feature selection was performed in the eight studies [24–26,29,33–36], with different algorithms specified in Table 2. Train–test split was the preferred method for training the model in 12 of the selected studies [24,26–32,34–37], with 80/20% being the most common partition. The remaining two studies performed a cross-validation [25,33]. The algorithm used for creating the model varied between studies, but classic machine learning algorithms were used for handcrafted radiomics studies, and deep neural networks were used for deep radiomic studies.

Tables 3 and 4 depict the overall results of the radiomic models, divided into studies that use handcrafted radiomics (in Table 3) or deep radiomics (in Table 4). In both tables, the validation strategy (i.e., internal or external validation) and the specific analysis (i.e., per index lesion) are detailed. The AUC, sensitivity, and specificity of the best radiomic model for csPCa prediction are also given, alongside the MRI sequences in which the image features were extracted that proved to be the most relevant for the prediction. For comparison, the metrics of the PI-RADS evaluation are also depicted if it was assessed, with the threshold considered as csPCa in such cases (i.e., csPCa is considered if PI-RADS ≥ 4).

In the studies based on handcrafted radiomics [24–26,29,33–36], index lesion was the preferred analysis except in one case in which the analysis was based on all the lesions [33]. Three of the eight studies (38%) performed an external validation [26,29,35]. The AUC was reported in all the studies and ranged from 0.72 to 0.98 for index lesions in the internal validation. The results for the external validation sets were similar to the ones obtained in the internal validation, being 0.75 and 0.95. Sensitivity and specificity were reported in five of the eight handcrafted radiomics studies [26,29,35,36]. In the studies based on deep radiomics [27,28,30–32,37], the preferred analysis was more diverse since it included the index lesion and all the lesions, as well as a sextant-level analysis in one study [30]. Three of the six studies (50%) conducted an external validation [27,28,31], albeit two [27,31] were based on the PROSTATEx public dataset [38]. The AUC was reported in all but one study [30], which ranged from 0.73 to 0.85 for index lesions and 0.73 to 0.89 for all lesions in internal validation. The values were 0.63 for index lesions and 0.86 and 0.87 for all lesions in the external validation.

The PI-RADS performance was evaluated in half of the studies [24,25,29–32,35,37], in which five reported the AUC, sensitivity, and specificity [29,31,32,35,37]. The statistical comparison between the radiomic model and PI-RADS was assessed in four studies [30–32,37]. Zhu et al. [30] reported no significant differences in sensitivity between both models (considering PI-RADS $\geq$ 3 as csPCa) at index lesion, sextant-level, and all-lesions-level analysis. Liu et al. [32] reported a similar performance between both models (considering PI-RADS $\geq$ 4 as csPCa) at index lesion based on AUC, but the radiomic model performed significantly better than PI-RADS in all lesion-level analysis. Zhong et al. [37] reported no significant differences between both models (considering PI-RADS $\geq$ 4 as csPCa) based on AUC at all lesion levels. In contrast, Jiang et al. [31] reported a significantly better performance of the PI-RADS model (considering PI-RADS $\geq$ 3 as csPCa) in the internal validation and similar in external validation, based on AUC.

Table 5 assesses other tested models such as clinical models and/or combined models (clinical variables with radiomic features), and it is displayed in a similar way to Tables 3 and 4 with the validation strategy, specific analysis, and metrics detailed.

In six studies [24–26,29,34,36], PSA density (PSA-D), clinical models, and combined models were also assessed. Dominguez et al. [24] reported a significantly better performance of the combined model in comparison to PI-RADS (cut-off not reported) and PSA-D in the cross-validation. Jing et al. [29] also reported a significantly better performance of the combined model in comparison to PI-RADS (cut-off not reported) in internal and external validation. Li et al. [36] showed no significant differences between the radiomic model and combined models, but both were better than the clinical model.

4. Discussion

This systematic review evaluated the current evidence of deep and handcrafted radiomics models in distinguishing csPCa from iPCa and benign lesions in prostate MRIs assessed with PI-RADS v2 and/or v2.1. The selected studies demonstrated good performance for index lesion classification, with handcrafted radiomics models achieving AUCs ranging from 0.72 to 0.98, and deep radiomics models achieving AUCs from 0.73 to 0.85. A meta-analysis was not conducted due to the significant heterogeneity in the datasets, methodologies, model development, and validation of the selected studies, preventing definitive conclusions. Nevertheless, there is no clear difference between the performance of both approaches, nor between internal and external validations, consistent with other reviews [39]. A meta-analysis published in 2019 favored handcrafted over deep radiomics models [40], although the authors noted that the low number of participants in the selected studies might have favored handcrafted methods. Developing deep learning models to achieve expert performance requires large amounts of data [41], so we believe that deep radiomic models will surpass handcrafted ones in the future as recent studies incorporate progressively more data. A recent review published in 2022 slightly favored deep radiomic methods over traditional ones, despite not being a meta-analysis [42].

The substantial heterogeneity of the included studies is also observed in other similar reviews [39,40,42–44]. Specific eligibility criteria were designed to mitigate this limitation. First, studies with preprocedure MRI were included to avoid misinterpretation due to hemorrhage, which can affect radiologist judgment and induce bias [45]. Second, only studies using PI-RADS v2 and/or v2.1 for lesion assignment were included, as these provide better interpretability than PI-RADS v1 or Likert score [46,47]. Third, targeted biopsies (combined or not with systematic biopsies) or radical prostatectomies were the chosen reference standards. Exclusive systematic biopsies were excluded due to their inferior performance compared to targeted biopsies [48], which has been a source of heterogeneity in past reviews [40,42]. Moreover, mixing targeted biopsies and radical prostatectomies was avoided to homogenize the data, despite no clear pathological upgrading of radical prostatectomy compared to targeted prostate biopsy [49]. A recent study showed no differences in model performance based on reference standard [50], but further assessment is needed. Studies involving men in active surveillance or with prior prostate cancer treatment were excluded to prevent bias towards higher-risk patients. Finally, studies based on public repository datasets were excluded to ensure multicentric and larger studies, addressing issues highlighted in past reviews [40,42]. However, public repositories will be crucial in the future due to the current lack of sufficient multicentric data. Significant efforts are being made in this area [51], which are beyond the scope of this review. Despite these efforts, significant heterogeneity and restrictions were found in the data extracted and the quality analysis using QUADAS-2 [22], RQS [15], and CLAIM [23] tools, which will be discussed in the following paragraphs, along with recommendations for future studies.

First, there were several methodological constraints that might introduce bias into radiomics models, starting with data issues. Most of the studies were based on single-center datasets and exhibited data imbalance, with an overrepresentation of csPCa cases and a predominance of peripheral zone lesions. Data imbalance and lack of multicentric datasets are common problems in AI in medical imaging, which can introduce bias [52,53]. Although this is intrinsic to the collected data and difficult to overcome in healthcare due to data scarcity, few of the selected studies applied techniques to address data imbalance [26,28,34,35,37] or used data augmentation techniques [27,30,31,35,37]. Moreover, some studies excluded lesions smaller than 5 mm or advanced stages, introducing a bias by reducing false positives and excluding high-risk patients [24,25,36]. This reduces data representativity and may lead to bias, contributing to high-risk assessments in the QUADAS-2 evaluation [22]. Similarly, most studies used images from only one or two different MRI vendors and a magnetic field strength of 3T, which also reduces data representativity. Some nonselected studies reported no significant differences in performance based on magnetic field strength or MRI vendor [50,54,55], but further assessment is needed. Additionally, despite efforts to mitigate bias due to the chosen reference standard, few studies reported the time between the MRI and the procedure, or exceeded three months, contributing to unclear and high-risk bias, respectively [24,27,28,32–37]. It is also important to emphasize the interobserver variability between pathologists when assessing the Gleason Score, so the pathologist's experience should be reported [56].

Secondly, the review highlighted sources of bias in the radiomic pipeline. One of the most notable was the limited data on interobserver/inter-reader agreement when segmenting lesions, as noted in the RQS [15] and CLAIM [23] evaluations. Manual segmentations performed by multiple radiologists introduce heterogeneity and influence model performance. Although radiologist experience was specified in all but one paper [37], there was limited evaluation of interobserver/inter-reader variability in most cases. Similarly, in studies based on handcrafted radiomics, feature robustness was rarely assessed. This is important because radiomic features have low reproducibility and repeatability [57,58], introducing clear bias. In contrast, feature selection was performed in all the handcrafted radiomic studies, and the top selected features were reported except in two studies [33,35]. Image preprocessing was also well defined in most of the included studies, allowing reproducibility. None of the studies extracted features from dynamic contrast-enhanced (DCE) sequences. There has been a progressive decline in the number of studies that extract features from DCE in favor of T2 and/or ADC, as noted in similar reviews [39,42]. There is no clear added value in comparison to T2 and ADC [39]. All the studies extracted features from T2 and/or ADC sequences, and four of them from high-b value DWI [26,27,31,35]. While high-b values are better than low-b values for detecting PCa [59], there is controversy about the added value of DWI if features are already extracted from ADC, leading to potential bias [60]. In the studies that included both sequences, there was no clear drop in performance, but further assessment is needed [26,31,35].

Thirdly, there were important limitations in the training/validation of the models. The most significant one is the lack of external validation cohorts. Past similar reviews also highlighted this problem [39,40,42–44], which limits model applicability and robustness [61]. Six studies used external validation sets [26–29,31,35], but two of them were from public repositories [25,29]. Calibration studies should also be performed in external cohorts, but only two studies reported them [26,29]. There were also other constraints regarding the training/validation of the models, such as no mention of the minimum sample size needed to detect a clinically significant effect size and make comparisons [62], as well as poor reporting of how thresholds were chosen or reported. Moreover, all the studies were retrospective, which inherently induces bias due to the design and limited data. Prospective studies are needed to better assess the potential of AI models in clinical practice. Efforts are being made in this regard, and some prospective studies are being published with encouraging results [63]. Additionally, open-source code should be used to favor transparency and reproducibility, as specified in the RQS [15] and CLAIM [23] tools. Only three studies used open-source code [27,31,33]. Potential clinical applications should also be discussed, such as using the models as a second reader [64]. Explainability methods are also required to facilitate clinical implementation. In this review, only one study used interpretability methods [27].

Lastly, other objectives of this review were to compare radiomic models, radiologists, and multivariable models. This issue has been noted in past reviews [39,40] since there is a lack of comparisons between AI-based models and current clinical practice [65]. In fact, only four studies conducted a statistical comparison between the radiomic model and the PI-RADS classification [30–32,37], using PI-RADS ≥ 3 or ≥ 4 as the thresholds for detecting csPCa. Overall, there was no clear difference between the performance of PI-RADS and the models. Liu et al. [32] reported significantly better performance of the radiomic model at all lesion levels but not at the index lesion level. Jiang et al. [31] reported a significantly better performance of PI-RADS in the internal validation set but found no differences at external validation. Future studies should assess this issue to favor clinical implementation, as well as comparing the performance based on radiologist expertise. Hamm et al. [27] reported better performance of nonexpert readers when using the AI assistance, especially in PI-RADS 3 lesions, which represents a challenge due to the overdiagnosis of iPCa [8]. It is important to consider that there is also inherent inter-reader variability in MRI interpretation with PI-RADS system among radiologists [12,13], as well as limitations of the PI-RADS v2.1 [11], but these limitations are beyond the scope of this review. Four studies created multivariable models that incorporated clinical variables (including PI-RADS in some cases) [24,25,29,36]. Dominguez et al. [24] and Jing et al. [29] reported significantly better performance of the combined model than the PI-RADS. Future studies are needed to better assess the role of radiomics in combined models to improve the current standard based on PI-RADS.

In the light of the above, we offer the following recommendations for future studies to assess the constraints and heterogeneity and encourage clinical applicability: (i) large and multicentric datasets with representative and balanced data for the clinical aim of the model should be used; (ii) clear inclusion and exclusion criteria should be well specified, avoiding criteria that make nonrepresentative or biased data such as exclusion of advanced stages; (iii) detailed methodology, preferably following published AI guidelines for medical imaging (such as CLAIM [23]); (iv) robust reference standard, such as targeted biopsy or radical prostatectomy; (v) prospective design is desired; (vi) assessment of interobserver/inter-reader variability in manual segmentations, as well as feature robustness; (vii) detailed statistical methods, including sample size calculation and appropriate discrimination metrics with statistical significance and information about selected thresholds; (viii) validation on external datasets; (ix) open source and explainability methods are encouraged; (x) comparison of the model with current PI-RADS version, as well as development of combined models with clinical variables (such as PSA-D, DRE or others).

This review had some limitations. First, the publication bias favors studies with good performance that might overestimate the results. Second, relevant studies published after the deadline of the review might have been missed. Third, the specific eligibility criteria might have discharged relevant studies in which the methodology was not properly defined. Lastly, no direct comparisons and analysis were possible due to the heterogeneity of the data.

5. Conclusions

This systematic review denotes promising results of radiomic models in the prediction of csPCa in the included studies. However, the quality evaluation highlights significant heterogeneity and constraints that limit the clinical application of these models. This includes limited data representativity and methodological errors in the radiomic pipeline such as proper evaluation of interobserver/inter-reader variability or feature robustness, as well as a lack of prospective studies and external validation to evaluate the real performance outside the internal dataset. Furthermore, more efforts are needed to compare these models with radiologists and the integration of radiomics in combined models with other clinical variables. Future studies should tackle these problems to better understand the potential of radiomics in this field and ensure proper implementation in routine clinical practice.

Supplementary Materials: The following supporting information can be downloaded at: https://www.mdpi.com/article/10.3390/cancers16172951/s1, Supplementary Table S1: Schematic representation of the eligible criteria extracted from the Population, Intervention, Comparator, Outcome (PICO) framework. Supplementary File S2: An explanation of the relevant data extracted from each selected study.

Author Contributions: Conceptualization, A.A. and J.M.; methodology and data curation, A.A. and J.M.; writing—original draft preparation, A.A., N.R., J.M. and E.T.; resources, A.A. and J.M.; writing—review and editing, all authors; visualization, A.A., N.R., J.M. and E.T.; supervision, A.A., N.R., J.M. and E.T.; project administration, A.A. and J.M. All authors have read and agreed to the published version of the manuscript.

Funding: This paper was funded by the European project FLUTE, which has received funding from HORIZON-HLTH2022-IND-13 action under the Horizon Europe Framework with grant agreement Nr.101095382.

Institutional Review Board Statement: Not applicable.

Informed Consent Statement: Not applicable.

Conflicts of Interest: The authors declare no conflicts of interest.

References

Sung, H.; Ferlay, J.; Siegel, R.L.; Laversanne, M.; Soerjomataram, I.; Jemal, A.; Bray, F. Global Cancer Statistics 2020: GLOBOCAN Estimates of Incidence and Mortality Worldwide for 36 Cancers in 185 Countries. *CA Cancer J Clin.* **2021**, *71*, 209–249. [CrossRef] [PubMed]

Epstein, J.I.; Egevad, L.; Amin, M.B.; Delahunt, B.; Srigley, J.R.; Humphrey, P.A.; Grading Committee. The 2014 International Society of Urological Pathology (ISUP) Consensus Conference on Gleason Grading of Prostatic Carcinoma: Definition of Grading Patterns and Proposal for a New Grading System. *Am. J. Surg. Pathol.* **2016**, *40*, 244–252. [CrossRef] [PubMed]

Van Poppel, H.; Roobol, M.J.; Chandran, A. Early Detection of Prostate Cancer in the European Union: Combining Forces with PRAISE-U. *Eur. Urol.* **2023**, *84*, 519–522. [CrossRef] [PubMed]

Van Poppel, H.; Hogenhout, R.; Albers, P.; van den Bergh, R.C.N.; Barentsz, J.O.; Roobol, M.J. A European Model for an Organised Risk-stratified Early Detection Programme for Prostate Cancer. *Eur. Urol. Oncol.* **2021**, *4*, 731–739. [CrossRef]

Van Poppel, H.; Albreht, T.; Basu, P.; Hogenhout, R.; Collen, S.; Roobol, M. Serum PSA-based Early Detection of Prostate Cancer in Europe and Globally: Past, Present and Future. *Nat. Rev. Urol.* **2022**, *19*, 562–572. [CrossRef]

Turkbey, B.; Rosenkrantz, A.B.; Haider, M.A.; Padhani, A.R.; Villeirs, G.; Macura, K.J.; Tempany, C.M.; Choyke, P.L.; Cornud, F.; Margolis, D.J.; et al. Prostate Imaging Reporting and Data System Version 2.1: 2019 Update of Prostate Imaging Reporting and Data System Version 2. *Eur. Urol.* **2019**, *76*, 340–351. [CrossRef]

Sathianathen, N.J.; Omer, A.; Harriss, E.; Davies, L.; Kasivisvanathan, V.; Punwani, S.; Moore, C.M.; Kastner, C.; Barrett, T.; Van Den Bergh, R.C.; et al. Negative Predictive Value of Multiparametric Magnetic Resonance Imaging in the Detection of Clinically Significant Prostate Cancer in the Prostate Imaging Reporting and Data System Era: A Systematic Review and Meta-analysis. *Eur. Urol.* **2020**, *78*, 402–414. [CrossRef]

Oerther, B.; Engel, H.; Bamberg, F.; Sigle, A.; Gratzke, C.; Benndorf, M. Cancer Detection Rates of the PI-RADS v2.1 Assessment Categories: Systematic Review and Meta-analysis on Lesion Level and Patient Level. *Prostate Cancer Prostatic Dis.* **2022**, *25*, 256–263. [CrossRef]

9. Drost, F.H.; Osses, D.; Nieboer, D.; Bangma, C.H.; Steyerberg, E.W.; Roobol, M.J.; Schoots, I.G. Prostate Magnetic Resonance Imaging, with or Without Magnetic Resonance Imaging-targeted Biopsy, and Systematic Biopsy for Detecting Prostate Cancer: Cochrane Systematic Review and Meta-analysis. *Eur. Urol.* **2020**, *77*, 78–94. [CrossRef]
10. Mottet, N.; van den Bergh, R.C.N.; Briers, E.; Van den Broeck, T.; Cumberbatch, M.G.; De Santis, M.; Fanti, S.; Fossati, N.; Gandaglia, G.; Gillessen, S.; et al. EAU-EANM-ESTRO-ESUR-SIOG Guidelines on Prostate Cancer-2020 Update. Part 1: Screening, Diagnosis, and Local Treatment with Curative Intent. *Eur. Urol.* **2021**, *79*, 243–262. [CrossRef]
11. Purysko, A.S.; Baroni, R.H.; Giganti, F.; Costa, D.; Renard-Penna, R.; Kim, C.K.; Raman, S.S. PI-RADS Version 2.1: A Critical Review, From the AJR Special Series on Radiology Reporting and Data Systems. *AJR Am. J. Roentgenol.* **2021**, *216*, 20–32. [CrossRef] [PubMed]
12. Bhayana, R.; O'Shea, A.; Anderson, M.A.; Bradley, W.R.; Gottumukkala, R.V.; Mojtahed, A.; Pierce, T.T.; Harisinghani, M. PI-RADS Versions 2 and 2.1: Interobserver Agreement and Diagnostic Performance in Peripheral and Transition Zone Lesions Among Six Radiologists. *AJR Am. J. Roentgenol.* **2021**, *217*, 141–151. [CrossRef] [PubMed]
13. Smith, C.P.; Harmon, S.A.; Barrett, T.; Bittencourt, L.K.; Law, Y.M.; Shebel, H.; An, J.Y.; Czarniecki, M.; Mehralivand, S.; Coskun, M.; et al. Intra- and Interreader Reproducibility of PI-RADSv2: A Multireader Study. *J. Magn. Reson. Imaging* **2019**, *49*, 1694–1703. [CrossRef] [PubMed]
14. Osses, D.F.; Roobol, M.J.; Schoots, I.G. Prediction Medicine: Biomarkers, Risk Calculators and Magnetic Resonance Imaging as Risk Stratification Tools in Prostate Cancer Diagnosis. *Int. J. Mol. Sci.* **2019**, *20*, 1637. [CrossRef]
15. Lambin, P.; Leijenaar, R.T.H.; Deist, T.M.; Peerlings, J.; de Jong, E.E.C.; van Timmeren, J.; Sanduleanu, S.; Larue, R.T.H.M.; Even, A.J.G.; Jochems, A.; et al. Radiomics: The Bridge Between Medical Imaging and Personalized Medicine. *Nat. Rev. Clin. Oncol.* **2017**, *14*, 749–762. [CrossRef]
16. Scapicchio, C.; Gabelloni, M.; Barucci, A.; Cioni, D.; Saba, L.; Neri, E. A Deep Look Into Radiomics. *Radiol Med.* **2021**, *126*, 1296–1311. [CrossRef]
17. Ferro, M.; de Cobelli, O.; Musi, G.; Del Giudice, F.; Carrieri, G.; Busetto, G.M.; Falagario, U.G.; Sciarra, A.; Maggi, M.; Crocetto, F.; et al. Radiomics in Prostate Cancer: An Up-to-Date Review. *Ther. Adv. Urol.* **2022**, *14*, 17562872221109020. [CrossRef]
18. Cutaia, G.; La Tona, G.; Comelli, A.; Vernuccio, F.; Agnello, F.; Gagliardo, C.; Salvaggio, L.; Quartuccio, N.; Sturiale, L.; Stefano, A.; et al. Radiomics and Prostate MRI: Current Role and Future Applications. *J. Imaging* **2021**, *7*, 34. [CrossRef]
19. Penzkofer, T.; Padhani, A.R.; Turkbey, B.; Haider, M.A.; Huisman, H.; Walz, J.; Salomon, G.; Schoots, I.G.; Richenberg, J.; Villeirs, G.; et al. ESUR/ESUI Position Paper: Developing Artificial Intelligence for Precision Diagnosis of Prostate Cancer Using Magnetic Resonance Imaging. *Eur. Radiol.* **2021**, *31*, 9567–9578. [CrossRef]
20. Page, M.J.; Moher, D.; Bossuyt, P.M.; Boutron, I.; Hoffmann, T.C.; Mulrow, C.D.; Shamseer, L.; Tetzlaff, J.M.; Akl, E.A.; Brennan, S.E.; et al. PRISMA 2020 Explanation and Elaboration: Updated Guidance and Exemplars for Reporting Systematic Reviews. *BMJ* **2021**, *372*, n160. [CrossRef]
21. Schardt, C.; Adams, M.B.; Owens, T.; Keitz, S.; Fontelo, P. Utilization of the PICO Framework to Improve Searching PubMed for Clinical Questions. *BMC Med. Inform. Decis. Mak.* **2007**, *7*, 16. [CrossRef] [PubMed]
22. QUADAS-2 | Bristol Medical School: Population Health Sciences | University of Bristol. Available online: https://www.bristol.ac.uk/population-health-sciences/projects/quadas/quadas-2/ (accessed on 1 June 2024).
23. Mongan, J.; Moy, L.; Kahn, C.E., Jr. Checklist for Artificial Intelligence in Medical Imaging (CLAIM): A Guide for Authors and Reviewers. *Radiol. Artif. Intell.* **2020**, *2*, e200029. [CrossRef]
24. Dominguez, I.; Rios-Ibacache, O.; Caprile, P.; Gonzalez, J.; San Francisco, I.F.; Besa, C. MRI-Based Surrogate Imaging Markers of Aggressiveness in Prostate Cancer: Development of a Machine Learning Model Based on Radiomic Features. *Diagnostics* **2023**, *13*, 2779. [CrossRef] [PubMed]
25. Prata, F.; Anceschi, U.; Cordelli, E.; Faiella, E.; Civitella, A.; Tuzzolo, P.; Iannuzzi, A.; Ragusa, A.; Esperto, F.; Prata, S.M.; et al. Radiomic Machine-Learning Analysis of Multiparametric Magnetic Resonance Imaging in the Diagnosis of Clinically Significant Prostate Cancer: New Combination of Textural and Clinical Features. *Curr. Oncol.* **2023**, *30*, 2021–2031. [CrossRef] [PubMed]
26. Jin, P.; Shen, J.; Yang, L.; Zhang, J.; Shen, A.; Bao, J.; Wang, X. Machine Learning-Based Radiomics Model to Predict Benign and Malignant PI-RADS v2.1 Category 3 Lesions: A Retrospective Multi-Center Study. *BMC Med. Imaging* **2023**, *23*, 47. [CrossRef]
27. Hamm, C.A.; Baumgärtner, G.L.; Biessmann, F.; Beetz, N.L.; Hartenstein, A.; Savic, L.J.; Froböse, K.; Dräger, F.; Schallenberg, S.; Rudolph, M.; et al. Interactive Explainable Deep Learning Model Informs Prostate Cancer Diagnosis at MRI. *Radiology* **2023**, *307*, e222276. [CrossRef]
28. Hong, S.; Kim, S.H.; Yoo, B.; Kim, J.Y. Deep Learning Algorithm for Tumor Segmentation and Discrimination of Clinically Significant Cancer in Patients with Prostate Cancer. *Curr. Oncol.* **2023**, *30*, 7275–7285. [CrossRef]
29. Jing, G.; Xing, P.; Li, Z.; Ma, X.; Lu, H.; Shao, C.; Lu, Y.; Lu, J.; Shen, F. Prediction of Clinically Significant Prostate Cancer with a Multimodal MRI-Based Radiomics Nomogram. *Front. Oncol.* **2022**, *12*, 918830. [CrossRef]
30. Zhu, L.; Gao, G.; Zhu, Y.; Han, C.; Liu, X.; Li, D.; Liu, W.; Wang, X.; Zhang, J.; Zhang, X.; et al. Fully Automated Detection and Localization of Clinically Significant Prostate Cancer on MR Images Using a Cascaded Convolutional Neural Network. *Front. Oncol.* **2022**, *12*, 958065. [CrossRef]
31. Jiang, K.W.; Song, Y.; Hou, Y.; Zhi, R.; Zhang, J.; Bao, M.L.; Li, H.; Yan, X.; Xi, W.; Zhang, C.X.; et al. Performance of Artificial Intelligence-Aided Diagnosis System for Clinically Significant Prostate Cancer with MRI: A Diagnostic Comparison Study. *J. Magn. Reson. Imaging* **2023**, *57*, 1352–1364. [CrossRef]

2. Liu, Y.; Zheng, H.; Liang, Z.; Miao, Q.; Brisbane, W.G.; Marks, L.S.; Raman, S.S.; Reiter, R.E.; Yang, G.; Sung, K. Textured-Based Deep Learning in Prostate Cancer Classification with 3T Multiparametric MRI: Comparison with PI-RADS-Based Classification. *Diagnostics* **2021**, *11*, 1785. [CrossRef] [PubMed]
3. Lim, C.S.; Abreu-Gomez, J.; Thornhill, R.; James, N.; Al Kindi, A.; Lim, A.S.; Schieda, N. Utility of Machine Learning of Apparent Diffusion Coefficient (ADC) and T2-Weighted (T2W) Radiomic Features in PI-RADS Version 2.1 Category 3 Lesions to Predict Prostate Cancer Diagnosis. *Abdom. Radiol.* **2021**, *46*, 5647–5658. [CrossRef] [PubMed]
4. Hectors, S.J.; Chen, C.; Chen, J.; Wang, J.; Gordon, S.; Yu, M.; Al Hussein Al Awamlh, B.; Sabuncu, M.R.; Margolis, D.J.A.; Hu, J.C. Magnetic Resonance Imaging Radiomics-Based Machine Learning Prediction of Clinically Significant Prostate Cancer in Equivocal PI-RADS 3 Lesions. *J. Magn. Reson. Imaging* **2021**, *54*, 1466–1473. [CrossRef] [PubMed]
5. Castillo, T.J.M.; Starmans, M.P.A.; Arif, M.; Niessen, W.J.; Klein, S.; Bangma, C.H.; Schoots, I.G.; Veenland, J.F. A Multi-Center, Multi-Vendor Study to Evaluate the Generalizability of a Radiomics Model for Classifying Prostate Cancer: High Grade vs. Low Grade. *Diagnostics* **2021**, *11*, 369. [CrossRef]
6. Li, M.; Chen, T.; Zhao, W.; Wei, C.; Li, X.; Duan, S.; Ji, L.; Lu, Z.; Shen, J. Radiomics Prediction Model for the Improved Diagnosis of Clinically Significant Prostate Cancer on Biparametric MRI. *Quant. Imaging Med. Surg.* **2020**, *10*, 368–379. [CrossRef]
7. Zhong, X.; Cao, R.; Shakeri, S.; Scalzo, F.; Lee, Y.; Enzmann, D.R.; Wu, H.H.; Raman, S.S.; Sung, K. Deep Transfer Learning-Based Prostate Cancer Classification Using 3 Tesla Multi-Parametric MRI. *Abdom. Radiol.* **2019**, *44*, 2030–2039. [CrossRef]
8. Litjens, G.; Debats, O.; Barentsz, J.; Karssemeijer, N.; Huisman, H. SPIE-AAPM PROSTATEx Challenge Data (Version 2) [dataset]. *Cancer Imaging Arch.* **2017**. [CrossRef]
9. Castillo, T.J.M.; Arif, M.; Niessen, W.J.; Schoots, I.G.; Veenland, J.F. Automated Classification of Significant Prostate Cancer on MRI: A Systematic Review on the Performance of Machine Learning Applications. *Cancers* **2020**, *12*, 1606. [CrossRef]
10. Cuocolo, R.; Cipullo, M.B.; Stanzione, A.; Romeo, V.; Green, R.; Cantoni, V.; Ponsiglione, A.; Ugga, L.; Imbriaco, M. Machine Learning for the Identification of Clinically Significant Prostate Cancer on MRI: A Meta-Analysis. *Eur. Radiol.* **2020**, *30*, 6877–6887. [CrossRef]
11. Hosseinzadeh, M.; Saha, A.; Brand, P.; Slootweg, I.; de Rooij, M.; Huisman, H. Deep Learning-Assisted Prostate Cancer Detection on Bi-Parametric MRI: Minimum Training Data Size Requirements and Effect of Prior Knowledge. *Eur. Radiol.* **2022**, *32*, 2224–2234. [CrossRef]
12. Sushentsev, N.; Moreira Da Silva, N.; Yeung, M.; Barrett, T.; Sala, E.; Roberts, M.; Rundo, L. Comparative Performance of Fully-Automated and Semi-Automated Artificial Intelligence Methods for the Detection of Clinically Significant Prostate Cancer on MRI: A Systematic Review. *Insights Imaging* **2022**, *13*, 59. [CrossRef] [PubMed]
13. Syer, T.; Mehta, P.; Antonelli, M.; Mallelet, S.; Atkinson, D.; Ourselin, S.; Punwani, S. Artificial Intelligence Compared to Radiologists for the Initial Diagnosis of Prostate Cancer on Magnetic Resonance Imaging: A Systematic Review and Recommendations for Future Studies. *Cancers* **2021**, *13*, 3318. [CrossRef] [PubMed]
14. Twilt, J.J.; van Leeuwen, K.G.; Huisman, H.J.; Fütterer, J.J.; de Rooij, M. Artificial Intelligence Based Algorithms for Prostate Cancer Classification and Detection on Magnetic Resonance Imaging: A Narrative Review. *Diagnostics* **2021**, *11*, 959. [CrossRef] [PubMed]
15. Rosenkrantz, A.B.; Taneja, S.S. Radiologist, Be Aware: Ten Pitfalls That Confound the Interpretation of Multiparametric Prostate MRI. *AJR Am. J. Roentgenol.* **2014**, *202*, 109–120. [CrossRef]
16. Tewes, S.; Mokov, N.; Hartung, D.; Schick, V.; Peters, I.; Schedl, P.; Pertschy, S.; Wacker, F.; Voshage, G.; Hueper, K. Standardized Reporting of Prostate MRI: Comparison of the Prostate Imaging Reporting and Data System (PI-RADS) Version 1 and Version 2. *PLoS ONE* **2016**, *11*, e0162879. [CrossRef]
17. Rudolph, M.M.; Baur, A.D.J.; Cash, H.; Haas, M.; Mahjoub, S.; Hartenstein, A.; Hamm, C.A.; Beetz, N.L.; Konietschke, F.; Hamm, B.; et al. Diagnostic Performance of PI-RADS Version 2.1 Compared to Version 2.0 for Detection of Peripheral and Transition Zone Prostate Cancer. *Sci. Rep.* **2020**, *10*, 15982. [CrossRef]
18. Kasivisvanathan, V.; Rannikko, A.S.; Borghi, M.; Panebianco, V.; Mynderse, L.A.; Vaarala, M.H.; Briganti, A.; Budäus, L.; Hellawell, G.; PRECISION Study Group Collaborators; et al. MRI-Targeted or Standard Biopsy for Prostate-Cancer Diagnosis. *N. Engl. J. Med.* **2018**, *378*, 1767–1777. [CrossRef]
19. Goel, S.; Shoag, J.E.; Gross, M.D.; Al Hussein Al Awamlh, B.; Robinson, B.; Khani, F.; Baltich Nelson, B.; Margolis, D.J.; Hu, J.C. Concordance Between Biopsy and Radical Prostatectomy Pathology in the Era of Targeted Biopsy: A Systematic Review and Meta-Analysis. *Eur. Urol. Oncol.* **2020**, *3*, 10–20. [CrossRef]
20. Sun, Z.; Wu, P.; Cui, Y.; Liu, X.; Wang, K.; Gao, G.; Wang, H.; Zhang, X.; Wang, X. Deep-Learning Models for Detection and Localization of Visible Clinically Significant Prostate Cancer on Multi-Parametric MRI. *J. Magn. Reson. Imaging* **2023**, *58*, 1067–1081. [CrossRef]
21. Bonmatí, L.M.; Miguel, A.; Suárez, A.; Aznar, M.; Beregi, J.P.; Fournier, L.; Neri, E.; Laghi, A.; França, M.; Sardanelli, F.; et al. CHAIMELEON Project: Creation of a Pan-European Repository of Health Imaging Data for the Development of AI-Powered Cancer Management Tools. *Front. Oncol.* **2022**, *12*, 742701. [CrossRef]
22. Leevy, J.L.; Khoshgoftaar, T.M.; Bauder, R.A.; Seliya, N. A Survey on Addressing High-Class Imbalance in Big Data. *J. Big Data* **2018**, *5*, 42. [CrossRef]
23. Varoquaux, G.; Cheplygina, V. Machine Learning for Medical Imaging: Methodological Failures and Recommendations for the Future. *NPJ Digit. Med.* **2022**, *5*, 48. [CrossRef]

54. Peng, Y.; Jiang, Y.; Antic, T.; Giger, M.L.; Eggener, S.E.; Oto, A. Validation of Quantitative Analysis of Multiparametric Prostate MR Images for Prostate Cancer Detection and Aggressiveness Assessment: A Cross-Imager Study. *Radiology* **2014**, *271*, 461–47. [CrossRef] [PubMed]
55. Transin, S.; Souchon, R.; Gonindard-Melodelima, C.; de Rozario, R.; Walker, P.; Funes de la Vega, M.; Loffroy, R.; Cormier, L.; Rouvière, O. Computer-Aided Diagnosis System for Characterizing ISUP Grade ≥2 Prostate Cancers at Multiparametric MRI: Cross-Vendor Evaluation. *Diagn. Interv. Imaging* **2019**, *100*, 801–811. [CrossRef] [PubMed]
56. Ozkan, T.A.; Eruyar, A.T.; Cebeci, O.O.; Memik, O.; Ozcan, L.; Kuskonmaz, I. Interobserver Variability in Gleason Histologic Grading of Prostate Cancer. *Scand. J. Urol.* **2016**, *50*, 420–424. [CrossRef]
57. Schwier, M.; van Griethuysen, J.; Vangel, M.G.; Pieper, S.; Peled, S.; Tempany, C.; Aerts, H.J.W.L.; Kikinis, R.; Fennessy, F.M.; Fedorov, A. Repeatability of Multiparametric Prostate MRI Radiomics Features. *Sci. Rep.* **2019**, *9*, 9441. [CrossRef]
58. Lee, J.; Steinmann, A.; Ding, Y.; Lee, H.; Owens, C.; Wang, J.; Yang, J.; Followill, D.; Ger, R.; MacKin, D.; et al. Radiomics Feature Robustness as Measured Using an MRI Phantom. *Sci. Rep.* **2021**, *11*, 3973. [CrossRef]
59. Rosenkrantz, A.B.; Hindman, N.; Lim, R.P.; Das, K.; Babb, J.S.; Mussi, T.C.; Taneja, S.S. Diffusion-Weighted Imaging of the Prostate: Comparison of b1000 and b2000 Image Sets for Index Lesion Detection. *J. Magn. Reson. Imaging* **2013**, *38*, 694–700. [CrossRef]
60. Peerlings, J.; Woodruff, H.C.; Winfield, J.M.; Ibrahim, A.; Van Beers, B.E.; Heerschap, A.; Jackson, A.; Wildberger, J.E.; Mottaghy, F.M.; DeSouza, N.M.; et al. Stability of Radiomics Features in Apparent Diffusion Coefficient Maps from a Multi-Centre Test-Retest Trial. *Sci. Rep.* **2019**, *9*, 4800. [CrossRef]
61. Bluemke, D.A.; Moy, L.; Bredella, M.A.; Ertl-Wagner, B.B.; Fowler, K.J.; Goh, V.J.; Halpern, E.F.; Hess, C.P.; Schiebler, M.L.; Weiss, C.R. Assessing Radiology Research on Artificial Intelligence: A Brief Guide for Authors, Reviewers, and Readers-From the Radiology Editorial Board. *Radiology* **2020**, *294*, 487–489. [CrossRef]
62. Park, S.H.; Han, K. Methodologic Guide for Evaluating Clinical Performance and Effect of Artificial Intelligence Technology for Medical Diagnosis and Prediction. *Radiology* **2018**, *286*, 800–809. [CrossRef] [PubMed]
63. Lin, Y.; Yilmaz, E.C.; Belue, M.J.; Harmon, S.A.; Tetreault, J.; Phelps, T.E.; Merriman, K.M.; Hazen, L.; Garcia, C.; Yang, D.; et al. Evaluation of a Cascaded Deep Learning-Based Algorithm for Prostate Lesion Detection at Biparametric MRI. *Radiology* **2024**, *31*, e230750. [CrossRef] [PubMed]
64. Jaouen, T.; Souchon, R.; Moldovan, P.C.; Bratan, F.; Duran, A.; Hoang-Dinh, A.; Di Franco, F.; Debeer, S.; Dubreuil-Chambardel, M.; Arfi, N.; et al. Characterization of High-Grade Prostate Cancer at Multiparametric MRI Using a Radiomic-Based Computer-Aided Diagnosis System as Standalone and Second Reader. *Diagn. Interv. Imaging* **2023**, *104*, 465–476. [CrossRef] [PubMed]
65. Liu, X.; Faes, L.; Kale, A.U.; Wagner, S.K.; Fu, D.J.; Bruynseels, A.; Mahendiran, T.; Moraes, G.; Shamdas, M.; Kern, C.; et al. Comparison of Deep Learning Performance Against Health-Care Professionals in Detecting Diseases from Medical Imaging: Systematic Review and Meta-Analysis. *Lancet Digit. Health* **2019**, *1*, e271–e297. [CrossRef] [PubMed]

Disclaimer/Publisher's Note: The statements, opinions and data contained in all publications are solely those of the individual author(s) and contributor(s) and not of MDPI and/or the editor(s). MDPI and/or the editor(s) disclaim responsibility for any injury to people or property resulting from any ideas, methods, instructions or products referred to in the content.

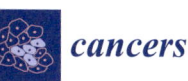

Article

A Multiparametric MRI and Baseline-Clinical-Feature-Based Dense Multimodal Fusion Artificial Intelligence (MFAI) Model to Predict Castration-Resistant Prostate Cancer Progression

Dianning He [1,†], Haoming Zhuang [2,†], Ying Ma [2], Bixuan Xia [2], Aritrick Chatterjee [3], Xiaobing Fan [3], Shouliang Qi [2], Wei Qian [2], Zhe Zhang [4,*] and Jing Liu [5,*]

1. School of Health Management, China Medical University, Shenyang 110122, China; hedn@cmu.edu.cn
2. College of Medicine and Biological Information Engineering, Northeastern University, Shenyang 110169, China; 2271371@stu.neu.edu.cn (H.Z.); xuanduth@gmail.com (Y.M.); 2271354@stu.neu.edu.cn (B.X.); qisl@bmie.neu.edu.cn (S.Q.); wqian@bmie.neu.edu.cn (W.Q.)
3. Department of Radiology, University of Chicago, 5841 S Maryland Ave, Chicago, IL 60637, USA; aritrick@uchicago.edu (A.C.); xfan@uchicago.edu (X.F.)
4. Department of Urology, First Hospital of China Medical University, Shenyang 110001, China
5. Department of Radiology, First Hospital of China Medical University, Shenyang 110001, China
* Correspondence: zzhang@cmu.edu.cn (Z.Z.); jrjj108@sina.com (J.L.)
† These authors contributed equally to this work.

Simple Summary: The majority of patients with advanced prostate cancer who receive hormone therapy ultimately progress to castration-resistant prostate cancer (CRPC), which is associated with a significantly poorer prognosis. The current methods to predict CRPC progression rely on invasive and highly time-consuming approaches. This study proposes a multimodal fusion artificial intelligence model that combines multiparametric magnetic resonance imaging data with baseline clinical characteristics of patients to predict whether prostate cancer patients could progress to CRPC after 12 months of hormone therapy. A dense multimodal fusion artificial intelligence (Dense-MFAI) model was developed and validated in this study using data from 96 patients. The model demonstrated a high degree of accuracy in predicting CRPC progression, with a prediction accuracy of 94.2%. This non-invasive approach has the potential to assist urologists in making more informed treatment decisions and developing appropriate prognostic measures for prostate cancer patents, thereby improving patient prognosis through early intervention and personalized treatment strategies.

Abstract: Objectives: The primary objective of this study was to identify whether patients with prostate cancer (PCa) could progress to denervation-resistant prostate cancer (CRPC) after 12 months of hormone therapy. Methods: A total of 96 PCa patients with baseline clinical data who underwent multiparametric magnetic resonance imaging (MRI) between September 2018 and September 2022 were included in this retrospective study. Patients were classified as progressing or not progressing to CRPC on the basis of their outcome after 12 months of hormone therapy. A dense multimodal fusion artificial intelligence (Dense-MFAI) model was constructed by incorporating a squeeze-and-excitation block and a spatial pyramid pooling layer into a dense convolutional network (DenseNet), as well as integrating the eXtreme Gradient Boosting machine learning algorithm. The accuracy, sensitivity, specificity, positive predictive value, negative predictive value, receiver operating characteristic curves, area under the curve (AUC) and confusion matrices were used as classification performance metrics. Results: The Dense-MFAI model demonstrated an accuracy of 94.2%, with an AUC of 0.945, when predicting the progression of patients with PCa to CRPC after 12 months of hormone therapy. The experimental validation demonstrated that combining radiomics feature mapping with baseline clinical characteristics significantly improved the model's classification performance, confirming the importance of multimodal data. Conclusions: The Dense-MFAI model proposed in this study has the ability to more accurately predict whether a PCa patient could progress to CRPC. This model can assist urologists in developing the most appropriate treatment plan and prognostic measures.

Keywords: prostate cancer; castration-resistant prostate cancer; mpMRI; deep learning; radiomics

1. Introduction

Prostate cancer (PCa) is the second most common cancer in men worldwide [1]. The prostate cancer screening rate is lower in China than in other developed countries [2]. Consequently, the majority of initial diagnoses occur in the middle or late clinical stages, resulting in a less favorable overall prognosis for prostate cancer patients [3]. Androgen deprivation therapy is currently the primary treatment for men diagnosed with advanced PCa [4]. However, after a median of 12 months of androgen deprivation therapy, almost all advanced PCa patients progress to castration-resistant prostate cancer (CRPC) and the time to progress to CRPC varies considerably between patients [5–7]. Once a patient reaches the CRPC stage, the disease rapidly progresses and the prognosis is extremely poor [8].

The clinical progression of CRPC is currently determined by the following three factors: serum testosterone reaching desmoplastic levels (i.e., <50 ng/dL or <1.7 nmol/L), persistent elevation of prostate-specific antigen (PSA) and tumor progression visible in images [9]. However, the use of single indicators such as PSA and serum testosterone for judgments is inherently unreliable [10]. Therefore, there is a pressing need for a method to predict at an early stage whether a patient could progress to CRPC within a specified period following hormone therapy to facilitate clinical decision-making.

Despite significant advancements in precision medicine, proactively and accurately predicting whether a patient could progress to CRPC within a specific time frame remains challenging. A number of studies have predicted PCa progression by fusing multiparametric magnetic resonance imaging (mpMRI) and clinical features. Roest et al. [11] utilized a U-Net model fusing these two modalities to predict clinically significant PCa progression. In contrast to the utilization of a solitary deep learning modeling approach, our study employed a staged and multi-module model design, accompanied by the further integration of information from radiomics. Currently, the majority of methods employed for CRPC prediction utilize biomarkers, the expression of specific genes or proteins and tumor immunohistochemistry [12–14]. Jun et al. [15] identified six genes, including NPEPL1 and VWF, to be predictive of CRPC using screening and a regression analysis of 287 genes. Scher et al. [12] demonstrated a strong correlation between the measured circulating tumor cell counts and the progression of CRPC (r = 0.84). However, these methods are associated with high costs, invasive procedures and additional time delays. In contrast, mpMRI—specifically, radiomics feature mapping—and clinical parameters were employed in the present study to construct a multimodal model for prediction. T2-weighted imaging provides anatomical information regarding PCa and dynamic contrast-enhanced MRI (DCE-MRI) aids in the detection of recurrent prostate disease by evaluating the characteristics of the prostate microvascular system [16,17]. Radiomics using tumor heterogeneity features can provide more comprehensive information to accurately predict tumor progression [18,19]. Furthermore, previous studies have demonstrated that baseline clinical features may also provide crucial prognostic information to monitor disease progression in prostate cancer patients [20]. Therefore, a quantitative analysis approach was employed in the present study to predict outcomes, thereby reducing the subjectivity inherent in traditional methods while circumventing the laborious process of the manual testing of genes and proteins that is needed.

Here, we propose an approach based on a multimodal fusion artificial intelligence (MFAI) model to predict whether PCa could progress to CRPC at an earlier time point, at a median of 12 months, on the basis of mpMRI, radiomic feature mapping and baseline clinical data. The implementation of this model by urologists could enable early intervention in high-risk patients and the development of more precise treatment and follow-up plans.

2. Materials and Methods

2.1. Patients

This retrospective study was approved by the Radiological Review Board of the First Hospital of China Medical University, Shenyang, and adhered to the principles and requirements of the Declaration of Helsinki. No further consent was required for the study. This study involved a retrospective analysis of previously collected data from PCa patients treated between September 2018 and September 2022 at our hospital. The following clinical information was recorded: age, baseline PSA level, Gleason score and clinical TNM stage. The following individuals were excluded from the study: (i) those who did not undergo DCE-MRI prior to hormone therapy and biopsy; (ii) those with an incomplete apparent diffusion coefficient sequence; (iii) those with a history of aggressive malignancy or serious complications in the absence of complete information; (iv) those with other tumor types, confirmed pathologically; (v) those lacking appropriate baseline clinicopathological information; and (vi) those who underwent treatment or tissue biopsy prior to MRI. A total of 96 patients (mean age = 65 years; range 45–88 years) were enrolled in this study; 58 patients did not progress to CRPC after 12 months of hormone therapy and 38 patients progressed to CRPC. The patient recruitment process is shown in Figure 1.

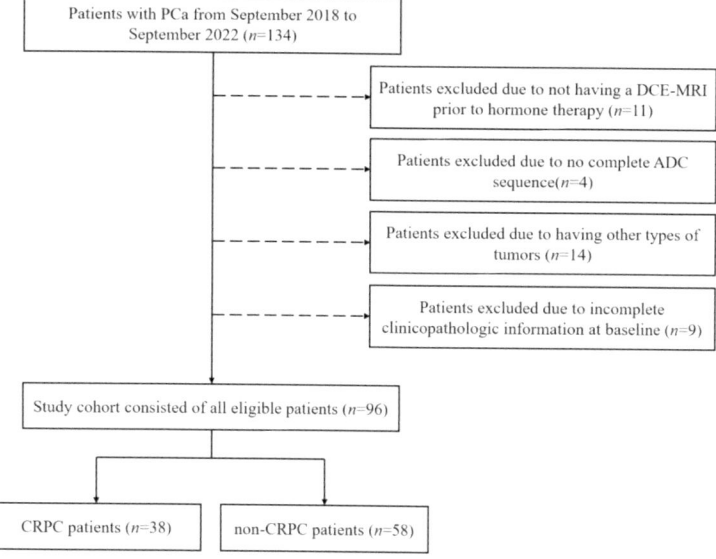

Figure 1. Flowchart of patient selection. PCa: prostate cancer; DCE-MRI: dynamic contrast-enhanced magnetic resonance imaging; ADC: apparent diffusion coefficient; CRPC: castration-resistant prostate cancer.

2.2. Image Acquisition

MRI was performed using a Siemens VIDA 3T MRI scanner (Siemens Healthineers, Erlangen, Germany). The mpMRI protocols included T2-weighted imaging, diffusion-weighted imaging (DWI) and DCE-MRI. DWI used SPAIR (SPectral Attenuated Inversion Recovery) fat suppression and b-values of 10, 50, 100, 150, 200, 400, 600, 800, 1000 and 1500 s/mm². DCE-MRI data were acquired at a temporal resolution of 7 s. The total amount of gadopentetate dimeglumine injected was calculated on the basis of the patient's weight (0.2 mmol/kg) and the imaging time was 4.3 min. The specific parameters of the MRI are presented in Table 1.

Table 1. Magnetic resonance imaging parameters.

Imaging Sequence	FOV (mm)	Scan Matrix Size	TE (ms)	TR (ms)	Slice Thickness (mm)	Interval (mm)	Flip Angle (°)
T2WI	200	512 × 512	128	500	3	0.6	90
DWI	260	120 × 96	72	400	3	0.6	/
DCE	340	203 × 320	1.3	3.4	3.5	0	9

FOV: field of view; TE: echo time; TR: repetition time; T2WI: T2-weighted imaging; DWI: diffusion-weighted imaging; DCE: dynamic contrast-enhanced.

2.3. Data Analysis

The DCE-MRI signal enhancement rate (α), apparent diffusion coefficient (ADC) values and T2 values were calculated on the basis of mpMRI. Previous studies have also demonstrated the effectiveness of these parameters at identifying lesions [21]. Consequently, the three quantitative parameters were selected for the purpose of predicting whether a patient could progress to CRPC.

2.3.1. α-Mapping Acquisition

The percentage signal enhancement (PSE) per pixel in DCE-MRI was calculated as shown in Equation (1), where $S(t)$ is the signal intensity curve and S_0 is the baseline signal before contrast-agent injection.

$$PSE(t) = \frac{S(t) - S_0}{S_0} \cdot 100 \tag{1}$$

Then, an empirical mathematical model was used to fit the $PSE(t)$ as follows:

$$PSE(t) = A\left(1 - e^{-\alpha t}\right)e^{-\beta t} \tag{2}$$

where A is the amplitude of the PSE, α is the rate of signal enhancement and β is the elution rate. Instead of performing overall averaging directly over the ROI, this process first calculates the percentage signal enhancement profile ($PSE(t)$) (Equation (1)) independently for each voxel of the DCE-MRI sequence and then fits the parameter α (Equation (2)) to that voxel based on an empirical mathematical model. Then, we averaged the values for all the voxels in the ROI for our analysis.

2.3.2. T2 Mapping Acquisition

The T2 value was calculated from multi-spin–echo images via a monoexponential signal model according to Equation (3), as follows:

$$S = S_0 \exp\left(-\frac{TE}{T2}\right) \quad (3)$$

where TE is the echo time, S is the signal strength corresponding with different echo times and S_0 is the signal strength at the moment when $TE = 0$.

2.3.3. Apparent Diffusion Coefficient Mapping Acquisition

The apparent diffusion coefficient value was calculated from diffusion-weighted imaging via Equation (4), as follows:

$$S = S_0 \exp(-b \cdot ADC) \quad (4)$$

where b is the diffusion weighting factor, S_0 is the undiffused spin–echo signal and S is the diffusion-weighted attenuated spin–echo signal. The b-values of this experiment were 10, 50, 100, 150, 200, 400, 600, 800, 1000 and 1500 s/mm^2.

2.3.4. Long-Run High Gray-Level Emphasis Mapping Acquisition

Our research team previously reported that the long-run high gray-level emphasis (LRHGLE) features calculated on the basis of the gray-level contour matrix in α-parameter mapping are significantly influencing factors for determining sensitive resistance to hormone therapy in prostate cancer [22]. Consequently, we also calculated the radiomic feature mapping. Each pixel was designated as the center of a matrix with a size of 5 × 5, which was used to calculate the LRHGLE features. The average value was then assigned to the center pixel. In this manner, the LRHGLE texture feature mapping was constructed.

2.4. Data Preparation

In this study, index lesions were manually and independently marked as regions of interest using a semi-automated method involving two experienced radiologists on the basis of the patient's diagnostic report. In the event of a Dice similarity coefficient for tumor contours less than 0.80 for two radiologists, the contour was considered to be significantly different, prompting a consultation to reach a consensus. To ensure consistency and reliability, the tumor contours delineated by a radiologist with greater experience were used for all subsequent analyses after a consensus was reached. Neither of the radiologists had access to the pathological reports. The regions of interest (ROIs) were based on the sequence that showed the greatest extent of the cancer. They were mapped using T2WI and transferred to other sequences [23]. The ROIs were subsequently mapped from the T2-weighted image to the ADC mapping and DCE-MRI via image alignment. Despite the demonstrated variability in ROI mapping across different MRI sequences, the relatively fixed position of the prostate and its limited mobility enhanced the reliability of the alignment process [24,25]. Moreover, the accuracy of ROIs has been validated by experienced radiologists following the alignment procedure. The protocol for tumor marking is delineated in Figure 2. Subsequently, following the execution of feature mapping calculations, the ROIs were extracted, normalized and combined using extraction. These were then input into the model. The data preparation process is depicted in Figure 3a.

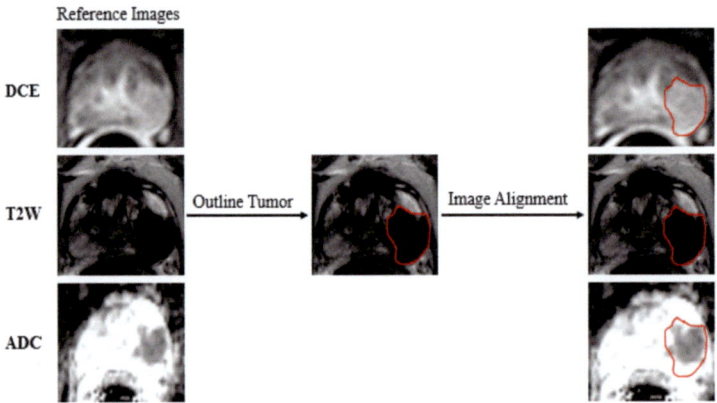

Figure 2. The protocol for tumor marking. The tumor-marking process was executed in T2W images and aligned with DCE and ADC images. T2W: T2-weighted; ADC: apparent diffusion coefficient; DCE: dynamic contrast-enhanced.

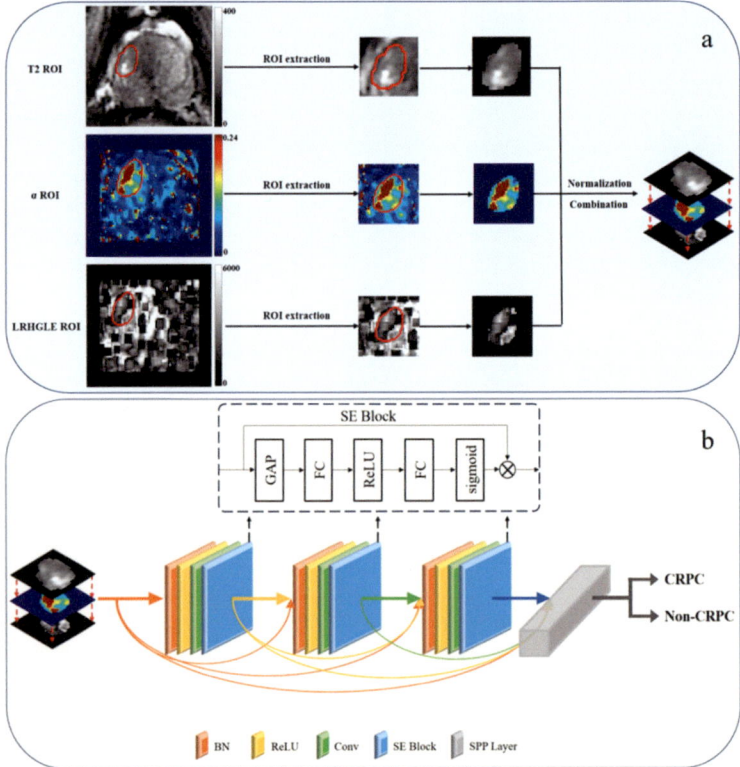

Figure 3. Data preparation process (**a**) and SE-SPP-DenseNet structure (**b**). (**a**) The preparation process included the extraction of ROIs from parametric mapping, normalization and the combination of ROIs. (**b**) The preprocessed images were input into SE-SPP-DenseNet, which uses DenseNet as the network skeleton, and the SE block and SPP layer were added to the model. ROI: region of interest; SE block: squeeze-and-excitation block; SPP layer: spatial pyramid pooling layer; BN: batch normalization; ReLU: rectified linear units; Conv: convolutional layer; GAP: global average pooling; FC: fully connected.

2.5. Deep Learning Model Construction

The deep learning models used in this study were implemented via the PyTorch 1.13.1 framework and Python 3.10 (Python Software Foundation, Fredericksburg, VA, USA) and were trained using a single workstation with an Intel Core i9-13900H processor (Intel, Santa Clara, CA, USA), an NVIDIA 4060 graphics card (NVIDIA, Santa Clara, CA, USA) and 8 GB of random-access memory.

In this study, we first constructed a pure deep learning classification model based on SE-SPP-DenseNet. The dataset was randomly divided into five equal-sized subsets. The dataset for each subset was divided into a training–validation–test set ratio of 0.8:0.1:0.1. The prediction accuracy was calculated from the average of five rounds of training and testing, which ensured the stability of the results and eliminated the effect of randomness. In each round, four subsets were utilized for the training set and one subset was allocated for the validation and testing sets. This approach was implemented once for each round until the entire cohort dataset, comprising 96 patients, was used as the testing set ($n = 50$) and validation set ($n = 46$). Data equalization and expansion were performed on the training and validation sets for both categories of patients (no data equalization or expansion were performed on the test set). The MedAugment algorithm was employed for data augmentation. This algorithm has been shown to be both efficient and effective in the context of automatic augmentation [26]. The framework used the following two transformation spaces: six pixel-level (photometric) transformations and eight spatial (geometric) transformations.

In this study, we employed the dense convolutional network (DenseNet) model, whose structure is depicted in Figure 3b [27]. The DenseNet architecture is predicated on a series of dense blocks, with each block comprising multiple convolutional layers. Each dense block receives the output of all preceding blocks, thereby establishing a dense pattern of connections between all the layers of the network. This configuration facilitates the efficient flow of information through the network. In selecting DenseNet121 as the backbone of the convolutional neural network, we considered the complexity of the data. Furthermore, in previous studies, we found that incorporating the squeeze-and-excitation block and spatial pyramid pooling layer into convolutional neural network models could markedly enhance the performance of deep learning models [28–30]. Consequently, we integrated them into the model. The structure of the squeeze-and-excitation block is illustrated in Figure 3b. The input convolutional layer was output after four operations. The squeeze-and-excitation block was applied to each convolutional block and its output was used as the input for the next convolutional block.

The pooling layer in the DenseNet output was replaced with the spatial pyramid pooling layer. The spatial pyramid pooling layer was implemented in three steps. First, the input feature maps were pooled using kernels of different sizes to obtain various output feature maps. Second, a fixed-size feature vector was obtained by merging the output feature maps of different sizes. Finally, the feature vectors were fed into the fully connected layer for classification, enabling the input of multiscale images that could then be processed and fed into a fixed-size fully connected layer. The multimodal image extracted 10,752 features following the spatial pyramid pooling layer. Notably, the images generated for this experiment were resized to 224 × 224 pixels utilizing the bilinear method for the interpolation of the images. The average size of the input ROIs was 54 × 48 pixels.

The more traditional deep residual network (ResNet)18 model and the Swin Transformer model were also used for training purposes [31–33]. The ResNet18 model is capable of capturing a greater range of features at varying depths within a dataset through the introduction of additional network layers. Concurrently, the ResNet18 model incorporates regularization to prevent gradient dispersion or explosion. The ResNet18 model was augmented with the squeeze-and-excitation block and spatial pyramid pooling layer. The squeeze-and-excitation block was employed as the output of each convolutional block and as the input of the subsequent convolutional layer. The spatial pyramid pooling layer replaced the global average pooling layer in the ResNet18 model and output the prediction results from its fully connected layer. The Swin Transformer model employs a hierarchical construction methodology and incorporates a sliding window mechanism, enabling information from multiple windows to be collected. Images undergo downsampling at 4, 8 and 16 times their original resolution as they pass through the patch partition block. This approach facilitates target classification and enables the model to process super-resolution images, focusing on both global and local information. The three-channel images were linearly transformed via the linear embedding layer in the model. The feature maps resulting from image chunking were doubled in depth and halved in width through the use of the patch merging layer.

2.6. Multimodal Fusion Artificial Intelligence Model Construction

Following the construction of a pure deep learning classification model, a multimodal fusion artificial intelligence model that used deep learning and machine learning to integrate patient image data and baseline clinical feature information is proposed in this study. Consequently, the Dense-MFAI model was constructed. Baseline clinical information (age, baseline PSA, Gleason score and clinical TNM stage) and the imaging data of each patient were input into the model. The Dense-MFAI model is shown in Figure 4. Fusion learning across two data streams is complex and involves the construction of two separate machine learning channels. One channel is employed to accept the image features predicted by the deep learning model as the input, whereas the other channel is utilized to transform the clinical feature information into a one-dimensional numerical matrix as the input. The outputs of the clinical data and image feature channels are subsequently concatenated into a matrix input into the eXtreme Gradient Boosting classifier, which can then predict whether a patient could progress to CRPC within a median time of 12 months [34]. This study employed a two-stage training approach, wherein the deep learning model was initially trained and the eXtreme Gradient Boosting model was subsequently trained for classification. The data division across the two phases was identical. The eXtreme Gradient Boosting model is an optimized distributed gradient boosting machine learning algorithm designed to solve classification and regression problems efficiently, flexibly and portably. The inputs into the image feature channel are transformed from the fully connected layer of the deep learning model. The fully connected layer acts as a classifier in a convolutional neural network, which maps the trained distributed features into the sample labeling space, which is also a one-dimensional numerical matrix. The three deep learning models in this experiment were exclusively trained on the imaging data. The clinical data were extracted directly from the data tables and subsequently used for the training of the machine learning model. Additionally, the integration of image features and clinical features was performed by label correspondence. A more detailed study of the deep learning model architectures involved in this research can be found on GitHub (https://github.com/2271371/Dense-MFAI-model.git (accessed on 26 January 2025)).

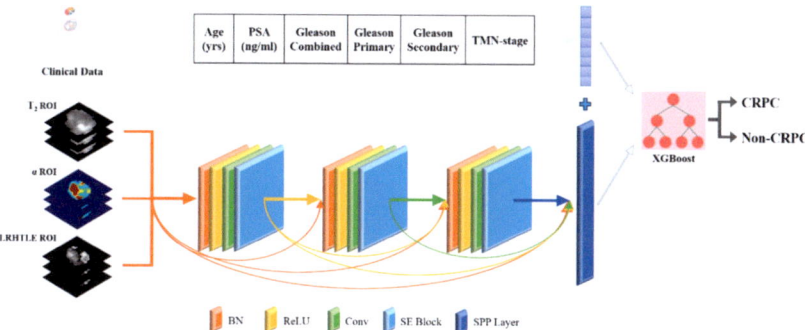

Figure 4. Dense-MFAI structure. The Dense-MFAI model comprises two components, SE-SPP-DenseNet and XGBoost. Images and clinical features are input into the multimodal fusion model and fused in the fully connected layer. PSA: prostate-specific antigen; XGBoost: eXtreme Gradient Boosting.

2.7. Quantitative Assessment Metrics

In this study, a Kaplan–Meier curve was used to illustrate the progression of CRPC in patients and comparisons between groups were made using the log-rank test. The accuracy, sensitivity, specificity, positive predictive value (PPV), negative predictive value (NPV), receiver operating characteristic (ROC) curves and confusion matrices were calculated for the purpose of predicting patient progression to CRPC within 12 months for the MFAI model described above using the test set. Additionally, the area under the curve (AUC) was calculated.

3. Results

3.1. Patient Characteristics

Following data equalization and expansion, the image data consisted of 2454 images (originally 270) for patients with CRPC and 3161 images (originally 391) for patients without CRPC. The final training set comprised approximately 4900 images per round, with 2200 images from CRPC patients and 2700 images from non-CRPC patients. The validation set comprised approximately 690 images per round, with 270 images from CRPC patients and 420 images from non-CRPC patients. The test set comprised approximately 60 images per round, with 25 images from CRPC patients and 35 images from non-CRPC patients. It is noteworthy that the delineation of all subsets and datasets was performed at the patient level.

3.2. Parameter Settings for Each Model

Following the comparison of the outcomes of a series of preliminary experiments, the specific hyperparameters of the DenseNet, ResNet18 and Swin Transformer models were established, as indicated in Table 2. The same hyperparameters were used for each model in the five rounds of training. The hyperparameters were optimized based on the changes in accuracy and loss during training and validation. The grid search method was selected for the optimization process. The parameter combinations that performed the best in the validation set were ultimately selected. During the training process, if the loss using the validation set did not decrease after 10 epochs, the learning rate was adjusted to 0.5 times the initial learning rate. During the preliminary experiments, all three deep learning models converged before 50 epochs were reached when training. Consequently, the number of epochs was fixed at 50. Furthermore, an early stopping strategy was implemented, whereby training was terminated if the loss of the validation set did not decrease within 20 epochs to prevent overfitting. The stochastic gradient descent algorithm and the binary cross-entropy loss function were selected as the network optimizer and loss function, respectively. Additionally, during the training process, image enhancement was conducted, including the reversal of the vertical orientation of the images and normalization of the images by calculating the mean and variance for each set of images. Notably, image enhancement was only applied to the training images; the images used for testing were not enhanced.

Table 2. Training parameters for the ResNet18, DenseNet and Swin Transformer models.

Parameter	Epoch	Learning Rate	Batch Size	Momentum	Weight Decay	Optimizer
ResNet18	50	0.001	48	0.9	0.0001	SGD
DenseNet	50	0.0001	48	0.9	0.0001	SGD
Swin Transformer	50	0.001	64	0.9	0.0001	SGD

SGD: stochastic gradient descent.

3.3. Predictive Performance of MFAI Models

This study proposes a multimodal fusion artificial intelligence detection framework based on deep learning and machine learning techniques to predict whether a PCa patient could progress to CRPC after 12 months of hormone therapy. This framework fused multimodal data with mpMRI parametric profiles, texture feature profiles and clinical feature information. The performance of three different MFAI models based on DenseNet, ResNet18 and the Swin Transformer was investigated. The receiver operating characteristic curves of the three models are shown in Figure 5b. The Dense-MFAI model achieved an accuracy of 94.2%, a sensitivity of 100.0%, a specificity of 82.1%, a positive predictive value of 89.6% and a negative predictive value of 100.0%. The Res-MFAI model achieved an accuracy of 92.7%, a sensitivity of 87.5%, a specificity of 96.4%, a positive predictive value of 97.5% and a negative predictive value of 84.1%. The Swin Transformer-MFAI model demonstrated an accuracy of 85.2%, a sensitivity of 87.8%, a specificity of 81.4%, a positive predictive value of 86.5% and a negative predictive value of 80.6%. The receiver operating characteristic curves of the aforementioned three models are presented in Figure 5b, where the AUCs of the Dense-MFAI, Res-MFAI and Swin Transformer-MFAI models were 0.945, 0.925 and 0.836, respectively. The confusion matrices to predict CRPC using the three models are shown in Figure 5c–e.

3.4. Effectiveness of Radiomics Feature Mapping at Predicting CRPC Progression

We also performed ablation experiments to validate the effectiveness of radiomics feature mapping at improving the prediction performance of the DenseNet, ResNet18 and Swin Transformer models. The results of the ablation experiments are shown in Table 3.

Table 3. Prediction results of a pure deep learning model for images using only mpMRI parameter mapping and after the fusion of radiomic feature mapping.

		Accuracy	Sensitivity	Specificity	PPV	NPV
SE-SPP-ResNet18	T2-ADC	76.3%	74.6%	80.3%	78.1%	75.7%
	T2-α	83.5%	80.3%	87.7%	87.3%	80.5%
	T2-ADC-α	85.2%	83.6%	87.0%	87.5%	83.6%
	T2-ADC-LRHGLE	80.4%	80.7%	86.4%	86.7%	81.8%
	T2-α-LRHGLE	90.3%	83.3%	100.0%	100.0%	81.6%

Table 3. Cont.

		Accuracy	Sensitivity	Specificity	PPV	NPV
SE-SPP-DenseNet	T2-ADC	77.6%	80.5%	75.1%	77.2%	78.5%
	T2-α	85.1%	90.4%	75.2%	80.4%	91.2%
	T2-ADC-α	87.7%	89.6%	87.8%	88.9%	88.7%
	T2-ADC-LRHGLE	83.8%	82.4%	80.7%	81.2%	81.8%
	T2-α-LRHGLE	91.2%	91.9%	87.3%	91.7%	87.8%
Swin Transformer	T2-ADC	67.9%	75.4%	54.7%	62.2%	69.3%
	T2-α	73.1%	71.4%	75.4%	75.8%	70.5%
	T2-ADC-α	75.5%	82.4%	68.7%	70.3%	76.7%
	T2-ADC-LRHGLE	71.5%	79.7%	62.7%	69.9%	74.0%
	T2-α-LRHGLE	78.9%	98.1%	51.7%	73.3%	96.8%

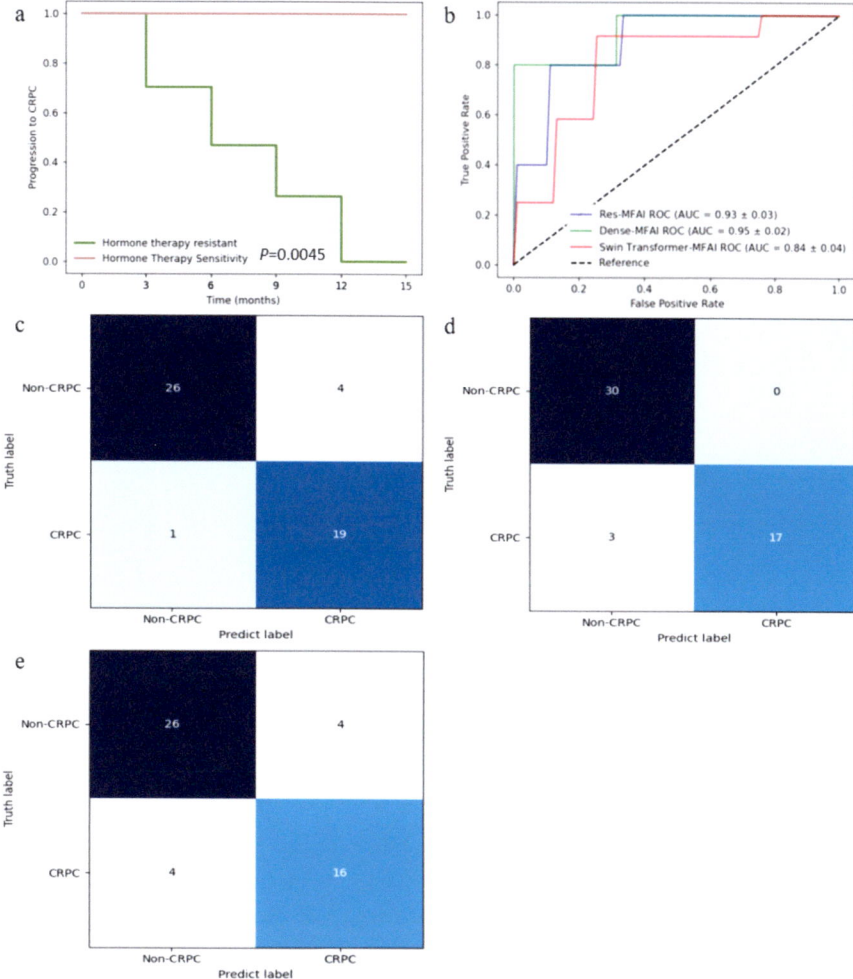

Figure 5. Performance evaluation of the MFAI models. (**a**) Kaplan–Meier curve for patients; (**b**) ROC curves for the prediction of CRPC via the Res-MFAI, Dense-MFAI and Swin Transformer-MFAI models; (**c**) confusion matrices for the Res-MFAI model; (**d**) confusion matrices for the Dense-MFAI model; (**e**) confusion matrices for the Swin Transformer-MFAI model.

3.5. Importance of Baseline Clinical Features in Predicting CRPC Progression and Validation of Visualization

Patient multimodal images fused with clinical features were used as multimodal data for training and testing. However, current studies using artificial intelligence (AI) approaches to predict patient CRPC progression have only used imaging data. To illustrate the importance of clinical features in predicting CRPC progression, we conducted experiments using the three aforementioned pure deep learning methods for training and testing.

The AUCs of the SE-SPP-DenseNet, SE-SPP-ResNet18 and Swin Transformer models were 0.906, 0.896 and 0.807, respectively. The receiver operating characteristic curves and quantitative results of the three models are shown in Table 4 and Figure 6a, respectively.

Table 4. Results of predictions using baseline clinical features, unimodal images composed of mpMRI parameter maps and multimodal images fused with baseline clinical features.

	Accuracy	Sensitivity	Specificity	PPV	NPV
Baseline Clinical Features	70.4%	87.1%	41.6%	72.5%	67.7%
SE-SPP-ResNet18	90.3%	83.3%	100.0%	100.0%	81.6%
SE-SPP-ResNet18 + MFAI	92.7%	87.5%	96.4%	97.5%	84.1%
SE-SPP-DenseNet	91.2%	91.9%	87.3%	91.7%	87.8%
SE-SPP-DenseNet + MFAI	94.2%	100.0%	82.1%	89.6%	100.0%
Swin Transformer	78.9%	98.1%	51.7%	73.3%	96.8%
Swin Transformer + MFAI	85.2%	87.8%	81.4%	86.5%	80.6%

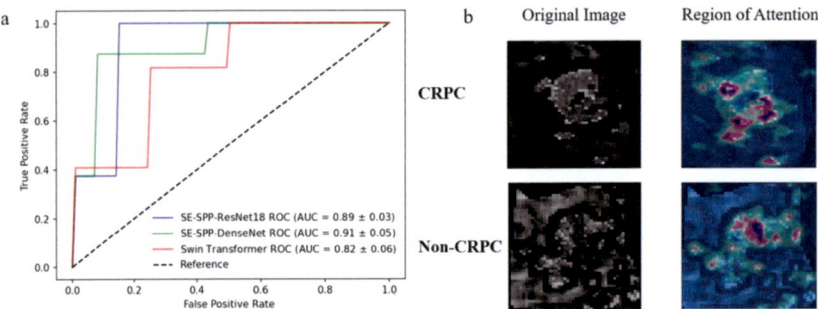

Figure 6. ROC curves and regions of attention. (**a**) ROC curves for CRPC prediction via the pure deep learning models SE-SPP-DenseNet, SE-SPP-ResNet18 and Swin Transformer; (**b**) predicted regions of attention using the SE-SPP-DenseNet model.

In addition, with regard to the validation study, the region of attention for the SE-SPP-DenseNet model, which demonstrated the optimal prediction performance, was visualized (see Figure 6b). The utilization of distinct colors indicated how much each region contributed to the model: red and yellow (warm colors) indicated that the region contributed the most to the final classification decision and the model "pays the most attention" to these locations; green indicated moderate activation and the region had some influence on the judgment but was not critical; and blue (cool colors) indicated that the region contributed little to the output and the model was not sensitive to this part of the model. It was observed that the attention region was predominantly concentrated in the inner region of the tumor, while no activation was observed in the surrounding tissues of the tumor.

4. Discussion

In this study, we developed a multimodal fusion AI model to predict whether PCa patients could progress to CRPC after 12 months of hormone therapy. To our knowledge, no previous study has used deep learning and machine learning to apply imaging profile and clinical feature fusion to predict whether PCa patients could progress to CRPC. The findings demonstrated that the Dense-MFAI model exhibited the highest accuracy (94.2%) when predicting whether patients could progress to CRPC.

As illustrated in Figure 6a and Table 4, the prediction accuracy of DenseNet exceeded that of ResNet because the DenseNet modules were interconnected with each other, leading to the collection of information included from previous modules and the integration of information from subsequent modules. In the construction of an MFAI model, the selection of the deep learning model should be contingent upon the complexity of the data. In this study, the ResNet18 and DenseNet121 models were utilized instead of a more complex model. In addition to the potential for high model complexity, resulting in overfitting, an increase in the network complexity leads to a more complex solution space, hindering the identification of the optimal solution by the optimizer.

With limited arithmetic power, the accuracy of model prediction can be enhanced by focusing the computational weights on the information of the regions that are more critical to the current classification task. Therefore, we incorporated the squeeze-and-excitation block into the model. Furthermore, the spatial pyramid pooling layer not only enabled the model to adapt to different sizes of input data but also enhanced the classification accuracy by addressing issues of object distortion and spatial layout variations through multilevel pooling [30]. Consequently, the spatial pyramid pooling layer was also incorporated into the model in this study.

In this study, we combined parametric and radiomic feature mapping and jointly output them from the fully connected layer. As illustrated in Table 3, the incorporation of radiomic feature mapping into the model input resulted in a notable enhancement in the prediction outcomes. This finding demonstrates that multimodal image inputs could provide more effective information to the model [35]. Furthermore, the ablation experiments presented in Table 3 demonstrate that the prediction accuracy decreased when α-mapping was replaced with apparent diffusion coefficient mapping. The observed decline in accuracy could be attributed to the limitations of apparent diffusion coefficient mapping, which is susceptible to higher image noise and a lower spatial resolution.

As illustrated in Figure 5 and Table 4, the Dense-MFAI model exhibited the highest accuracy rate. The improved results could be attributed to the fact that the majority of the clinical information selected for this study was based on current clinical measures to determine whether a PCa patient has progressed to CRPC, as well as the assessment metrics of the prostate cancer risk classification developed by the National Comprehensive Cancer Network. Although it is essential to consider evolving patient data over time in clinical diagnoses, experimental evidence has demonstrated that the utilization of baseline clinical information can also provide valid insights to predict the progression of a patient to CRPC to a certain extent.

Compared with existing prediction models, we utilized a distinct prediction methodology and made further enhancements. Ali et al. [36] evaluated the performance of MR image radiomics analyses for the detection of prostate cancer and constructed a robust predictive model using a sophisticated hybrid descriptive inference approach. Zhou et al. [37] extracted 2553 texture features based on mpMRI parametric mapping via radiomics, resulting in an AUC of 0.768 for the prediction of patient progression to CRPC. In our study, the Dense-MFAI model was capable of extracting and learning features directly from raw image data, in contrast to machine learning models that utilize radiomics. This approach enabled the construction of an end-to-end model. In a study by Park et al. [6], a phased long short-term memory deep learning model was used for the prediction, with a final accuracy of 88.6%. In a study by Jin and Zhang et al. [38,39], the prediction of prostate cancer bone metastasis using clinical information, mpMRI and pathology images demonstrated that multimodal data can effectively improve prediction accuracy. In a study by Zhou et al. [37], a ResNet50 deep learning model combining radiomics and pathomics was used to predict the progression of CRPC in patients, with a final AUC of 0.86. The Dense-MFAI model proposed in this study employed patient clinical information in combination with imaging data, thereby enhancing the predictive performance in this specific dataset when compared with the other two methods and their respective datasets. Jun et al. [15] identified six gene signatures to predict the risk of patient progression. However, this method was unable to accurately identify patients. Furthermore, the study by Cairone et al. [40] demonstrated that physicians can be assisted in radiomics analyses by semi-automated segmentation methods. In a subsequent study, the semi-automatic segmentation method will be employed to enhance the annotation efficiency and alleviate the workload of physicians.

Our study had several limitations. First, as we performed a retrospective study, only patient cases within a four year period were selected as experimental data, which may have resulted in biased results. Second, due to the limitation with the sample size, this work was not validated with an independent test set. In the future, an external test set will be required to validate the work robustness of the model in a multi-institutional setting. Further research with larger datasets is needed to investigate the impact of the tumor location on the model's performance and to explore how the structural information from different anatomical regions of the prostate influences quantitative imaging analyses. Third, the mpMRI equipment utilized in this study was identical, which reduced the variability of the data to some extent. Consequently, the results of this study require validation using a wider range of PCa patients and MRI from multiple vendors. Fourthly, the implementation of ROI delineation based on the sequence showing the maximum extent of cancer in this study resulted in a local volume effect. In future studies, we will perform systematic comparisons of different ROI delineation strategies (maximum, minimum or semi-automatic segmentation) to further optimize the accuracy and reproducibility of the model. Furthermore, subsequent studies could entail the ongoing development of regression models as a complement to existing classification models. This could furnish urologists with more comprehensive predictive information.

5. Conclusions

In this study, we proposed a multimodal fusion artificial intelligence model, Dense-MFAI, for the prediction of whether a PCa patient could progress to CRPC after 12 months of hormone therapy. This approach utilized the patient's mpMRI parametric profile, radiomic feature mapping and baseline clinical features. The ablation experiments demonstrated that constructing a pure deep learning model via parametric mapping and radiomics feature mapping could enhance the classification performance of the original model. Moreover, the ablation experiments demonstrated that the fusion model constructed using baseline clinical features and imaging data exhibited an enhanced prediction ability compared with the pure deep learning model. The Dense-MFAI model accurately predicted whether PCa patients could progress to CRPC after 12 months of hormone therapy, with a final accuracy of 94.2% and an AUC of 0.945. We believe that urologists can use this model to assist with diagnoses to determine the most appropriate treatment plan and prognostic measures on the basis of whether a patient could progress to CRPC.

Author Contributions: Conceptualization: D.H. and Z.Z.; data curation: J.L.; funding acquisition: D.H.; methodology: D.H. and H.Z.; software: D.H., H.Z., Y.M. and B.X.; supervision: X.F., A.C., S.Q.,

W.Q., Z.Z. and J.L.; writing—original draft: H.Z.; writing—review and editing: D.H. and X.F. All authors have read and agreed to the published version of the manuscript.

Funding: This work was partly supported by the National Natural Science Foundation of China under Grant 82001781, the Science and Technology Foundation of Liaoning Province under Grant 2023 MSBA-096 and the Fundamental Research Funds for the Central Universities under Grant N2419003.

Institutional Review Board Statement: All subjects gave their informed consent for inclusion before they participated in the study. The study was conducted in accordance with the Declaration of Helsinki and the protocol was approved by the Radiological Review Board of the First Hospital of China Medical University, Shenyang (AF-SOP-07-1, 1-01), at its meeting held on 18 November 2021, after an assessment of the procedures as well as the consent and patient information documents that the researchers provided.

Informed Consent Statement: Informed consent was obtained from all subjects involved in the study.

Data Availability Statement: Data generated or analyzed during the study are available from the corresponding author upon request.

Acknowledgments: The authors wish to thank all patients, staff and clinicians for their contributions.

Conflicts of Interest: The authors declare no conflicts of interest.

Abbreviations

PCa	Prostate cancer
CRPC	Castration-resistant prostate cancer
PSA	Prostate-specific antigen
mpMRI	Multiparametric magnetic resonance imaging
DCE-MRI	Dynamic contrast-enhanced MRI
MFAI	Multimodal fusion artificial intelligence
DWI	Diffusion-weighted imaging
ADC	Apparent diffusion coefficient
FOV	Field of view
TE	Echo time
TR	Repetition time
T2WI	T2-weighted imaging
PSE	Percentage signal enhancement
LRHGLE	Long-run high gray-level emphasis
ROI	Region of interest
SE block	Squeeze-and-excitation block
SPP layer	Spatial pyramid pooling layer
BN	Batch normalization
ReLU	Rectified linear units
Conv	Convolutional layer
GAP	Global average pooling
FC	Fully connected
DenseNet	Dense convolutional network
ResNet	Deep residual network
PPV	Positive predictive value
NPV	Negative predictive value
ROC	Receiver operating characteristic
AUC	Area under the curve
AI	Artificial intelligence

References

1. Sung, H.; Ferlay, J.; Siegel, R.L.; Laversanne, M.; Soerjomataram, I.; Jemal, A.; Bray, F. Global cancer statistics 2020: GLOBOCAN estimates of incidence and mortality worldwide for 36 cancers in 185 countries. *CA Cancer J. Clin.* **2021**, *71*, 209–249. [CrossRef]
2. Sharma, R. The burden of prostate cancer is associated with human development index: Evidence from 87 countries, 1990–2016. *EPMA J.* **2019**, *10*, 137–152. [CrossRef]
3. Khauli, R.; Ferrigno, R.; Guimarães, G.; Bulbulan, M.; Uson Junior, P.L.S.; Salvajoli, B.; Palhares, D.M.F.; Racy, D.; Gil, E.; de Arruda, F.F.; et al. Treatment of localized and locally advanced, high-risk prostate cancer: A report from the First Prostate Cancer Consensus Conference for Developing Countries. *JCO Glob. Oncol.* **2021**, *7*, 530–537. [CrossRef] [PubMed]
4. Pernigoni, N.; Zagato, E.; Calcinotto, A.; Troiani, M.; Mestre, R.P.; Calì, B.; Attanasio, G.; Troisi, J.; Minini, M.; Mosole, S.; et al. Commensal bacteria promote endocrine resistance in prostate cancer through androgen biosynthesis. *Science* **2021**, *374*, 216–224. [CrossRef] [PubMed]
5. Nagappa, A.N.; Bhatt, S.; Kanoujia, J. Studies on Structures and Functions of Kinases leading to Prostate Cancer and Their Inhibitors. *Curr. Enzym. Inhib.* **2020**, *16*, 90–105. [CrossRef]
6. Park, J.; Rho, M.J.; Moon, H.W.; Lee, J.Y. Castration-Resistant Prostate Cancer Outcome Prediction Using Phased Long Short-Term Memory with Irregularly Sampled Serial Data. *Appl. Sci.* **2020**, *10*, 2000. [CrossRef]
7. Ryan, C.J.; Smith, M.R.; Fizazi, K.; Saad, F.; Mulders, P.F.; Sternberg, C.N.; Miller, K.; Logothetis, C.J.; Shore, N.D.; Small, E.J.; et al. Abiraterone acetate plus prednisone versus placebo plus prednisone in chemotherapy-naive men with metastatic castration-resistant prostate cancer (COU-AA-302): Final overall survival analysis of a randomised, double-blind, placebo-controlled phase 3 study. *Lancet Oncol.* **2015**, *16*, 152–160. [CrossRef]
8. de Jong, A.C.; Danyi, A.; van Riet, J.; de Wit, R.; Sjöström, M.; Feng, F.; de Ridder, J.; Lolkema, M.P. Predicting response to enzalutamide and abiraterone in metastatic prostate cancer using whole-omics machine learning. *Nat. Commun.* **2023**, *14*, 196. [CrossRef]
9. Cornford, P.; Bellmunt, J.; Bolla, M.; Briers, E.; De Santis, M.; Gross, T.; Henry, A.M.; Joniau, S.; Lam, T.B.; Mason, M.D.; et al. EAU-ESTRO-SIOG guidelines on prostate cancer. Part II: Treatment of relapsing, metastatic, and castration-resistant prostate cancer. *Eur. Urol.* **2017**, *71*, 630–642. [CrossRef]
10. Cornford, P.; van den Bergh, R.C.; Briers, E.; Van den Broeck, T.; Cumberbatch, M.G.; De Santis, M.; Fanti, S.; Fossati, N.; Gandaglia, G.; Gillessen, S.; et al. EAU-EANM-ESTRO-ESUR-SIOG guidelines on prostate cancer. Part II—2020 update: Treatment of relapsing and metastatic prostate cancer. *Eur. Urol.* **2021**, *79*, 263–282. [CrossRef]
11. Roest, C.; Kwee, T.C.; de Jong, I.J.; Schoots, I.G.; van Leeuwen, P.; Heijmink, S.W.; van der Poel, H.G.; Fransen, S.J.; Saha, A.; Huisman, H.; et al. Development and Validation of a Deep Learning Model Based on MRI and Clinical Characteristics to Predict Risk of Prostate Cancer Progression. *Radiol. Imaging Cancer* **2025**, *7*, e240078. [CrossRef] [PubMed]
12. Scher, H.; Armstrong, A.; Schonhoft, J.; Gill, A.; Zhao, J.; Barnett, E.; Carbone, E.; Lu, J.; Antonarakis, E.; Luo, J.; et al. Development and validation of circulating tumour cell enumeration (Epic Sciences) as a prognostic biomarker in men with metastatic castration-resistant prostate cancer. *Eur. J. Cancer* **2021**, *150*, 83–94. [CrossRef] [PubMed]
13. Jeong, S.-H.; Kyung, D.; Yuk, H.D.; Jeong, C.W.; Lee, W.; Yoon, J.-K.; Kim, H.-P.; Bang, D.; Kim, T.-Y.; Lim, Y.; et al. Practical Utility of Liquid Biopsies for Evaluating Genomic Alterations in Castration-Resistant Prostate Cancer. *Cancers* **2023**, *15*, 2847. [CrossRef] [PubMed]
14. McGrath, S.; Christidis, D.; Perera, M.; Hong, S.K.; Manning, T.; Vela, I.; Lawrentschuk, N. Prostate cancer biomarkers: Are we hitting the mark? *Prostate Int.* **2016**, *4*, 130–135. [CrossRef]
15. A, J.; Zhang, B.; Zhang, Z.; Hu, H.; Dong, J.-T. Novel Gene Signatures Predictive of Patient Recurrence-Free Survival and Castration Resistance in Prostate Cancer. *Cancers* **2021**, *13*, 917. [CrossRef]
16. Turkbey, B.; Rosenkrantz, A.B.; Haider, M.A.; Padhani, A.R.; Villeirs, G.; Macura, K.J.; Tempany, C.M.; Choyke, P.L.; Cornud, F.; Margolis, D.J.; et al. Prostate imaging reporting and data system version 2.1: 2019 update of prostate imaging reporting and data system version 2. *Eur. Urol.* **2019**, *76*, 340–351. [CrossRef]
17. Hara, N.; Okuizumi, M.; Koike, H.; Kawaguchi, M.; Bilim, V. Dynamic contrast-enhanced magnetic resonance imaging (DCE-MRI) is a useful modality for the precise detection and staging of early prostate cancer. *Prostate* **2005**, *62*, 140–147. [CrossRef]
18. Lambin, P.; Leijenaar, R.T.; Deist, T.M.; Peerlings, J.; De Jong, E.E.; Van Timmeren, J.; Sanduleanu, S.; Larue, R.T.; Even, A.; Jochems, A.; et al. Radiomics: The bridge between medical imaging and personalized medicine. *Nat. Rev. Clin. Oncol.* **2017**, *14*, 749–762. [CrossRef]
19. Liberini, V.; Laudicella, R.; Balma, M.; Nicolotti, D.G.; Buschiazzo, A.; Grimaldi, S.; Lorenzon, L.; Bianchi, A.; Peano, S.; Bartolotta, T.V.; et al. Radiomics and artificial intelligence in prostate cancer: New tools for molecular hybrid imaging and theragnostics. *Eur. Radiol. Exp.* **2022**, *6*, 27. [CrossRef]
20. Esteva, A.; Feng, J.; van der Wal, D.; Huang, S.-C.; Simko, J.P.; DeVries, S.; Chen, E.; Schaeffer, E.M.; Morgan, T.M.; Sun, Y.; et al. Prostate cancer therapy personalization via multi-modal deep learning on randomized phase III clinical trials. *npj Digit. Med.* **2022**, *5*, 71. [CrossRef]

1. Chatterjee, A.; He, D.; Fan, X.; Antic, T.; Jiang, Y.; Eggener, S.; Karczmar, G.S.; Oto, A. Diagnosis of prostate cancer by use of MRI-derived quantitative risk maps: A feasibility study. *Am. J. Roentgenol.* **2019**, *213*, W66–W75. [CrossRef] [PubMed]
2. Ma, Y.; He, D. Multiparametric MRI-based artificial intelligence analysis to predict hormone therapy effectiveness for prostate cancer: A clustering-driven ensemble-learning approach. In Proceedings of the China Biomedical Engineering Conference & Innovative Healthcare Summit, Shenzhen, China, 20–22 September 2024; p. 2825.
3. Sun, C.; Chatterjee, A.; Yousuf, A.; Antic, T.; Eggener, S.; Karczmar, G.S.; Oto, A. Comparison of T2-weighted imaging, DWI, and dynamic contrast-enhanced MRI for calculation of prostate cancer index lesion volume: Correlation with whole-mount pathology. *Am. J. Roentgenol.* **2019**, *212*, 351–356. [CrossRef] [PubMed]
4. Heerkens, H.; Hall, W.; Li, X.; Knechtges, P.; Dalah, E.; Paulson, E.; van den Berg, C.; Meijer, G.; Koay, E.; Crane, C.; et al. Recommendations for MRI-based contouring of gross tumor volume and organs at risk for radiation therapy of pancreatic cancer. *Pract. Radiat. Oncol.* **2017**, *7*, 126–136.
5. Dalah, E.; Moraru, I.; Paulson, E.; Erickson, B.; Li, X.A. Variability of target and normal structure delineation using multimodality imaging for radiation therapy of pancreatic cancer. *Int. J. Radiat. Oncol. Biol. Phys.* **2014**, *89*, 633–640. [CrossRef]
6. Liu, Z.; Lv, Q.; Li, Y.; Yang, Z.; Shen, L. Medaugment: Universal Automatic Data Augmentation Plug-in for Medical Image Analysis. *arXiv* **2023**, arXiv:2306.17466.
7. Huang, G.; Liu, Z.; Van Der Maaten, L.; Weinberger, K.Q. Densely connected convolutional networks. In Proceedings of the IEEE Conference on Computer Vision and Pattern Recognition, Honolulu, HI, USA, 21–26 July 2017; pp. 4700–4708.
8. Zhuang, H.; Li, B.; Ma, J.; Monkam, P.; Qian, W.; He, D. An attention-based deep learning network for predicting Platinum resistance in ovarian cancer. *IEEE Access* **2024**, *12*, 41000–41008. [CrossRef]
9. Hu, J.; Shen, L.; Sun, G. Squeeze-and-excitation networks. In Proceedings of the IEEE Conference on Computer Vision and Pattern Recognition, Salt Lake City, UT, USA, 18–23 June 2018; pp. 7132–7141.
10. He, K.; Zhang, X.; Ren, S.; Sun, J. Spatial pyramid pooling in deep convolutional networks for visual recognition. *IEEE Trans. Pattern Anal. Mach. Intell.* **2015**, *37*, 1904–1916. [CrossRef]
11. He, K.; Zhang, X.; Ren, S.; Sun, J. Deep residual learning for image recognition. In Proceedings of the IEEE Conference on Computer Vision and Pattern Recognition, Las Vegas, NV, USA, 27–30 June 2016; pp. 770–778.
12. Liu, Z.; Lin, Y.; Cao, Y.; Hu, H.; Wei, Y.; Zhang, Z.; Lin, S.; Guo, B. Swin transformer: Hierarchical vision transformer using shifted windows. In Proceedings of the IEEE/CVF International Conference on Computer Vision, Montreal, QC, Canada, 10–17 October 2021; pp. 10012–10022.
13. Xu, X.; Feng, Z.; Cao, C.; Li, M.; Wu, J.; Wu, Z.; Shang, Y.; Ye, S. An improved swin transformer-based model for remote sensing object detection and instance segmentation. *Remote Sens.* **2021**, *13*, 4779. [CrossRef]
14. Chen, T.; Guestrin, C. Xgboost: A scalable tree boosting system. In Proceedings of the 22nd Acm Sigkdd International Conference on Knowledge Discovery and Data Mining, San Francisco, CA, USA, 13–17 August 2016; pp. 785–794.
15. Zheng, X.; Yao, Z.; Huang, Y.; Yu, Y.; Wang, Y.; Liu, Y.; Mao, R.; Li, F.; Xiao, Y.; Wang, Y.; et al. Deep learning radiomics can predict axillary lymph node status in early-stage breast cancer. *Nat. Commun.* **2020**, *11*, 1236. [CrossRef]
16. Ali, M.; Benfante, V.; Cutaia, G.; Salvaggio, L.; Rubino, S.; Portoghese, M.; Ferraro, M.; Corso, R.; Piraino, G.; Ingrassia, T.; et al. Prostate Cancer Detection: Performance of Radiomics Analysis in Multiparametric MRI. In *Image Analysis and Processing-ICIAP 2023 Workshops*; Springer: Berlin/Heidelberg, Germany, 2023; pp. 83–92.
17. Zhou, C.; Zhang, Y.-F.; Guo, S.; Huang, Y.-Q.; Qiao, X.-N.; Wang, R.; Zhao, L.-P.; Chang, D.-H.; Zhao, L.-M.; Da, M.-X.; et al. Multimodal data integration for predicting progression risk in castration-resistant prostate cancer using deep learning: A multicenter retrospective study. *Front. Oncol.* **2024**, *14*, 1287995. [CrossRef]
18. Jin, T.; An, J.; Wu, W.; Zhou, F. Development and validation of a machine learning model for bone metastasis in prostate cancer: Based on inflammatory and nutritional indicators. *Urology* **2024**, *190*, 63–70. [CrossRef] [PubMed]
19. Zhang, Y.-F.; Zhou, C.; Guo, S.; Wang, C.; Yang, J.; Yang, Z.-J.; Wang, R.; Zhang, X.; Zhou, F.-H. Deep learning algorithm-based multimodal MRI radiomics and pathomics data improve prediction of bone metastases in primary prostate cancer. *J. Cancer Res. Clin. Oncol.* **2024**, *150*, 78. [CrossRef] [PubMed]
20. Cairone, L.; Benfante, V.; Bignardi, S.; Marinozzi, F.; Yezzi, A.; Tuttolomondo, A.; Salvaggio, G.; Bini, F.; Comelli, A. Robustness of radiomics features to varying segmentation algorithms in magnetic resonance images. In *Image Analysis and Processing-ICIAP 2023 Workshops*; Springer: Berlin/Heidelberg, Germany, 2022; pp. 462–472.

Disclaimer/Publisher's Note: The statements, opinions and data contained in all publications are solely those of the individual author(s) and contributor(s) and not of MDPI and/or the editor(s). MDPI and/or the editor(s) disclaim responsibility for any injury to people or property resulting from any ideas, methods, instructions or products referred to in the content.

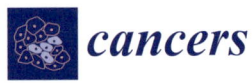

Article

Development and Validation of an Explainable Radiomics Model to Predict High-Aggressive Prostate Cancer: A Multicenter Radiomics Study Based on Biparametric MRI

Giulia Nicoletti [1,2], Simone Mazzetti [3], Giovanni Maimone [3], Valentina Cignini [2], Renato Cuocolo [4], Riccardo Faletti [2], Marco Gatti [2], Massimo Imbriaco [5], Nicola Longo [6], Andrea Ponsiglione [5], Filippo Russo [3], Alessandro Serafini [2], Arnaldo Stanzione [5], Daniele Regge [3,7] and Valentina Giannini [2,3,*]

[1] Department of Electronics and Telecommunications, Polytechnic of Turin, Corso Duca degli Abruzzi, 24, 10129 Turin, Italy; giulia.nicoletti@polito.it

[2] Department of Surgical Sciences, University of Turin, Corso Dogliotti, 14, 10126 Turin, Italy; valentina.cignini@unito.it (V.C.); riccardo.faletti@unito.it (R.F.); alessandro.serafini@unito.it (A.S.)

[3] Radiology Unit, Candiolo Cancer Institute, FPO-IRCCS, Strada Provinciale, 142—KM 3.95, 10060 Candiolo, Italy; simone.mazzetti@ircc.it (S.M.); giovanni.maimone@unito.it (G.M.); filippo.russo@ircc.it (F.R.); daniele.regge@ircc.it (D.R.)

[4] Department of Medicine, Surgery, and Dentistry, University of Salerno, Via Salvador Allende, 43, 84081 Baronissi, Italy; rcuocolo@unisa.it

[5] Department of Advanced Biomedical Sciences, University of Naples "Federico II", Via Pansini, 5, 80131 Naples, Italy; massimo.imbriaco@unina.it (M.I.); a.ponsiglionemd@gmail.com (A.P.)

[6] Department of Neurosciences, Reproductive Sciences and Odontostomatology, University of Naples "Federico II", Via Pansini, 5, 80131 Naples, Italy; nicola.longo@unina.it

[7] Department of Translational Research, Via Risorgimento, 36, University of Pisa, 56126 Pisa, Italy

* Correspondence: valentina.giannini@unito.it

Simple Summary: Prostate cancer (PCa) is one of the leading causes of mortality for men worldwide. PCa aggressiveness affects the patient's prognosis, with less aggressive tumors, i.e., Grade Group (GG) 1 and 2, having lower mortality and better outcomes. For this reason, the aim of this study is to distinguish between GG ≤ 2 and ≥ 3 PCa using an automatic and noninvasive approach based on artificial intelligence methods. The results obtained are promising, as the system achieved robust results on a multicenter external dataset. If further validated, this approach, combined with the expert knowledge of urologists, could help identify PCa patients who have a better prognosis and may benefit from less invasive treatments.

Abstract: In the last years, several studies demonstrated that low-aggressive (Grade Group (GG) ≤ 2) and high-aggressive (GG ≥ 3) prostate cancers (PCas) have different prognoses and mortality. Therefore, the aim of this study was to develop and externally validate a radiomic model to noninvasively classify low-aggressive and high-aggressive PCas based on biparametric magnetic resonance imaging (bpMRI). To this end, 283 patients were retrospectively enrolled from four centers. Features were extracted from apparent diffusion coefficient (ADC) maps and T2-weighted (T2w) sequences. A cross-validation (CV) strategy was adopted to assess the robustness of several classifiers using two out of the four centers. Then, the best classifier was externally validated using the other two centers. An explanation for the final radiomics signature was provided through Shapley additive explanation (SHAP) values and partial dependence plots (PDP). The best combination was a naïve Bayes classifier trained with ten features that reached promising results, i.e., an area under the receiver operating characteristic (ROC) curve (AUC) of 0.75 and 0.73 in the construction and external validation set, respectively. The findings of our work suggest that our radiomics model could help distinguish between low- and high-aggressive PCa. This noninvasive approach, if further validated and integrated into a clinical decision support system able to automatically detect PCa, could help clinicians managing men with suspicion of PCa.

Keywords: radiomics; prostate cancer; magnetic resonance imaging; feature extraction; explainable artificial intelligence; tumor aggressiveness

1. Introduction

Prostate cancer (PCa) is the most common cancer in men in Western countries, accounting for about 25% of new cancer diagnoses [1,2]. Since 2020, the European Association of Urology added a strong recommendation to perform multiparametric magnetic resonance imaging (mpMRI) in PCa patients before either planning a re-biopsy or in biopsy-naïve men [3] to better identify PCa suspicion and to target the biopsy to retrieve more precise information about cancer aggressiveness [4]. However, biopsies are known to suffer from limitations that negatively impact the therapeutic path and patients' outcomes [5]. Indeed, they are known to be invasive, affected by large inter-observer variability, and not able to provide information on spatial tumor heterogeneity [6,7].

In the last years, radiomics analysis to characterize PCa has been demonstrated as a potential alternative to overcome the main biopsy drawbacks [8,9]. The radiomics approach is challenging, and researchers have mainly focused on the identification of clinically significant ones (GG $\geq$ 2) [10], reaching considerably high performances [11]. However, a more precise separation between GG2 and GG3 is necessary since GG3 PCas show more aggressive behavior, with higher rates of biochemical failure, systemic recurrence, cancer-specific death [12–14], and lower probability of 5-year biochemical risk-free survival [4]. Only a few studies have classified GG $\leq$ 2 and GG $\geq$ 3 PCas [15–18] through radiomics analyses, but the generalization of their results has not been fully addressed yet. Moreover, these studies did not adopt an explainable approach [15–18]. A not-explained approach limits transparency, trustworthiness, and, therefore, application in real-world clinical practice [19]. To our knowledge, there is no study validating a machine learning classifier to predict GG $\leq$ 2 and GG $\geq$ 3 PCas on an external validation set and proposing an explainable AI approach.

The aims of this study are to develop a model to noninvasively distinguish between GG $\leq$ 2 and GG $\geq$ 3 PCa through a radiomics signature based on bpMRI and to validate this model on a multicenter dataset composed of images acquired with different MRI manufacturers, including both 1.5T and 3T scanners, also providing an explanation for the signature. The proposed pipeline is noninvasive, as it uses already available acquisitions from MRI without endorectal coil and contrast agent administration. Our model showed robust results on the external validation set, suggesting that, if further validated, it could be used as a noninvasive tool to select low-aggressive PCas, which, if confirmed by additional clinical evaluations, could avoid destructive and invasive treatments.

2. Materials and Methods

2.1. Patients

This is a multicenter retrospective study that includes four institutes: University Hospital "Città della Salute e della Scienza" of Turin (center A), "Mauriziano Umberto I" Hospital of Turin (center B), Candiolo Cancer Institute (center C), and Federico II Hospital of Naples (center D). Patients who underwent prostate MRI between November 2015 and October 2018 at sites A, B, and D and between May 2017 and February 2020 at site C were included in the study. The following inclusion criteria were applied: (1) patients with suspicion of PCa; (2) patients who underwent MRI examination before biopsy, including at least diffusion-weighted (DWI) and T2-weighted (T2w) axial images; and (3) imaging performed without endorectal coil. Exclusion criteria were as follows: (1) the presence of strong artifacts on the MRI examination; (2) patients who underwent transurethral resection of the prostate (TURP); (3) no match between the tumor location detected by the biopsy and the MRI's findings; and (4) absence of pathologically confirmed (either biopsy or prostatectomy) PCa.

2.2. MRI Acquisition and Reference Standard

MRI examinations were performed using 1.5T scanners at centers A, B, and C (Achieva Philips Medical Systems, Ingenia Philips Medical Systems, and Optimae GE Healthcare, respectively) and a 3T scanner at center D (Magnetom Trio Siemens Medical Solutions). The reference standard for this study was the GG obtained after targeted biopsy or prostatectomy, when available, on the lesions detected on MRI. More information on scanner parameters can be found in Supplementary Section S1. For patients with available prostatectomy results, the exact location of the tumor was found by comparing the MRI with the microscopic slices of the surgical specimen [19]. When the results of the prostatectomy were not available, the tumor was localized on MRI using the detailed report provided by uropathologists [20]. Dedicated uropathologists examined the hematoxylin- and eosin-stained slides and recorded the GG. Finally, PCas were dichotomized into low-(GG $\leq$ 2) and high-(GG $\geq$ 3) aggressive cancers, hereafter considered as the negative and positive class, respectively.

2.3. Tumor Segmentation and Feature Extraction

Four radiologists (one for each of the recruiting centers) with more than 5 years of experience manually segmented on T2w imaging all PCas using ITK Snap 3.8 [21] (www.itksnap.org, accessed on 29 December 2023), and the available contouring or report provided by uropathologists as a reference, as previously described in [22]. During the segmentation step, the radiologist checked that the mask of the tumor also matched the tumor on the ADC maps, and in case of misalignment, they reviewed the mask to segment only the common areas, as previously reported [22]. Then, an experienced senior radiologist reviewed and eventually corrected all the segmentations from the four centers. After a step of image preprocessing where both T2w sequences and ADC maps were normalized and pixels showing outlier signal intensities were removed, 169 first and second-order features were extracted (more details are available in Supplementary Section S2). Features were extracted in Python 3.8 using the open-source Python package Pyradiomics 3.0.1 [23], compliant with the Image Biomarker Standardization Initiative [24]. Figure 1A reports the main steps from image acquisition to feature extraction.

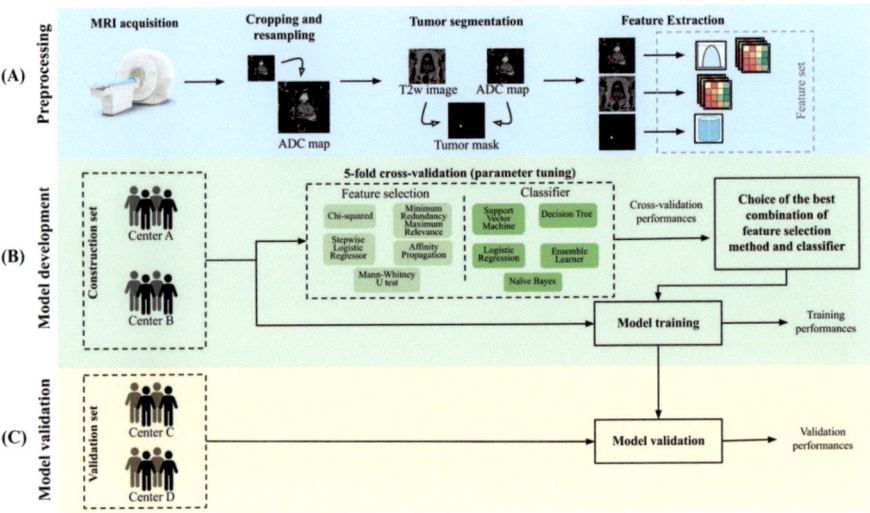

Figure 1. Pipeline of the study including (**A**) preprocessing, (**B**) model development, and (**C**) validation steps. ADC = apparent diffusion coefficient, T2w = T2-weighted, MRI = magnetic resonance imaging.

2.4. Model Development and Validation

During the development of the radiomics signature, 26 combinations of feature selection (FS) methods and classifiers/regressors were fine-tuned using only patients from centers A and B (construction dataset). Specifically, the feature selection methods included (1) minimum redundancy maximum relevance, (2) affinity propagation, feature ranking based on (3) chi-squared test or (4) Mann–Whitney U test, and (5) stepwise binomial logistic regressor. These 5 FS methods were combined with the following classifiers/regressors: (1) decision tree, (2) support vector machine, (3) ensemble learner (e.g., random forest), (4) naïve Bayes, and (5) binomial logistic regression. In addition, we evaluated the LASSO logistic regressor. Before performing the FS step, all features were normalized between 0 and 1 using the min-max scaling. The radiomics pipeline is reported in Figure 1. All algorithms were implemented in MATLAB® 2021b.

To select the best-performing model, a cross-validation (CV) strategy has been adopted, in which 4 folds (training a stratified 5-fold cross-set) were iteratively used to train a model that was subsequently tested on the left-out fold (test set). During the CV, all the combinations of FS and classifiers were evaluated. The parameters of the models were tuned, and models not reaching a mean area under the receiver operating characteristic (ROC) curve (AUC) ≥ 0.6 on the left-out folds were discarded. More details about the FS methods and classifiers are described in Supplementary Section S3.

Once all the FS/classifier/parameters combinations were tested, the one reaching the highest mean AUC on the left-out folds was selected and re-trained using the whole construction set (Figure 1B).

The validation step was performed by applying the previously selected model on the validation set, which included only patients that were left out from the model development phase, i.e., from centers C and D (Figure 1C). We decided to use centers A and B as the construction set to develop the model on a strong reference standard since all their patients had the prostatectomy results available and to train a model on 1.5T MRI images and evaluate its generalization capability on both 1.5T and 3T (center D) MRI images. The validation set was normalized using the min-max scaling, with the maximum and minimum values of the construction set.

2.5. Statistical Analysis

Correlation between all pairs of features employed in the best model was computed using Spearman's correlation test (MATLAB® 2022b). Balanced accuracy, sensitivity, specificity, positive predictive value (PPV), and negative predictive value (NPV) obtained using the cut-off corresponding to the Youden Index on the construction set were computed as an example of general model performances. Sensitivity was defined as the number of correctly classified high-aggressive PCas over the total number of high-aggressive PCas; specificity was defined as the number of correctly classified low-aggressive PCas over the total number of low-aggressive PCas; NPV was defined as the number of correctly classified low-aggressive PCas over the total number of patients classified as low-aggressive PCas; and PPV was defined as the number of correctly classified high-aggressive PCas over the total number of patients classified as high-aggressive PCas.

For the 5-fold CV, the difference in the mean of the six performance indexes between train and test sets was calculated to evaluate the robustness of the models and exclude those combinations that tend to overfit. Since in the literature, there is no commonly accepted criterion to identify overfitting models, in this analysis, a decrease in performances from the training set to the test set greater than 30% was considered overfitting. For the final classifier, changes in the performances obtained between the construction set and the validation set and between centers C and D were evaluated using the N−1 chi-squared test performed for each of the performance metrics, while AUCs were compared based on the DeLong test. A *p*-value < 0.05 was considered statistically significant. All the statistical analyses were computed on MedCalc Statistical Software version 20.105 (MedCalc Software bv, Ostend, Belgium).

2.6. Explanation of the Classification Model

To better understand the signature of the final radiomics model and the role of the selected features in the classification task, Shapley additive explanation (SHAP) values were computed for the external validation set. The SHAP values of a feature explain the role of that feature in "pushing" the model output toward positive or negative predictions [25]. Then, the feature importance was calculated as the average of the absolute SHAP values per feature across the external validation set. In addition to features explanation, we provided a global interpretation of the signature by computing the partial dependence plot (PDP) of each feature employed in the model. The PDP displays the marginal effect that a feature has on the predicted outcome, showing whether the relationship between the output and that feature is linear or more complex (see also Supplementary Section S4).

3. Results

3.1. Patient Characteristics

The multicenter dataset included a total of 299 PCas from 283 patients. The construction set included 175 PCas (132 from A and 43 from B, 77 low- and 98 high-aggressive), while the validation set was composed of 124 PCas (78 from C and 46 from D, 69 low- and 55 high-aggressive). More details are described in Figure 2. GG was derived from prostatectomy in 86% (243/283) of patients, while in the remaining patients, we used the GG provided by targeted biopsy. The review of the segmentations performed by the expert senior radiologist resulted in less than 10% of changes in the tumor masks provided by the four centers.

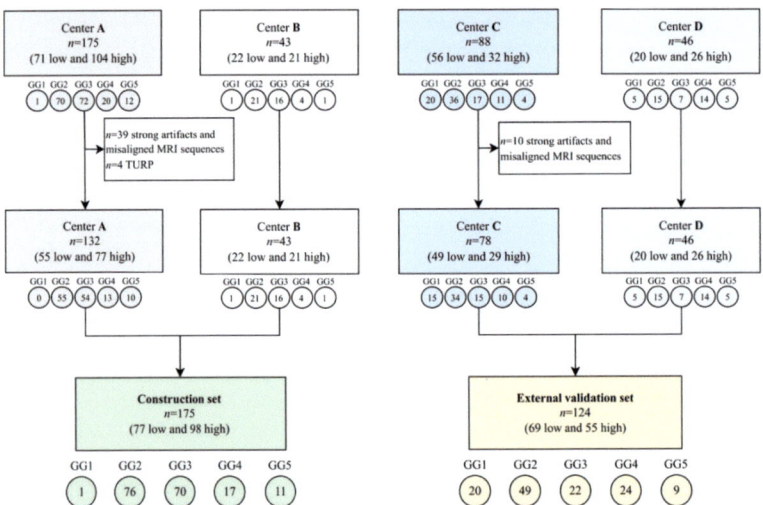

Figure 2. Flowchart of dataset division. In each box: N is the total number of PCas; in parentheses are reported the number of low-and high-aggressive PCas. Under each box: the number of lesions for each of the 5 GGs is reported in the circles. GG = grade group, MRI = magnetic resonance imaging, TURP = transurethral resection of the prostate.

3.2. Best Model

The naïve Bayes classifier trained using ten features selected by the affinity propagation algorithm was chosen as the best model based on its AUC of the left-out folder (Section 2.4) (see Supplementary Sections S5 and S6 for more details). The Spearman correlation coefficient (r) for the different combinations of the ten selected features showed a fair correlation ($r \leq 0.50$) [26] for 40/45 pairs and a moderate correlation ($0.50 < r \leq 0.70$) only in 5/45 pair comparisons. No highly correlated features, i.e., higher than 0.70, were found in the selected subset. The results of the final classifier trained with all patients enrolled from centers A and B and then externally validated with the cases from centers C and D are reported in Table 1. On the validation set, the classifier achieved results comparable to those obtained on the construction set, i.e., AUC of 0.75 and 0.73, respectively. No significant differences were found in the performance metrics between the construction and external validation sets (Table 1). In the comparison of the performances between centers C and D, only specificity was significantly lower in center D (p-value < 0.05) (Table 1). Figure 3 shows the discrete non-smoothed ROC curves of the construction and validation set. For completeness and transparency of reports of the diagnostic accuracy of this study, we reported the Standards for Reporting of Diagnostic Accuracy Studies (STARD) diagram [27] in Supplementary Section S7. The waterfall plots of the output signature of the classifier for the construction and validation sets are displayed in Figure 3. As we can see, the classifier is highly accurate when assigning a likelihood of a high-aggressive tumor equal to zero (<1%). Indeed, 11 out of 15 lesions of the training set (Figure 4A) and all 15 lesions of the validation set (Figure 4B) with assigned likelihood equal to zero are true low-aggressive PCas.

Table 1. Performances of the best model and results of the N−1 chi-squared test for the comparison of two proportions and of the DeLong test for the comparison of AUCs. Numbers in brackets represent the number of correctly classified cases over the total number of each class. Specifically, the resulting p-value, performances, and their differences are reported for centers A + B (construction set) and centers C + D (validation set) and individually for center C and center D. In bold, p-value < 0.05.

	Construction Set (Sample 1) vs. Validation Set (Sample 2)						Center C (Sample 1) vs. Center D (Sample 2)					
	AUC (95%CI)	Balanced Accuracy (%)	Sensitivity (%) (95%CI)	Specificity (%) (95%CI)	PPV (%) (95%CI)	NPV (%) (95%CI)	AUC (95%CI)	Balanced Accuracy (%)	Sensitivity (%) (95%CI)	Specificity (%) (95%CI)	PPV (%) (95%CI)	NPV (%) (95%CI)
Sample 1	0.75 (0.68–0.81)	72.2	70.4 [69/98] (60.3–79.2)	74.0 [57/77] (62.8–83.4)	77.5 [69/89] (69.8–83.7)	66.3 [57/86] (58.5–73.3)	0.77 (0.67–0.86)	69.4	55.2 [16/29] (35.7–73.5)	83.7 [41/49] (70.3–92.7)	66.7 [16/24] (49.5–80.3)	75.9 [41/54] (67.4–82.8)
Sample 2	0.73 (0.65–0.81)	67.9	61.8 [34/55] (47.7–74.6)	73.9 [51/69] (61.9–83.7)	65.4 [34/52] (54.7–74.7)	70.8 [51/72] (62.8–77.7)	0.63 (0.56–0.77)	59.6	69.2 [18/26] (48.2–85.7)	50.0 [10/20] (27.2–72.8)	64.3 [18/28] (52.0–74.9)	55.6 [10/18] (37.7–72.1)
p-value	0.731	0.423	0.278	0.989	0.120	0.546	0.143	0.274	0.290	**0.004**	0.857	0.103
|Diff| (95% CI)	0.02 (−0.1–0.1)	4.3 (−6.0–14.9)	8.6 (−6.5–24.1)	0.1 (−13.9–14.3)	12.1 (−2.9–27.6)	4.5 (−10.0–18.5)	0.15 (−0.1–0.3)	9.8 (−7.3–26.9)	14.0 (−11.3–36.7)	33.7 (9.95–55.2)	2.4 (−22.6–26.4)	20.3 (−3.4–44.1)

AUC = area under the receiver operating characteristic curve, CI = confidence interval, Diff = difference, PPV = positive predictive value, NPV = negative predictive value.

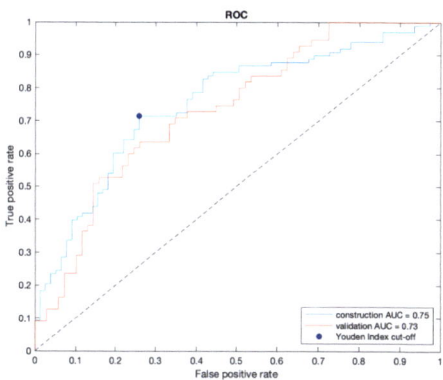

Figure 3. Receiver operating characteristic (ROC) curve of construction (blue) and validation set (red). The blue point corresponds to the cut-off based on the Youden Index. AUC = area under the ROC curve.

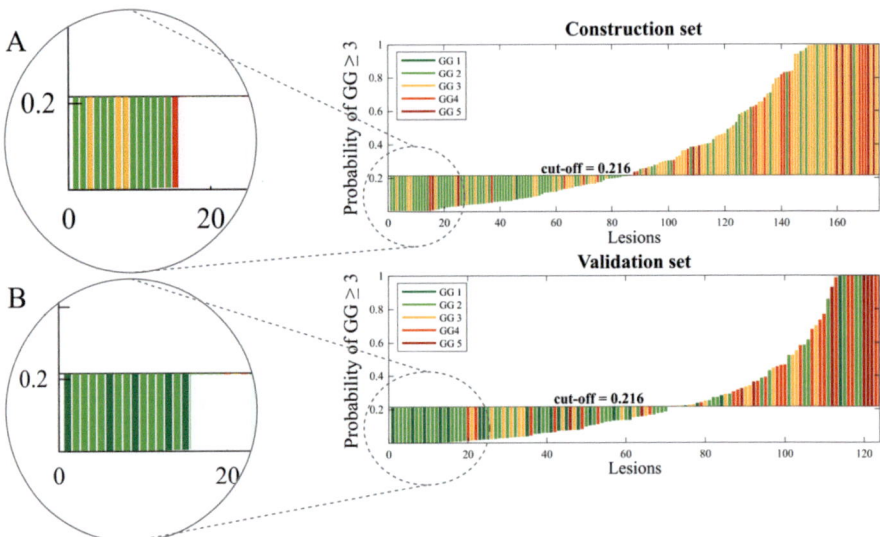

Figure 4. Waterfall plot of the output probabilities of the final classifier for construction set and validation set. The circles (**A**,**B**) highlight the lesions with zero likelihood of being high-aggressive. GG = grade group.

3.3. Explanation of the Best Model

Figure 5 displays the bar diagram reporting features in decreasing order of importance. The 'ADC-GLRLM- Run Length Non-Uniformity' was the most important feature, changing the predicted high-aggressive PCa probability, on average, by 14.5 percentage points, followed by the 'ADC-GLRLM- Run entropy' changing the prediction, on average, by 7.2 percentage points. The SHAP summary plot is reported in Figure 6, displaying on the y-axis all features of the NB classifier ordered by importance and on the x-axis their corresponding SHAP values, with color representing the value assumed by the feature, from low (red) to high (blue). It can be seen how the highest absolute SHAP values of the first most important feature were positive, meaning that the feature contributed more to the high-aggressive PCa predictions than to the low-aggressive ones. Vice versa, the second most important feature is characterized mainly by negative SHAP values, highlighting that it mainly contributed to the low-aggressive PCa predictions. Interestingly, low values of 'ADC-GLRLM- Run entropy' reduce the predicted high-aggressive PCa risk. In Figure 7, a local visualization of the SHAP values of a true positive and true negative prediction randomly selected from the external validation set is shown. As a corroboration of what has been deduced from the SHAP summary plot, the local visualization shows how, in the case of a true positive prediction (Figure 7a), the most important feature in Figure 5 has the highest SHAP value (0.434), thus highlighting its relevant contribution to that final prediction of a high-aggressive PCa. Similarly, for the true negative prediction example (Figure 7b), the second most important feature contributed far more than the others to the final classification, decreasing the predicted high-aggressive PCa probability of 24 percentage points, thus pushing the predictions toward the low-aggressive class.

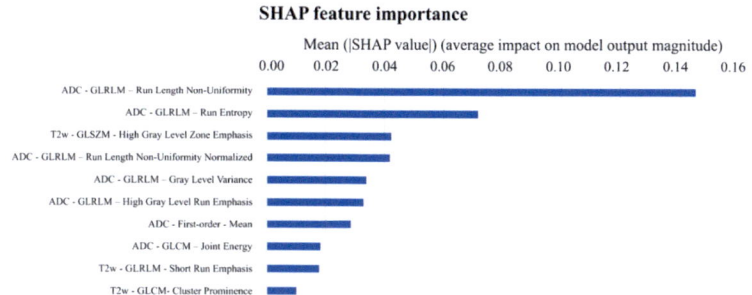

Figure 5. Ten features employed in the model ranked by their impact on model output. ADC = apparent diffusion coefficient, GLCM = grey-level co-occurrence matrix, GLRLM = grey-level run length matrix, GLSZM = grey-level size zone matrix, SHAP = Shapley additive explanation, T2w = T2-weighted.

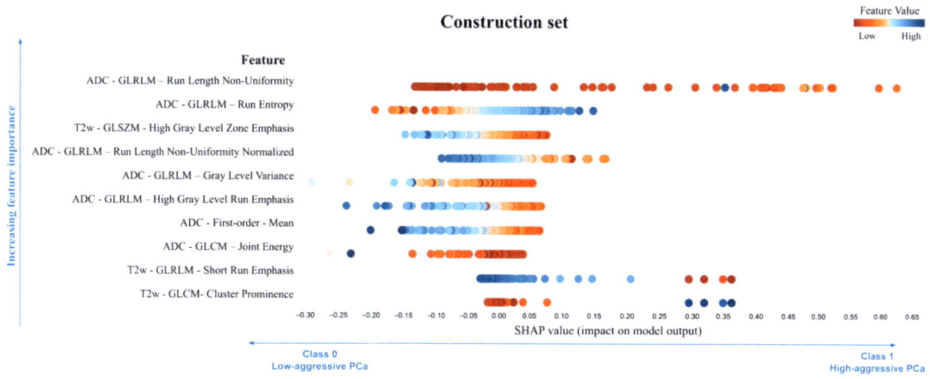

Figure 6. Shapley additive explanation (SHAP) summary plot for the construction (**a**) and validation (**b**) sets. ADC = apparent diffusion coefficient, GLCM = grey-level co-occurrence matrix, GLRLM = grey-level run length matrix, GLSZM = grey-level size zone matrix, SHAP = Shapley additive explanation, T2w = T2-weighted.

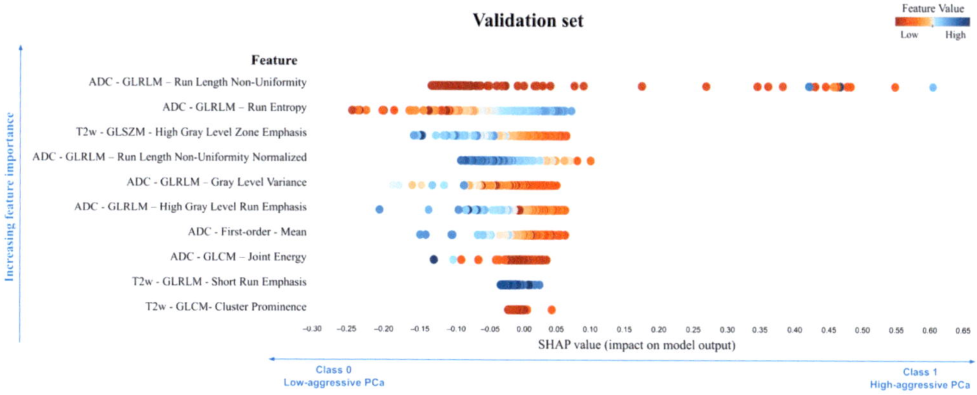

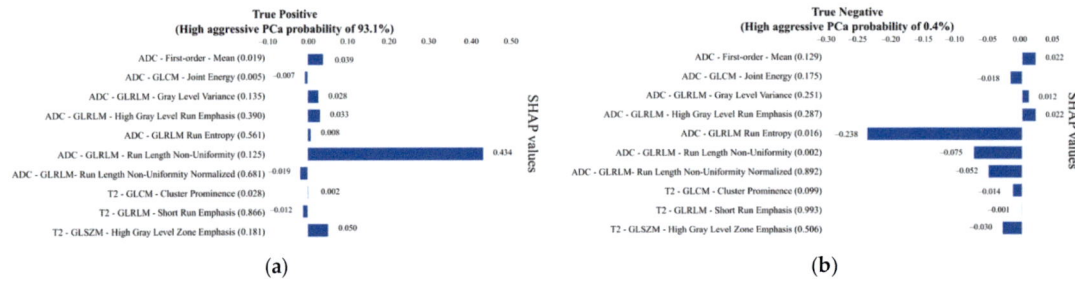

Figure 7. Shapley values of a true positive prediction (**a**) and a true negative prediction (**b**), randomly selected from the validation set. For each feature, the corresponding value is reported in parentheses. ADC = apparent diffusion coefficient, GG = grade group, GLCM = grey-level co-occurrence matrix, GLRLM = grey-level run length matrix, GLSZM = grey-level size zone matrix, SHAP = Shapley additive explanation, T2w = T2-weighted.

4. Discussion

In this study, we developed and validated a radiomics model to distinguish between GG $\leq$ 2 and GG $\geq$ 3 PCas using bpMRI. Regarding the classification GG $\leq$ 2 and GG $\geq$ 3, to the best of our knowledge, this is the first study that externally validated a classification model and that provided an explanation for the model's output. External validation is a challenging task since MRI suffers from high variability due to differences in scanners and acquisition protocols and researchers are struggling to develop AI-based models dealing with multicenter datasets. However, thanks to the engineering of the pipeline that we used to obtain the most robust and generalizable model, we reached promising results on both the construction and the external validation set, which included different scanners and magnetic field strengths. An important element of our system is that we provided, together with the binary classification, the likelihood of the tumor being high-aggressive. The latter can be considered to tune the classification output to maximize either NPV or PPV. Considering the value of this score, our studies showed an important result: all 15 lesions in the validation set having a likelihood of being high-aggressive equal to zero were indeed either GG1 or GG2 lesions. If further validated on a larger dataset, this might impact the management of this subgroup of patients for whom an invasive procedure might be avoided.

In the literature, several studies developed AI-based algorithms to characterize PCa aggressiveness, mainly focusing on distinguishing clinically significant PCas (GG1 vs. GG $\geq$ 2) [10] and reaching promising results in multicenter datasets [11]. However, only a few studies focused on the distinction of GG1/GG2 lesions from higher aggressive PCas, obtaining a cross-validated AUC from 0.75 to 0.77 using different machine learning algorithms [16,17]. Cuocolo et al. [18] evaluated the relationship between shape features and low/high aggressive tumors through a multivariable logistic analysis, reaching an AUC of 0.78 with a specificity and sensitivity of 97% and 56%, respectively, on the training set. Bertelli et al. [15] developed an ensemble learner classifier obtaining an AUC of 0.79 on an internal validation set, i.e., using a monocenter dataset. However, all these studies included only one center in their dataset, and none of them validated their results on an external set. Our results are comparable to those in the literature but with the remarkable advantage of keeping two centers as an external validation set, demonstrating the generalization capability of the radiomics classifier (no significant differences were found in the performances of the construction and validation set). As an additional strength of this work, we obtained a radiomics quality score (RQS) [8] of 11 (Supplementary Section S8), which is higher than the average RQS score of 7.93 previously calculated for prostate radiomics studies [28].

Finally, the innovative side of this study is that we have provided an explainable model, deriving relevant information about the importance of selected features. More specifically, seven out of ten features used by the best model were extracted from the ADC map, including the ADC mean, whose value was demonstrated to have a negative relationship with the probability of high-aggressive PCa (Figure 6 and Supplementary Section S5). This is consistent with the literature since ADC values are demonstrated to be moderately correlated to GG of peripheral zone lesions [29] and to have a role in differentiating GG2 and PCa with higher grades [16,30–32]. Moreover, it was demonstrated that high-aggressive peripheral zone tumors are associated, on the ADC map, with high values of entropy and low values of energy [33]. Interestingly, considering features individually, we found that entropy plays a crucial role in distinguishing between low and high aggressive PCas, also in our algorithm. Indeed, the 'ADC–GLRLM–Run Entropy', the second feature in decreasing order of importance (Figure 5) that measures the uncertainty/randomness in the distribution of run lengths, i.e., sequences in a straight scan direction of pixels with identical image value, and gray levels, was found to play a relevant role in the prediction of low-aggressive PCas. Low values of this feature, i.e., high homogeneity, were found to push predictions towards a lower probability of high-aggressive PCas (Figure 6). Conversely, the most important feature of the model, the 'ADC-GLRLM- Run Length Non-Uniformity' (Figure 5), drives the classification of PCa towards the high-aggressive class.

Nevertheless, our study has some limitations. The first limitation regards the limited sample size of the four centers, which affected several aspects of the results of this study. First, the sample size of center D not only impacts the robustness of the results of center D, but it might also be responsible for the significant difference in specificities that we found between centers C and D of the validation set. Indeed, it is important to notice that center D includes only 20 low-aggressive lesions, and therefore, the obtained p-value, close to 0.05, is highly influenced by the sample size. An increase in the number of low-aggressive lesions acquired with a 3T scanner would be beneficial to either confirm or reject the hypothesis that specificities between 1.5T and 3T datasets are significantly different. Second, an increase in the sample size of all four centers would have allowed us to perform cross-validation, permuting two centers in the construction set and then externally validating the models on the two remaining ones. This permutation strategy was implemented as our first attempt at the radiomic pipeline, but it did not result in acceptable performances, probably due to the low sample size and the unbalanced number of patients per class across the different centers. Third, we found that all of the 15 lesions of the validation set with a null likelihood of being high-aggressive were indeed GG $\leq$ 2; however, this was not true in the construction set, where 4/15 lesions with a null likelihood of being high-aggressive were misclassified. This difference may be due to the number of GG1 PCa in the validation set (n = 20), which was higher than in the construction set (n = 1). Therefore, an increase in the sample size of the centers would be of key importance to confirm the generalizability of the model in classifying low-aggressive PCas. A second limitation is that we did not perform a preliminary step of detection of outliers, which affected the values of some features. As can be seen in the colors of the SHAP plot of the construction and validation sets, since the construction set contained some elements with particularly high or low values of some features, after min-max normalization, these features were skewed towards, respectively, low or high values. However, we believe that this does not affect the predictions since for those methods using the distribution of values (e.g., Bayesian), the distribution is not impacted by the presence of one/two outliers, while for those methods using hyperplanes (e.g., SVM), again, the position of the hyperplanes is not influenced by the presence of a few outliers. A third limitation is that the reference standard of 14% of patients was based on target biopsy. However, the model was trained using only patients having prostatectomy as the reference standard; therefore, bias might be introduced only in the validation set. Finally, we did not account for intra-lesion heterogeneity to stratify GG2 and GG3 PCas according to the percentage of Gleason pattern 4. In the future, it would be useful to provide a probability map of tumor grade heterogeneity together with the aggressiveness index to spatially characterize different tissue characteristics.

5. Conclusions

In this study, we developed a radiomics model, based on texture features from bpMRI, that automatically assigns a PCa aggressiveness class to selected suspicious lesions, distinguishing tumors with a good prognosis, i.e., low-aggressive PCas, from more aggressive ones. Predicting high-aggressive PCa with radiomics remains very challenging; however, this noninvasive approach, if further validated and integrated into a clinical decision support system, could help clinicians to manage men with suspicion of PCa, suggesting personalized treatments and selecting patients that might benefit from radical treatment and those that could enter surveillance protocols or undergo less destructive treatments, avoiding biopsy discomfort and related complications.

Supplementary Materials: The following supporting information can be downloaded at https://www.mdpi.com/article/10.3390/cancers16010203/s1. Supplementary Section S1 Reporting Guidelines: from image acquisition to data conversion; Supplementary Section S2 Reporting Guidelines: from image preprocessing to features calculation steps; Supplementary Section S3 Feature selection algorithms and classifiers; Supplementary Section S4 Partial dependence plot; Supplementary Section S5 Comparison of feature selection techniques and classifiers; Supplementary Section S6 List of features selected by the affinity propagation algorithm and used to train the final classifier; Supplementary Section S7 Standards for Reporting of Diagnostic Accuracy Studies (STARD) diagram; Supplementary Section S8 Radiomics quality score (RQS).

Author Contributions: Conceptualization, G.N. and V.G.; methodology, G.N. and V.G.; software, G.N. and G.M.; validation, G.N.; formal analysis, G.N., S.M. and V.G.; investigation, G.N.; data curation, V.C., R.C., R.F., M.G., M.I., N.L., A.P., F.R., A.S. (Alessandro Serafini) and A.S. (Arnaldo Stanzione); writing—original draft preparation, G.N.; writing—review and editing, S.M. and V.G.; visualization, G.N.; supervision, V.G.; funding acquisition, D.R. All authors have read and agreed to the published version of the manuscript.

Funding: This work has received funding from the Fondazione AIRC under IG2017–ID.20398 project—P.I. Regge Daniele and from the European Union's Horizon 2020 research and innovation program under grant agreement no 952159.

Institutional Review Board Statement: The study was conducted in accordance with the Declaration of Helsinki and approved by the Institutional Review Board of A.O.U. Città della Salute e della Scienza of Turin, Mauriziano Umberto I Hospital of Turin, and Federico II Hospital of Naples (in date 27/04/2020 with Protocol number 0041332) and by the Ethical Committee of Candiolo Cancer Institute IRCCS (in date 29/06/2018 with protocol number 192/2018).

Informed Consent Statement: The ethical committees from all centers approved the study and waived the requirement to obtain informed consent, as only de-identified, completely anonymized data were used.

Data Availability Statement: The data presented in this study are available on request from the corresponding author. The data are not publicly available due to ethical reasons.

Conflicts of Interest: The authors declare no conflicts of interest. The funders had no role in the design of the study, in the collection, analyses, or interpretation of data, in the writing of the manuscript, or in the decision to publish the results.

References

1. Siegel, R.L.; Miller, K.D.; Fuchs, H.E.; Jemal, A. Cancer Statistics, 2022. *CA Cancer J. Clin.* **2022**, *72*, 7–33. [CrossRef] [PubMed]
2. Ferlay, J.; Colombet, M.; Soerjomataram, I.; Dyba, T.; Randi, G.; Bettio, M.; Gavin, A.; Visser, O.; Bray, F. Cancer Incidence and Mortality Patterns in Europe: Estimates for 40 Countries and 25 Major Cancers in 2018. *Eur. J. Cancer* **2018**, *103*, 356–3. [CrossRef] [PubMed]
3. Mottet, N.; Conford, P.; van den Bergh, R.C.N.; Briers, E. EAU Guidelines. Edn. Presented at the EAU Annual Congress Amsterdam. In *European Urology*; EAU Guidelines Office: Arnhem, The Netherlands, 2020; ISBN 978-94-92671-07-3.
4. Epstein, J.I.; Egevad, L.; Amin, M.B.; Delahunt, B.; Srigley, J.R.; Humphrey, P.A. The 2014 International Society of Urologic Pathology (ISUP) Consensus Conference on Gleason Grading of Prostatic Carcinoma: Definition of Grading Patterns and Proposal for a New Grading System. *Am. J. Surg. Pathol.* **2016**, *40*, 244–252. [CrossRef] [PubMed]

Flach, R.N.; Willemse, P.-P.M.; Suelmann, B.B.M.; Deckers, I.A.G.; Jonges, T.N.; van Dooijeweert, C.; van Diest, P.J.; Meijer, R.P. Significant Inter- and Intralaboratory Variation in Gleason Grading of Prostate Cancer: A Nationwide Study of 35,258 Patients in The Netherlands. *Cancers* **2021**, *13*, 5378. [CrossRef] [PubMed]

Goel, S.; Shoag, J.E.; Gross, M.D.; Al Hussein Al Awamlh, B.; Robinson, B.; Khani, F.; Baltich Nelson, B.; Margolis, D.J.; Hu, J.C. Concordance Between Biopsy and Radical Prostatectomy Pathology in the Era of Targeted Biopsy: A Systematic Review and Meta-Analysis. *Eur. Urol. Oncol.* **2020**, *3*, 10–20. [CrossRef] [PubMed]

Epstein, J.I.; Feng, Z.; Trock, B.J.; Pierorazio, P.M. Upgrading and Downgrading of Prostate Cancer from Biopsy to Radical Prostatectomy: Incidence and Predictive Factors Using the Modified Gleason Grading System and Factoring in Tertiary Grades. *Eur. Urol.* **2012**, *61*, 1019–1024. [CrossRef] [PubMed]

Lambin, P.; Leijenaar, R.T.H.; Deist, T.M.; Peerlings, J.; de Jong, E.E.C.; van Timmeren, J.; Sanduleanu, S.; Larue, R.T.H.M.; Even, A.J.G.; Jochems, A.; et al. Radiomics: The Bridge between Medical Imaging and Personalized Medicine. *Nat. Rev. Clin. Oncol.* **2017**, *14*, 749–762. [CrossRef]

Ghezzo, S.; Bezzi, C.; Presotto, L.; Mapelli, P.; Bettinardi, V.; Savi, A.; Neri, I.; Preza, E.; Samanes Gajate, A.M.; De Cobelli, F.; et al. State of the Art of Radiomic Analysis in the Clinical Management of Prostate Cancer: A Systematic Review. *Crit. Rev. Oncol. Hematol.* **2022**, *169*, 103544. [CrossRef]

Cuocolo, R.; Cipullo, M.B.; Stanzione, A.; Romeo, V.; Green, R.; Cantoni, V.; Ponsiglione, A.; Ugga, L.; Imbriaco, M. Machine Learning for the Identification of Clinically Significant Prostate Cancer on MRI: A Meta-Analysis. *Eur. Radiol.* **2020**, *30*, 6877–6887. [CrossRef]

Bleker, J.; Yakar, D.; van Noort, B.; Rouw, D.; de Jong, I.J.; Dierckx, R.A.J.O.; Kwee, T.C.; Huisman, H. Single-center versus multi-center biparametric MRI radiomics approach for clinically significant peripheral zone prostate cancer. *Insights Imaging* **2021**, *12*, 150. [CrossRef]

Kane, C.J.; Eggener, S.E.; Shindel, A.W.; Andriole, G.L. Variability in Outcomes for Patients with Intermediate-Risk Prostate Cancer (Gleason Score 7, International Society of Urological Pathology Gleason Group 2-3) and Implications for Risk Stratification: A Systematic Review. *Eur. Urol. Focus* **2017**, *3*, 487–497. [CrossRef] [PubMed]

Wright, J.L.; Salinas, C.A.; Lin, D.W.; Kolb, S.; Koopmeiners, J.; Feng, Z.; Stanford, J.L. Prostate Cancer Specific Mortality and Gleason 7 Disease Differences in Prostate Cancer Outcomes between Cases with Gleason 4 + 3 and Gleason 3 + 4 Tumors in a Population Based Cohort. *J. Urol.* **2009**, *182*, 2702–2707. [CrossRef] [PubMed]

Tollefson, M.K.; Leibovich, B.C.; Slezak, J.M.; Zincke, H.; Blute, M.L. Long-Term Prognostic Significance of Primary Gleason Pattern in Patients with Gleason Score 7 Prostate Cancer: Impact on Prostate Cancer Specific Survival. *J. Urol.* **2006**, *175*, 547–551. [CrossRef] [PubMed]

Bertelli, E.; Mercatelli, L.; Marzi, C.; Pachetti, E.; Baccini, M.; Barucci, A.; Colantonio, S.; Gherardini, L.; Lattavo, L.; Pascali, M.A.; et al. Machine and Deep Learning Prediction Of Prostate Cancer Aggressiveness Using Multiparametric MRI. *Front. Oncol.* **2021**, *11*, 802964. [CrossRef] [PubMed]

Bernatz, S.; Ackermann, J.; Mandel, P.; Kaltenbach, B.; Zhdanovich, Y.; Harter, P.N.; Döring, C.; Hammerstingl, R.; Bodelle, B.; Smith, K.; et al. Comparison of Machine Learning Algorithms to Predict Clinically Significant Prostate Cancer of the Peripheral Zone with Multiparametric MRI Using Clinical Assessment Categories and Radiomic Features. *Eur. Radiol.* **2020**, *30*, 6757–6769. [CrossRef] [PubMed]

Chaddad, A.; Niazi, T.; Probst, S.; Bladou, F.; Anidjar, M.; Bahoric, B. Predicting Gleason Score of Prostate Cancer Patients Using Radiomic Analysis. *Front. Oncol.* **2018**, *8*, 630. [CrossRef] [PubMed]

Cuocolo, R.; Stanzione, A.; Ponsiglione, A.; Romeo, V.; Verde, F.; Creta, M.; La Rocca, R.; Longo, N.; Pace, L.; Imbriaco, M. Clinically Significant Prostate Cancer Detection on MRI: A Radiomic Shape Features Study. *Eur. J. Radiol.* **2019**, *116*, 144–149. [CrossRef]

Giannini, V.; Mazzetti, S.; Defeudis, A.; Stranieri, G.; Calandri, M.; Bollito, E.; Bosco, M.; Porpiglia, F.; Manfredi, M.; De Pascale, A.; et al. A Fully Automatic Artificial Intelligence System Able to Detect and Characterize Prostate Cancer Using Multiparametric MRI: Multicenter and Multi-Scanner Validation. *Front. Oncol.* **2021**, *11*, 718155. [CrossRef]

Giannini, V.; Mazzetti, S.; Armando, E.; Carabalona, S.; Russo, F.; Giacobbe, A.; Muto, G.; Regge, D. Multiparametric Magnetic Resonance Imaging of the Prostate with Computer-Aided Detection: Experienced Observer Performance Study. *Eur. Radiol.* **2017**, *27*, 4200–4208. [CrossRef]

Yushkevich, P.A.; Piven, J.; Hazlett, H.C.; Smith, R.G.; Ho, S.; Gee, J.C.; Gerig, G. User-Guided 3D Active Contour Segmentation of Anatomical Structures: Significantly Improved Efficiency and Reliability. *Neuroimage* **2006**, *31*, 1116–1128. [CrossRef]

Nicoletti, G.; Barra, D.; Defeudis, A.; Mazzetti, S.; Gatti, M.; Faletti, R.; Russo, F.; Regge, D.; Giannini, V. Virtual Biopsy in Prostate Cancer: Can Machine Learning Distinguish Low and High Aggressive Tumors on MRI? *Annu. Int. Conf. IEEE Eng. Med. Biol. Soc. IEEE Eng. Med. Biol. Soc. Annu. Int. Conf.* **2021**, *2021*, 3374–3377. [CrossRef]

van Griethuysen, J.J.M.; Fedorov, A.; Parmar, C.; Hosny, A.; Aucoin, N.; Narayan, V.; Beets-Tan, R.G.H.; Fillion-Robin, J.-C.; Pieper, S.; Aerts, H.J.W.L. Computational Radiomics System to Decode the Radiographic Phenotype. *Cancer Res.* **2017**, *77*, e104–e107. [CrossRef] [PubMed]

Zwanenburg, A.; Vallières, M.; Abdalah, M.A.; Aerts, H.J.W.L.; Andrearczyk, V.; Apte, A.; Ashrafinia, S.; Bakas, S.; Beukinga, R.J.; Boellaard, R.; et al. The Image Biomarker Standardization Initiative: Standardized Quantitative Radiomics for High-Throughput Image-Based Phenotyping. *Radiology* **2020**, *295*, 328–338. [CrossRef] [PubMed]

25. Lundberg, S.M.; Lee, S.-I. A Unified Approach to Interpreting Model Predictions. In Proceedings of the 31st International Conference on Neural Information Processing Systems, Long Beach, CA, USA, 4–9 December 2017; Curran Associates Inc.: Red Hook, NY, USA, 2017; pp. 4768–4777.
26. Akoglu, H. User's Guide to Correlation Coefficients. *Turk. J. Emerg. Med.* **2018**, *18*, 91–93. [CrossRef] [PubMed]
27. Bossuyt, P.M.; Reitsma, J.B.; Bruns, D.E.; Gatsonis, C.A.; Glasziou, P.P.; Irwig, L.; Lijmer, J.G.; Moher, D.; Rennie, D.; de Vet, H.C.W.; et al. STARD 2015: An Updated List of Essential Items for Reporting Diagnostic Accuracy Studies. *BMJ* **2015**, *351*, h5527. [CrossRef] [PubMed]
28. Stanzione, A.; Gambardella, M.; Cuocolo, R.; Ponsiglione, A.; Romeo, V.; Imbriaco, M. Prostate MRI Radiomics: A Systematic Review and Radiomic Quality Score Assessment. *Eur. J. Radiol.* **2020**, *129*, 109095. [CrossRef]
29. Surov, A.; Meyer, H.J.; Wienke, A. Correlations between Apparent Diffusion Coefficient and Gleason Score in Prostate Cancer: Systematic Review. *Eur. Urol. Oncol.* **2020**, *3*, 489–497. [CrossRef]
30. Karaarslan, E.; Altan Kus, A.; Alis, D.; Karaarslan, U.C.; Saglican, Y.; Argun, O.B.; Kural, A.R. Performance of Apparent Diffusion Coefficient Values and Ratios for the Prediction of Prostate Cancer Aggressiveness across Different MRI Acquisition Settings. *Diagn. Interv. Radiol.* **2022**, *28*, 12–20. [CrossRef]
31. Alessandrino, F.; Taghipour, M.; Hassanzadeh, E.; Ziaei, A.; Vangel, M.; Fedorov, A.; Tempany, C.M.; Fennessy, F.M. Predictive Role of PI-RADSv2 and ADC Parameters in Differentiating Gleason Pattern 3 + 4 and 4 + 3 Prostate Cancer. *Abdom. Radiol.* **2019**, *44*, 279–285. [CrossRef]
32. Tamada, T.; Prabhu, V.; Li, J.; Babb, J.S.; Taneja, S.S.; Rosenkrantz, A.B. Assessment of Prostate Cancer Aggressiveness Using Apparent Diffusion Coefficient Values: Impact of Patient Race and Age. *Abdom. Radiol.* **2017**, *42*, 1744–1751. [CrossRef]
33. Wibmer, A.; Hricak, H.; Gondo, T.; Matsumoto, K.; Veeraraghavan, H.; Fehr, D.; Zheng, J.; Goldman, D.; Moskowitz, C.; Fine, S.W.; et al. Haralick Texture Analysis of Prostate MRI: Utility for Differentiating Non-Cancerous Prostate from Prostate Cancer and Differentiating Prostate Cancers with Different Gleason Scores. *Eur. Radiol.* **2015**, *25*, 2840–2850. [CrossRef] [PubMed]

Disclaimer/Publisher's Note: The statements, opinions and data contained in all publications are solely those of the individual author(s) and contributor(s) and not of MDPI and/or the editor(s). MDPI and/or the editor(s) disclaim responsibility for any injury to people or property resulting from any ideas, methods, instructions or products referred to in the content.

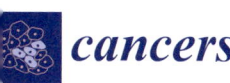

MRI Radiomics-Based Machine Learning Models for Ki67 Expression and Gleason Grade Group Prediction in Prostate Cancer

Xiaofeng Qiao [1,†], Xiling Gu [1,†], Yunfan Liu [1], Xin Shu [1], Guangyong Ai [1], Shuang Qian [2], Li Liu [2], Xiaojing He [1,*] and Jingjing Zhang [3,4,*]

1. Department of Radiology, The Second Affiliated Hospital of Chongqing Medical University, Chongqing 400010, China; qiaoxiaofeng@hospital.cqmu.edu.cn (X.Q.); guxiling@cqmu.edu.cn (X.G.); szpm515@163.com (Y.L.); bryant0824sx@163.com (X.S.); 303701@hospital.cqmu.edu.cn (G.A.)
2. Big Data and Software Engineering College, Chongqing University, Chongqing 400000, China; 202024131068@cqu.edu.cn (S.Q.); dcsliuli@cqu.edu.cn (L.L.)
3. Departments of Diagnostic Radiology, National University of Singapore, Singapore 119074, Singapore
4. Clinical Imaging Research Centre, Centre for Translational Medicine, National University of Singapore, Singapore 117599, Singapore
* Correspondence: he_xiaojing@hospital.cqmu.edu.cn (X.H.); j.zhang@nus.edu.sg (J.Z.); Tel.: +65-84353534 (J.Z.)
† These authors contributed equally to this work.

Simple Summary: Given the variable aggressiveness of PCa, patients with indolent PCa do not require intervention, but rather require active surveillance and close lifelong follow-up, while those with invasive PCa require surgery, various types of radiation therapy, androgen-deprivation therapy (ADT), or multimodal treatment. Hence, it is critical to accurately distinguish indolent from invasive PCa for prognosis evaluation and treatment decision-making. The aim of the present study was to investigate the value of MR radiomics feature-based machine learning (ML) models in predicting the Ki67 index and Gleason grade group (GGG) of PCa. Biparametric magnetic resonance imaging (bpMRI) radiomics-based ML models to predict immuno-histochemically-determined Ki67 expression and the GGG demonstrated the ability to identify aggressive PCa. A preliminary exploration was performed in the conjoint analysis, laying the theoretical foundation for models predicting two or more variables; such models are expected to provide more comprehensive pathological information and provide valuable guidance for clinical decision-making in a noninvasive, synchronous, and objective manner.

Abstract: Purpose: The Ki67 index and the Gleason grade group (GGG) are vital prognostic indicators of prostate cancer (PCa). This study investigated the value of biparametric magnetic resonance imaging (bpMRI) radiomics feature-based machine learning (ML) models in predicting the Ki67 index and GGG of PCa. Methods: A total of 122 patients with pathologically proven PCa who had undergone preoperative MRI were retrospectively included. Radiomics features were extracted from T2-weighted imaging (T2WI), diffusion-weighted imaging (DWI), and apparent diffusion coefficient (ADC) maps. Then, recursive feature elimination (RFE) was applied to remove redundant features. ML models for predicting Ki67 expression and GGG were constructed based on bpMRI and different algorithms, including logistic regression (LR), support vector machine (SVM), random forest (RF), and K-nearest neighbor (KNN). The performances of different models were evaluated with receiver operating characteristic (ROC) analysis. In addition, a joint analysis of Ki67 expression and GGG was performed by assessing their Spearman correlation and calculating the diagnostic accuracy for both indices. Results: The ML model based on LR and ADC + T2 (LR_ADC + T2, AUC = 0.8882) performed best in predicting Ki67 expression, and ADC_wavelet-LHH_firstorder_Maximum had the highest feature weighting. The SVM_DWI + T2 (AUC = 0.9248) performed best in predicting GGG, and DWI_wavelet HLL_glcm_SumAverage had the highest feature weighting. The Ki67 and GGG exhibited a weak positive correlation ($r = 0.382$, $p < 0.001$), and LR_ADC + DWI had the highest diagnostic accuracy in predicting both (0.6230). Conclusion: The proposed ML models are suitable for predicting both Ki67 expression and GGG in PCa. This algorithm could be used to identify indolent or invasive PCa with a noninvasive, repeatable, and accurate diagnostic method.

Keywords: prostate cancer; MRI; Gleason grade group; Ki67; machine learning

1. Introduction

Prostate cancer (PCa) accounts for an estimated 29% of all new incident cases and has become the second leading cause of cancer-related deaths (11%), according to the American Cancer Society (ACS) [1]. Given the variable aggressiveness of PCa, patients with indolent PCa do not require intervention, but rather require active surveillance (AS) and close lifelong follow-up, while those with invasive PCa require surgery, various types of radiation therapy, androgen-deprivation therapy (ADT), or multimodal treatment [2–4]. Hence, it is critical to accurately distinguish indolent from invasive PCa for prognosis evaluation and treatment decision-making.

The Gleason score (GS), as a widely recognized indicator of PCa aggressiveness, reflects the differentiation degree and heterogeneity of prostate tumor cells [5–7]. Tumors with lower GSs are predominantly associated with indolent PCa, whereas tumors with higher GSs exhibit greater aggressiveness due to dysplastic, fused, or cribriform glands. The new Gleason grade group (GGG) scale reflects PCa biology and predicts tumor progression more accurately than the Gleason score system, according to the International Society of Urological Pathology (ISUP). Studies have demonstrated that the hazard ratios of GGG 2, 3, 4, and 5 relative to GGG 1 are 2.2, 7.3, 12.3, and 23.9, respectively, and the corresponding 5-year biochemical risk-free survival rates are 96%, 88%, 63%, 48%, and 26%. The GGG is an important indicator for prognostic assessment, treatment regimen formulation, and survival prediction in PCa [7].

The nuclear protein Ki67 is a nonspecific marker of cell proliferation expressed only in the cell proliferation cycle, which contributes to evaluating the tumor growth fraction [8]. The assessment of Ki67 has made great contributions to the evaluation of tumor proliferation and invasion, especially in breast cancer, since it was first applied to lymphoma in 1984. Higher Ki67 expression is strongly associated with a higher GS, more advanced cancer, seminal vesicle invasion, extracapsular extension, poorer survival, and a higher risk of fatal cancer [9–17]; Matthew K. Tollefson et al. found that, in PCa, the risk of disease-specific death increased by nearly 12% with each 1% increase in Ki67 expression after adjusting for perineural invasion and GS [18].

Although Ki67 expression and the GGG are important indicators for assessing tumor invasiveness, there are limitations to their independent application. For instance, PCa is usually a multifocal tumor, and the GS is determined by the highest score among the tumors, which may lead to an overestimation of the overall GGG. Ki67 evaluation alone is not recommended for outcome prediction due to the high heterogeneity and variability of PCa, although it has great value in low-risk/indolent PCa [13]. Ki67 is, however, considered a good supplement to the GS [14–16]. The combination of Ki67 and GSs may be the best indicator for long-term PCa outcome assessment [18] and may offer more comprehensive preoperative information. Nevertheless, both the GGG and Ki67 expression are obtained through histopathology, which requires an invasive procedure that may result in complications such as postsurgical hemorrhage, pain, infection, and prolonged hospital stay. Therefore, noninvasive methods for Ki67 and GGG assessment need to be explored. Biomarker analysis and magnetic resonance imaging (MRI) were recommended as alternatives to conventional biopsy at the 23rd Annual Conference of the National Comprehensive Cancer Network (NCCN) [19].

Considering the demonstrated advantages of MRI, it is widely used for tumor characterization, staging, treatment planning, targeted therapy, treatment response assessment, and surveillance. However, interobserver differences are a nonnegligible limitation of the technique [20]. With the development of artificial intelligence, radiomics combined with machine learning (ML) has become a novel approach in medical image analysis, by which a large amount of high-quality and quantitative data are obtained noninvasively and objectively. Therefore, radiomics-based ML has emerged as a field of high research interest in recent years, and great achievements have been made in numerous areas, especially in the assessment of malignant tumors [21–27]. There have been relatively few studies on predicting Ki67 and GGG. Duc Fehr et al. presented an ML-based automatic classification of GS that combines apparent diffusion coefficient (ADC)- and T2-weighted imaging (T2WI)-based texture features [28]. Fan et al. constructed innovative ML models for predicting Ki67 based on T2WI, diffusion-weighted imagine (DWI) and dynamic contrast-enhanced (DCE) MRI, which contributed to the risk stratification evaluation of PCa [29]. However, most studies to date have focused on the use of single clinical or pathological variables. Considering the great clinical value of the GGG combined with Ki67, the ultimate goal of this study is to shift the prognostic assessment and treatment decision-making paradigm in PCa from an invasive, subjective process to a noninvasive, objective process by predicting Ki67 expression and the GGG through ML-based image analysis.

2. Materials and Methods

2.1. Patients

The institutional review board of our hospital approved this retrospective study and waived the requirement for informed consent (decision number (2019) 289). Patients who underwent prostate MRI scanning between August 2016 and May 2021 were screened for inclusion according to the following criteria: (1) PCa confirmed by pathology, (2) sufficient tissue samples for immunohistochemical Ki67 and GGG analyses, and (3) systematic biopsy performed within 3 months after the MRI examination. The exclusion criteria were as follows: (1) operation or endocrine treatment before MRI examination (n = 16) and (2) poor MR image quality (n = 2). The details are summarized in Figure 1.

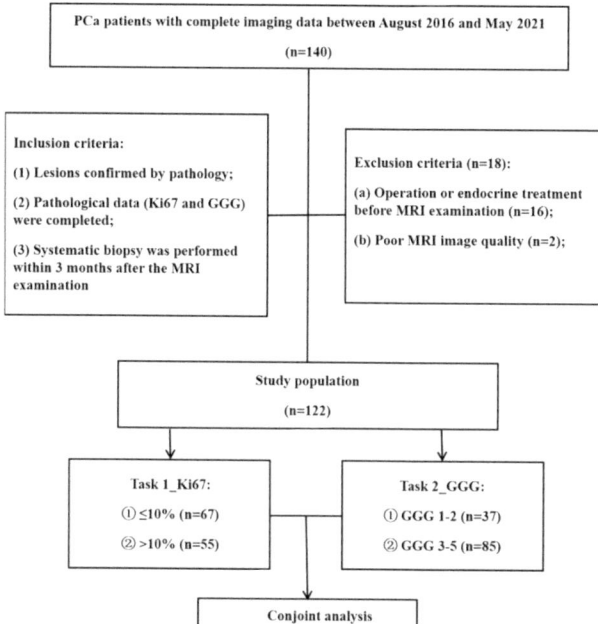

Figure 1. Flowchart of patient selection. PCa = prostate cancer, GGG = Gleason grade group.

2.2. MRI Protocol

The biparametric magnetic resonance (bpMR) images were acquired using a 3.0 T MRI scanner (MAGNETOM Prisma; SIEMENS A Tim Dot System) and an 8-channel phased-array software coil. The scan covered the prostate gland, the seminal vesicles, and as many adjoining structures as possible. The parameters for fat suppression (FS) axial T2WI were as follows: repetition time (TR)—3090 ms; echo time (TE)—77 ms; slice thickness—3 mm; number of excitations (NEX)—2; field of view (FOV)—20 × 20 cm; and acquisition matrix—320 × 240. Axial DWI was performed in the same orientation and location as in axial T2WI using axial echo-planar imaging (EPI) sequences as follows: TR—3800 ms; TE—84 ms; slice thickness—3 mm; NEX—2; FOV—20 × 20 cm; acquisition matrix—118 × 118; and b value—1400 s/mm^2. ADC maps were automatically generated from intravoxel incoherent motion (IVIM) imaging on a designated workstation (Version syngo MR E11; Siemens software packages (syngo.via VB20A_HF06); NUMARIS/4), in which the low b-value was 0 s/mm^2 and the intermediate b-value was 1000 s/mm^2.

2.3. Pathology

All patients underwent transrectal ultrasound (TRUS)-guided 12-core systematic biopsy within 3 months after the MRI examinations. The Ki67 expression of all prostatic parenchymal tissue samples was re-evaluated by a pathologist with more than 15 years of experience. To determine the immunohistochemical evaluation standard for Ki67, the percentage of stained cells in three hotspots (the areas with the most intense proliferation) was calculated, and the average value was taken. When there were multiple tumors, the maximum value was taken [16,17]. The data were classified into 2 subgroups in task 1 and task 2 according to the pathological results: (1) Task 1_Ki67—the patients were divided into a high-expression group (>10%) and a low-expression group ($\leq$10%), using the median value as the cutoff [12,29]; (2) Task 2_GGG—the patients were classified into low-grade (GGG 1-2) and high-grade (GGG 3-5) groups according to strict evaluation using the Gleason Grade Conference standards of the 2019 ISUP [7].

2.4. Radiomics Feature Extraction

All original T2W, DW, and ADC images, stored in DICOM format, were imported into Artificial Intelligence Kit software (A.K. software; GE Healthcare) for delineating the region of interest (ROI) of tumor areas and extracting features. Two doctors (a radiologist with 5 years of experience in abdominal imaging and an attending doctor with 10 years of experience in urinary imaging) read the original images together and then drafted the lesion ROI segmentation plan by discussion until a consensus was reached. If any disagreements could not be resolved, the final judgment was conducted by a third reviewer with extensive seniority, possessing over 15 years of experience in urinary system imaging. The ROI delineation encompassed the entire tumor while excluding the invasion of the urethra and adjacent structures. For multifocal tumors, only the largest lesion was segmented. An example of ROI segmentation and the corresponding pathological images (GGG and Ki67) are shown in Figure 2. Following the application of gray-level discretization with a bin size of 5, a total of 107 radiomics features were extracted, including first-order features (n = 18), shape features (n = 14), and texture features (n = 75); the latter, used to describe the internal and surface textures of the lesions, consisted of the gray-level cooccurrence matrix (GLCM) (n = 24), the gray-level size zone matrix (GLSZM) (n = 16), the gray-level dependence matrix (GLDM) (n = 5), the gray-level run length matrix (GLRLM) (n = 16), and the neighborhood gray tone difference matrix (NGTDM) (n = 14) features. Subsequently, by employing wavelet transformation (level = 1), 851 radiomic features were extracted from each of the T2WI, DWI, and ADC images. In total, 2553 radiomic features were ultimately obtained.

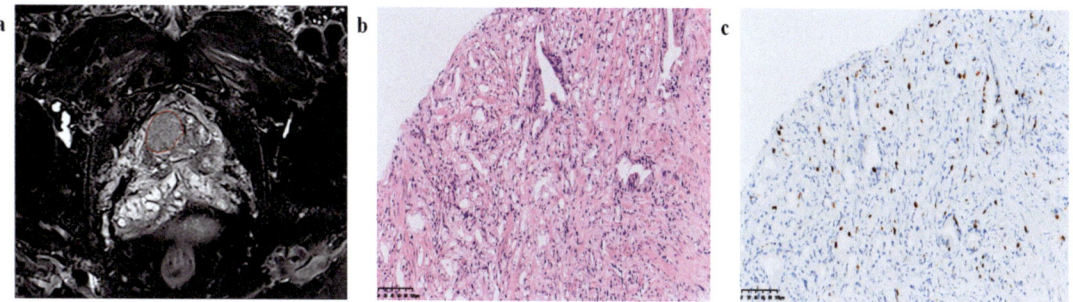

Figure 2. Region of interest (ROI) segmentation and corresponding pathological pictures. (**a**) ROI segmentation, (**b**) Loupe image of hematoxylin–eosin stain shows the GS = 4 + 3 (×20), (**c**) Loupe image of immunohistochemical stain shows the percentage.

2.5. Preprocessing of Radiomic Features

The data were normalized, scaled, and dimensionally reduced for subsequent comparison. Recursive feature elimination (RFE) was conducted to eliminate redundant and irrelevant features by fitting a given ML algorithm used in the core model, computing and ranking the importance of each feature, and discarding the least important features. This process was repeated until the optimal combination of radiomic features was obtained. Following feature elimination, each model was constructed using a selected set of 20 features. The synthetic minority oversampling technique (SMOTE) was used to resolve data imbalance problems, and 5-fold cross-validation was applied to validate the performance of the ML models. The dataset was randomly divided into a training and testing set with an 8:2 ratio. The code for models training and testing was implemented on Python 3.6, and the common libraries included numpy 1.19.2, cv 2 4.5.1, SimpleITK 2.0.2, pandas 1.1.5, and scikit-learn 0.24.2. This process was repeated five times, and the average of the five iterations was taken as the final experimental result of this study.

2.6. Construction of ML Models

Twenty-eight ML models were established to predict Ki67 expression and GGG based on four ML algorithms and seven different sequences or sequence combinations. The classification algorithms included logistic regression (LR), support vector machine (SVM), random forest (RF), and K-nearest neighbor (KNN). The sequences included T2WI, DWI, ADC, and 4 combinations thereof (T2+DWI, T2+ADC, ADC+DWI, ADC+DWI+T2). Subsequently, the feature compositions of the best models for the two tasks were analyzed. A technical flowchart of this study is presented in Figure 3.

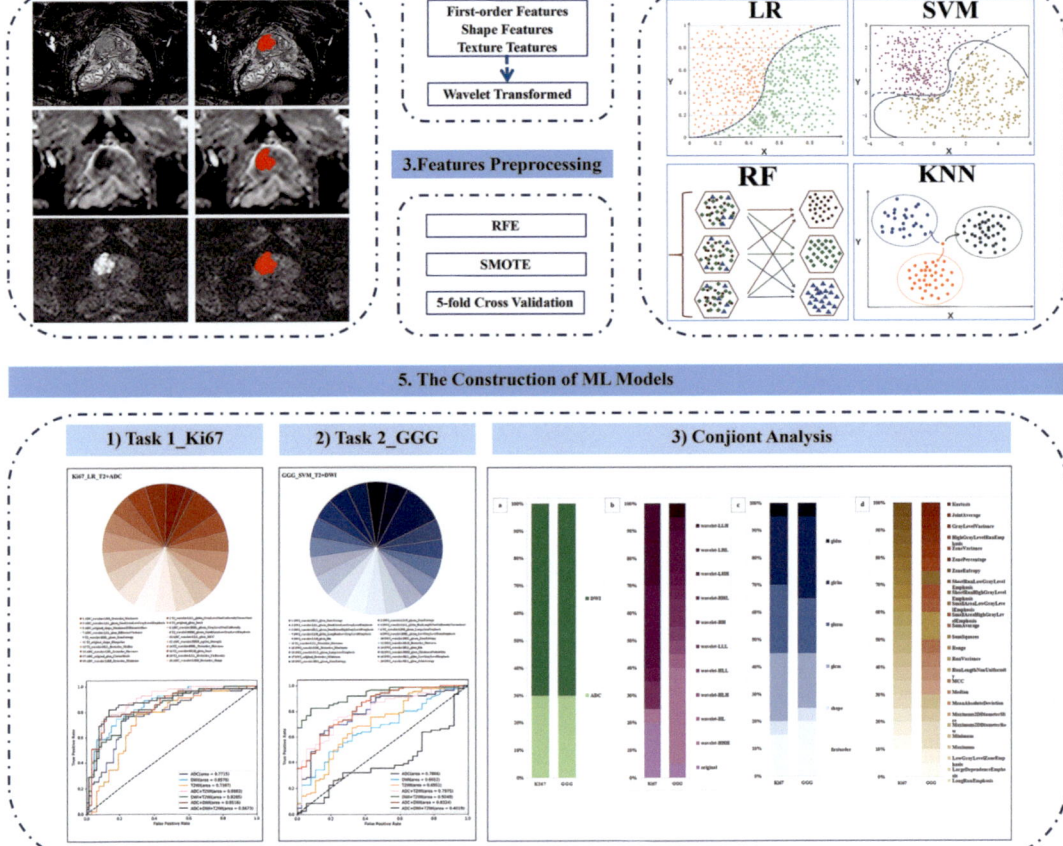

Figure 3. Technical flowchart. RFE = recursive feature elimination, SMOTE = synthetic minority oversampling technique, LR = logistic regression, SVM = support vector machine, RF = random forest, KNN = K-nearest neighbor, ML = machine learning, GGG = Gleason grade group.

2.7. Statistical Analysis

All statistical analyses were performed with SPSS software (version 25; IBM Corporation, Armonk, NY, USA) and Python codes. Comparisons among groups were performed by the independent-sample t-test. Normally distributed variables are shown as the mean ± standard deviation (SD). Non-normally distributed variables are expressed as the median with the interquartile range in parentheses (25th and 75th percentiles). $p < 0.05$ was considered statistically significant. The performance of the ML models was evaluated by using receiver operating characteristic (ROC) curve analysis, including calculation of the area under the curve (AUC), sensitivity, and specificity. The Spearman correlation test was applied to analyze the correlation between Ki67 expression and GGGs. Finally, a joint analysis of the two tasks was performed by calculating the diagnostic accuracy.

3. Results

3.1. Baseline Characteristics

A total of 122 patients were enrolled in this study, including 31 with tumors located in the peripheral zone (PZ), 27 with tumors located in the transition zone (TZ), and 64 with cross-zone tumors, occupying both the PZ and TZ. For task 1, the Ki67 ≤ 10% group included 67 patients (average age 72.7 ± 8.6 years), and the Ki67 > 10% group included 55 patients (average age 71.4 ± 8.7 years). For task 2, the GGG 1-2 group had 37 patients (average age 72.4 ± 8.8 years), and the GGG 3-5 group had 85 patients (average age 72.0 ± 8.6 years). There was no statistically significant age difference between the subgroups in either task 1 ($t = 0.801$, $p = 0.425$) or task 2 ($t = 0.213$, $p = 0.832$). The median (25th–75th percentile) prostate-specific antigen (PSA) and free PSA (fPSA) levels were 47.3 (16.4–136.5) ng/mL and 4.00 (1.37–13.35) ng/mL, respectively.

3.2. Task 1: ML Models for Predicting Ki67 Expression

The comparisons of the 28 ML models are displayed in Table 1 and Figure 4. LR had the best performance, especially for the combination sequences. LR_T2+ADC (AUC = 0.8882, sensitivity = 0.7636, specificity = 0.8657) achieved the optimal performance among the 28 ML models.

Table 1. Ki67 prediction based on four machine learning algorithms and seven sequences *.

Images	LR			SVM			RF			KNN		
	AUC	Sens.	Spec.	AUC	Sens.	Spec.	AUC	Sens.	Spec.	AUC	Sens.	Spec.
T2	0.7383	0.6364	0.7463	0.7913	0.7091	0.7463	0.6946	0.5455	0.6567	0.6425	0.6000	0.6119
DWI	0.8578	0.7091	0.8209	0.8152	0.7455	0.7612	0.5273	0.5455	0.7910	0.6832	0.6182	0.7164
ADC	0.7715	0.7273	0.7612	0.7449	0.7273	0.6716	0.6689	0.5455	0.6866	0.5986	0.4364	0.6716
T2 + DWI	0.8285	0.7273	0.7761	0.7984	0.7455	0.7015	0.6634	0.5455	0.7015	0.6408	0.5455	0.6716
T2 + ADC	0.8882	0.7636	0.8657	0.8475	0.7091	0.7910	0.6965	0.5818	0.7164	0.6650	0.5818	0.7612
ADC + DWI	0.8516	0.7636	0.8209	0.7874	0.7091	0.7164	0.7115	0.5636	0.7015	0.6837	0.6000	0.7164
ADC + DWI + T2	0.8673	0.8182	0.8358	0.8336	0.8727	0.7463	0.6925	0.5636	0.7015	0.6794	0.5818	0.7015

* LR = logistic regression, SVM = support vector machine, RF = random forest, KNN = K-nearest neighbor, AUC = area under the curve, Sens. = sensitivity, Spec. = specificity, T2WI = T2-weighted imaging, DWI = diffusion-weighted imaging, ADC = apparent diffusion coefficient.

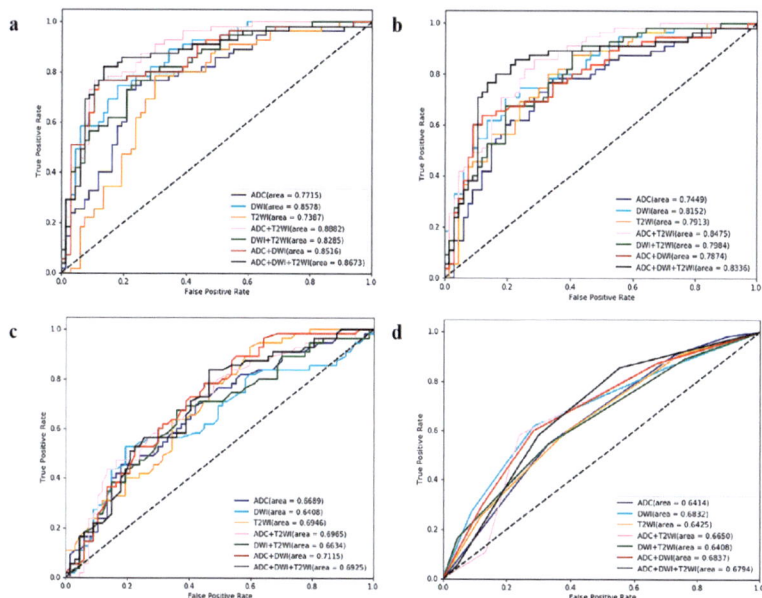

Figure 4. ROC curves of the twenty-eight ML models (based on four algorithms and seven sequences) for predicting Ki67 expression *. (**a**) Logistic regression-, (**b**) support vector machine-, (**c**) random forest-, and (**d**) K-nearest neighbor-based model ROC curves. * ROC = receiver operating characteristic, ML = machine learning, T2WI = T2-weighted imaging, DWI = diffusion-weighted imaging, ADC = apparent diffusion coefficient.

The radiomics features of LR_T2+ADC are illustrated in Figure 5. Of the 20 features, 11 were derived from ADC imaging, and the other 9 were from T2WI, including 7 first-order features, 2 shape features, and 11 texture features. Among them, ADC_wavelet-LHH_first-order_Maximum had the highest weight in predicting Ki67 expression.

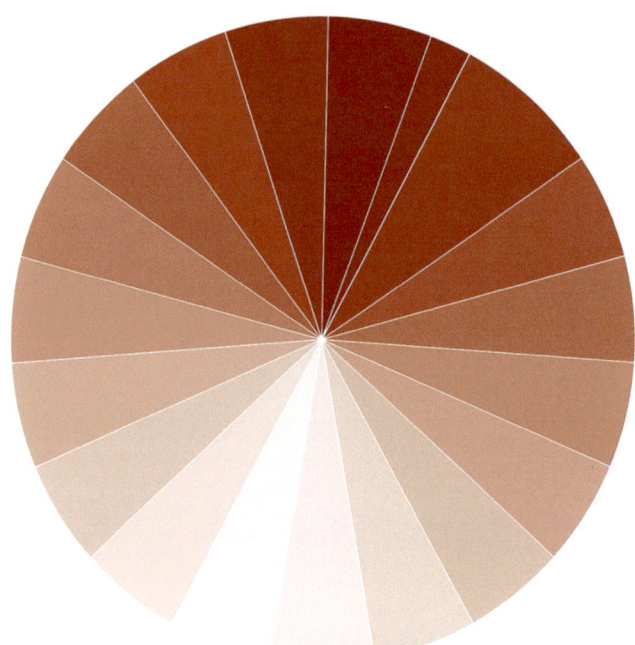

Figure 5. Optimal combined ML model (LR_T2+ADC) for task 1 (Ki67 expression prediction). Different colors represent different radiomics features, and the area represents the weighted contribution of each radiomics feature in the ML model. The feature with the highest weight for Ki67 expression prediction was ADC_wavelet-LHH_first-order_Maximum. ML = machine learning, LR = logistic regression, T2 = T2-weighted imaging, ADC = apparent diffusion coefficient.

3.3. Task 2: ML Models for Predicting GGG

The comparison results for the four ML algorithms and seven sequences are displayed in Table 2 and Figure 6. SVM and LR performed better than KNN and RF. Among the 28 ML models, the optimal model was SVM_T2+DWI (AUC = 0.9248, sensitivity = 0.8588, specificity = 0.7838).

Table 2. GGG prediction based on four machine learning algorithms and seven sequences *.

Images	LR			SVM			RF			KNN		
	AUC	Sens.	Spec.	AUC	Sens.	Spec.	AUC	Sens.	Spec.	AUC	Sens.	Spec.
T2	0.7994	0.8706	0.5946	0.6951	0.7765	0.5946	0.7690	0.8824	0.4595	0.7041	0.8471	0.4054
DWI	0.7736	0.8824	0.4595	0.6652	0.7294	0.4324	0.6060	0.9059	0.2973	0.6068	0.7765	0.3243
ADC	0.8016	0.8706	0.5135	0.7866	0.8000	0.6216	0.6835	0.8824	0.6835	0.6490	0.8941	0.3784
T2 + DWI	0.9072	0.8706	0.6216	0.9248	0.8588	0.7838	0.7232	0.8000	0.3514	0.7065	0.8353	0.4054
T2 + ADC	0.8006	0.8471	0.4865	0.7975	0.7529	0.6757	0.7078	0.9059	0.4595	0.6701	0.9059	0.2703
ADC + DWI	0.8658	0.8824	0.5946	0.8324	0.7765	0.6757	0.6466	0.8235	0.2432	0.6677	0.8471	0.3243
ADC + DWI + T2	0.6162	0.7765	0.1892	0.4019	0.6353	0.3514	0.6013	0.8118	0.2973	0.6073	0.7647	0.3514

* GGG = Gleason grade group, LR = logistic regression, SVM = support vector machine, RF = random forest, KNN = K-nearest neighbor, AUC = area under the curve, Sens. = sensitivity, Spec. = specificity, T2WI = T2-weighted imaging, DWI = diffusion-weighted imaging, ADC = apparent diffusion coefficient.

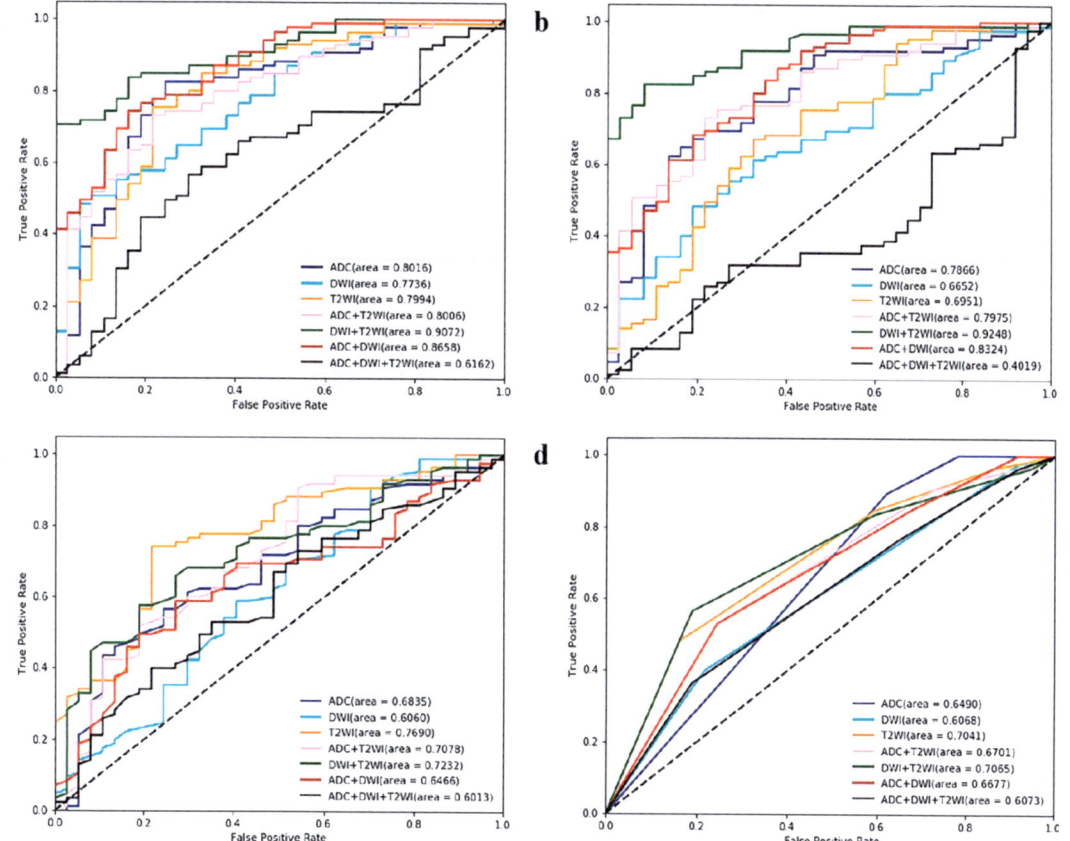

Figure 6. ROC curves of the twenty-eight ML models (based on four algorithms and seven sequences) for GGG prediction. (**a**) Logistic regression-, (**b**) support vector machine-, (**c**) random forest-, and (**d**) K-nearest neighbor-based model ROC curves. ROC = receiver operating characteristic, ML = machine learning, GGG = Gleason grade group, T2WI = T2-weighted imaging, DWI = diffusion-weighted imaging, ADC = apparent diffusion coefficient.

The radiomics feature analysis of SVM_T2 + DWI is presented in Figure 7. The 20 radiomics features consisted of 4 first-order features and 16 texture features, with 18 from DWI and 2 from T2WI. The radiomics feature with the highest weight was DWI_wavelet-HLL_glcm_SumAverage.

GGG_SVM_T2+DWI

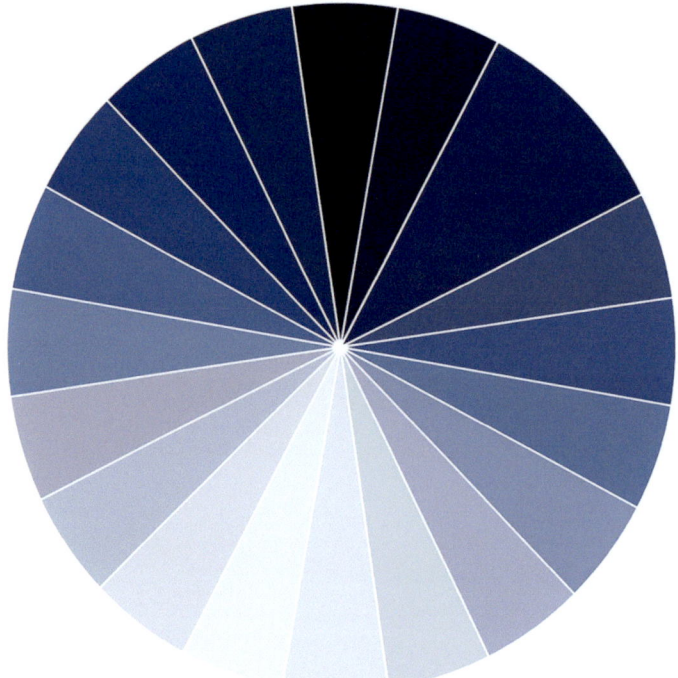

- 1 DWI_wavelet-HLL_glcm_SumAverage
- 2 DWI_wavelet-LLH_glszm_ZoneEntropy
- 3 DWI_wavelet-LLL_glszm_SmallAreaLowGrayLevelEmphasis
- 4 DWI_wavelet-LLL_glrlm_RunLengthNonUniformityNormalized
- 5 DWI_wavelet-HLL_glszm_SmallAreaHighGrayLevelEmphasis
- 6 T2_wavelet-LHH_glszm_LargeAreaEmphasis
- 7 DWI_wavelet-LLH_glrlm_LongRunLowGrayLevelEmphasis
- 8 DWI_wavelet-HHL_glszm_LowGrayLevelZoneEmphasis
- 9 DWI_wavelet-LLH_glcm_Idn
- 10 DWI_wavelet-HHL_glszm_ZoneEntropy
- 11 T2_wavelet-LLL_firstorder_Skewness
- 12 DWI_wavelet-HLH_firstorder_Skewness
- 13 DWI_wavelet-LHL_firstorder_Maximum
- 14 DWI_wavelet-HLL_glcm_Idn
- 15 DWI_wavelet-LLL_glszm_LargeAreaEmphasis
- 16 DWI_wavelet-HHH_glcm_MaximumProbability
- 17 DWI_original_firstorder_Minimum
- 18 DWI_wavelet-HLL_gldm_LowGrayLevelEmphasis
- 19 DWI_wavelet-HLL_glszm_ZoneEntropy
- 20 DWI_wavelet-HLL_glcm_JointAverage

Figure 7. Optimal combined ML model (SVM_T2+DWI) for task 2 (GGG prediction). Different colors represent different radiomics features, and the area indicates the weighted contribution of each radiomics feature in the ML model. DWI_wavelet-HLL_glcm_SumAverage had the highest weight of all the radiomics features. ML = machine learning, SVM = support vector machine, T2WI = T2-weighted imaging, DWI = diffusion-weighted imaging, GGG = Gleason grade group.

3.4. Conjoint Analysis of the Ki67 and GGG Tasks

The Ki67 and GGG exhibited a weak positive correlated ($r = 0.382$, $p < 0.001$). Then, the diagnostic accuracies of the combined task (task 1 and task 2) were calculated. LR_ADC + DWI performed best, with an accuracy of 0.6230, in making correct predictions in both task 1 and task 2, as illustrated in Table 3.

A detailed feature comparison for LR_ADC+DWI in the combined task is shown in Figure 8. The feature comparison consisted of four parts, which yielded the following findings. First, the features were extracted from both ADC ($n = 6$) and DWI ($n = 14$) in two tasks with the same extraction ratio. Second, most of the features were subjected to a wavelet transform (Ki67 = 16/20, GGG = 19/20). Third, the proportions of first-order, shape, and texture features are similar (Ki67 = 3/1/16, GGG = 4/1/15). Fourth, seven features were shared between the two tasks.

Table 3. Prediction accuracy of the combined task *.

Images	LR	SVM	RF	KNN
T2	0.5080	0.4670	0.4340	0.4340
DWI	0.5820	0.4840	0.4920	0.4670
ADC	0.5660	0.5570	0.4590	0.4260
T2+DWI	0.5900	0.6230	0.4260	0.4430
T2+ADC	0.6070	0.5820	0.5250	0.4670
ADC+DWI	0.6230	0.5490	0.4020	0.4670
ADC+DWI+T2	0.5000	0.4340	0.3850	0.4020

* LR = logistic regression, SVM = support vector machine, RF = random forest, KNN = K-nearest neighbor, T2WI = T2-weighted imaging, DWI = diffusion-weighted imaging, ADC = apparent diffusion coefficient.

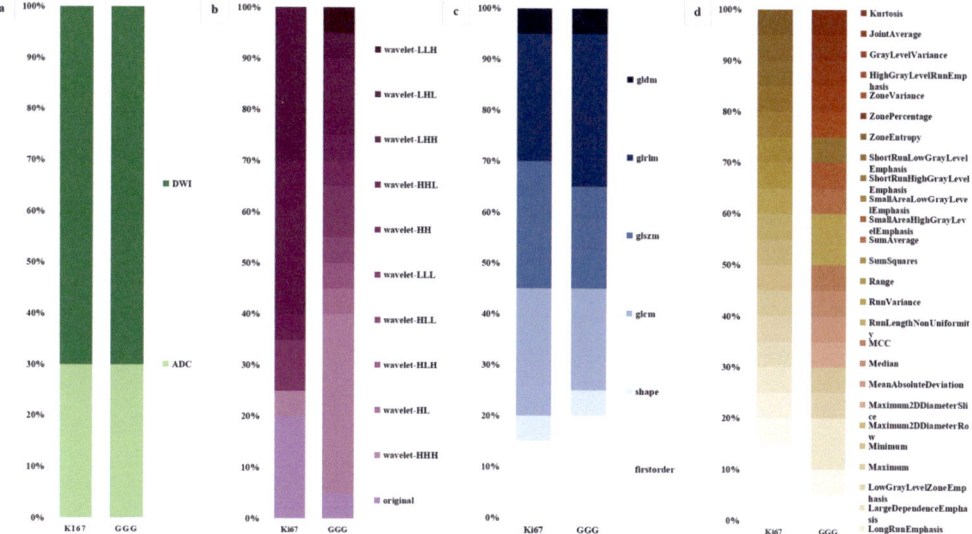

Figure 8. Comparative analysis of the radiomic features of LR_ADC+DWI. (a) The sources of the radiomics features. (b) Use of wavelet transformation for the radiomics feature. (c) Radiomics feature categories (first-order, shape, or texture). (d) Radiomics feature similarity between Ki67 expression and GGG prediction. LR = logistic regression, ADC = apparent diffusion coefficient, DWI = diffusion-weighted imaging, GGG = Gleason grade group.

4. Discussion

In this study, we constructed bpMRI radiomics-based ML models to predict Ki67 expression and GGGs in PCa, and we performed a conjoint analysis of the two corresponding tasks, establishing a foundation for the prediction of multiple pathological indicators. The results demonstrated that the best model for predicting Ki67 expression (task 1) was LR_T2+ADC, the best model for predicting GGGs (task 2) was SVM_T2+DWI, and the highest-performing model in the conjoint analysis was LR_ADC+DWI. These bpMRI radiomics ML models could be applied in clinical practice to obtain pathology information noninvasively and objectively for PCa assessment and treatment-related decision-making.

Four ML algorithms were used in this study to predict Ki67 and GGGs. Overall, the LR- and SVM-based models were superior to the KNN- and RF-based models. LR (AUC = 0.8882) was the best-performing classification algorithm in task 1. However, Xuhui Fan et al. found that RF was the best-performing algorithm in their study (AUC = 0.87) [29].

We speculate that the reason for this discrepancy is that LR, as a supervised classifier, is adept at binary classification tasks, and the training result is mainly influenced by feature weights. The use of adequate high-weight radiomic features in our study might have improved the performance of the LR model. This speculation was confirmed by Lili Zhou et al. [30], who indicated that LR yielded superior results when the key information in the sample was sufficient for predicting Ki67 in medulloblastoma. SVM (AUC = 0.9248) had the best predictive performance in task 2, consistent with the results from D.F. and H.V. et al. [28] SVM considers the interactions among all features and removes features whose effects might offset each other during each iteration in the training until the best performance is achieved.

The images of bpMRI (T2, DWI, ADC) were included individually and in different combinations in this study to comprehensively evaluate the predictive ability of the models. T2+ADC (AUC = 0.8882) was the highest-performing model in task 1, followed by ADC+DWI+T2 (AUC = 0.8673). In a study by Xuhui Fan et al., the T2+DWI+DCE-based model (AUC = 0.87) significantly outperformed the T2 + DWI model (AUC = 0.8285) [29]. We speculate that DCE exerts a large effect associated with neovascularization in PCa. However, our T2+ADC-based model achieved comparable or even better performance without the use of contrast agents. One potential explanation for this outcome could be the fourth dimension (time) present in DCE, which poses challenges in aligning and matching two-dimensional anatomical images like T2WI and DWI. Additionally, extracting information on contrast media arrival and distribution, serving as a surrogate marker for microvascular density, requires the use of semi-quantitative or quantitative pharmacokinetic models, thereby introducing further complexity in post-processing [31]. BpMRI offers the advantage of avoiding potential harmful effects associated with gadolinium contrast agents while also enhancing confidence in the additional value of bpMRI in radiomics research [32]. In contrast to the results for the Ki67 task, the T2+DWI (AUC = 0.9248) was the highest-performing model in the GGG task. Previous studies have placed greater emphasis on T2 and ADC sequences [28,33–36]. Ahmad Chaddad et al. constructed a predictive model for predicting GS based on T2+ADC, with an AUC value of 0.8235 [34]. We surmise that finer grouping may lead to slightly decreased performance. On the other hand, most of the features were from DWI ($n = 18$) rather than T2 ($n = 2$) in this study. One of the reasons might be that some heavily weighted radiomic features from DWI better represented the characteristics of cell atypia and increased tumor cell density with increasing GGG. Frustratingly, ADC+DWI+T2 had the worst performance in predicting GGG, even lower than that of any of the individual sequences. A potential explanation is that the higher-weight features might cancel each other out, but this possibility remains to be studied thoroughly.

We further analyzed the radiomic features and found that wavelet features had a particularly high proportion among the best models for all tasks ($\geq 80\%$), similar to the research of Xu Huifan et al. [29]. Another study on rectal cancer reported that wavelet features accounted for the highest proportion of features in models predicting Ki67 (75%), HER-2 (70%), and lymph node metastasis (80%) [37]. It appears to us that wavelet features have strong predictive ability, effectively representing tumor heterogeneity. In the feature-type analyses, texture features were the most common, comprising 55.5% of all features for the Ki67 task, 80% for the GGG task, and 80% for the Ki67+GGG task. First-order and shape features represent the distribution of voxel intensities and 3D shapes, which are more or less reliant on manual segmentation, an inevitable source of bias. Studies have demonstrated that texture features can be used to accurately classify GGGs [34] and can be stably extracted from the original image.

The best ML algorithms in the conjoint analysis were LR and SVM, but the highest accuracy was only 0.6230. We speculate that the reason may be as follows. First, Ki67 and GGG are excellent predictors of the invasiveness of PCa, but they are essentially different, with Ki67 representing the proliferative capacity of tumor cells and GGG representing cell atypia and differentiation capacity. The five texture features that overlapped between the two tasks (SmallAreaLowGrayLevelEmphasis, Maximum, Minimum, ZoneEntropy, and Skewness) are the most frequently mentioned features in the literature [28,29,33,34]. Second, the complexity of the calculation increased when the tasks were superimposed. Particularly in patients with high Ki67/low GGG and low Ki67/high GGG, even small changes in proportions may affect the calculations of the models. Much more research and analysis is necessary to achieve the prediction of two or more variables.

This study had some limitations that should be noted. First, ROI segmentation could be optimized in follow-up studies using semiautomatic or automatic methods instead of manual segmentation. Second, the pathological specimens in this study were derived from systematic biopsy, which might lead to underestimation, sampling errors, and bias. This shortcoming may be improved by performing radical prostatectomy and targeted biopsy. Third, while Ki67 and GGG are of significant importance in preoperative and prognostic assessments, their inherent limitations and inability to encompass all clinical information suggest that utilizing 5-year overall survival (OS) or disease-free survival (DFS) as prognostic indicators might be a more optimal choice. Furthermore, our study received a radiomics quality score (RQS) of 8 according to the assessment [38], which is comparable to the reported score for prostate imaging (7.93) [39] and slightly higher than the general one (7.56) [40]. However, the main factor affecting the RQS of this study is the lack of external validation. By introducing external validation, the credibility of this single-center retrospective observational study can be significantly enhanced. Each of these points is worthy of further study.

5. Conclusions

In this study, nonenhanced MRI radiomics-based ML models that were used to predict immunohistochemically determined Ki67 expression and the GGG demonstrated the ability to identify aggressive PCa. A preliminary exploration was performed in the conjoint analysis, laying the theoretical foundation for models predicting two or more variables; such models are expected to provide more comprehensive pathological information and provide valuable guidance for clinical decision-making in a noninvasive, synchronous, and objective manner.

Author Contributions: Conceptualization, X.H. and X.Q.; Data curation, X.G., Y.L., X.S., S.Q. and L.L.; Methodology, X.G., Y.L., X.S. and G.A.; Software, S.Q. and L.L.; Formal analysis, X.Q.; Investigation, X.G., Y.L. and X.S.; Resources, X.G. and G.A.; Validation, S.Q. and L.L.; Visualization, S.Q. and L.L.; Supervision, X.H. and J.Z.; Project administration, J.Z.; Funding acquisition, X.H.; Writing—original draft, X.Q.; Writing—review & editing, X.H. and J.Z. All authors have read and agreed to the published version of the manuscript.

Funding: This work was supported by grants from the General Program of the Joint Project of Chongqing Health Commission and Science and Technology Bureau (2019GDRC011), the High-Level Medical Reserved Personnel Training Project of Chongqing and the Kuanren Talents Program of the Second Affiliated Hospital of Chongqing Medical University.

Institutional Review Board Statement: The study was conducted in accordance with the Declaration of Helsinki. The institutional review board of our hospital approved this retrospective study and waived the requirement for informed consent (decision number (2019) 289), approval date (14 May 2019). This article does not contain any studies with human participants or animals performed by any of the authors.

Informed Consent Statement: Informed consent was obtained from all subjects involved in the study.

Data Availability Statement: Data are contained within the article.

Conflicts of Interest: The authors declare no conflict of interest.

References

1. Siegel, R.; Miller, K.; Wagle, N.; Jemal, A. Cancer statistics, 2023. *CA Cancer J. Clin.* **2023**, *73*, 17–48. [CrossRef] [PubMed]
2. Schaeffer, E.; Srinivas, S.; Antonarakis, E.; Armstrong, A.; Bekelman, J.; Cheng, H.; D'Amico, A.; Davis, B.; Desai, N.; Dorff, et al. NCCN Guidelines Insights: Prostate Cancer, Version 1.2021. *J. Natl. Compr. Cancer Netw.* **2021**, *19*, 134–143. [CrossRef]
3. Mottet, N.; van den Bergh, R.C.; Briers, E.; Van den Broeck, T.; Cumberbatch, M.G.; De Santis, M.; Fanti, S.; Fossati, N.; Gandaglia, G.; Gillessen, S.; et al. EAU-EANM-ESTRO-ESUR-SIOG Guidelines on Prostate Cancer-2020 Update. Part 1: Screening, Diagnosis and Local Treatment with Curative Intent. *Eur. Radiol.* **2021**, *79*, 243–262. [CrossRef]
4. Loeb, S.; Folkvaljon, Y.; Curnyn, C.; Robinson, D.; Bratt, O.; Stattin, P. Uptake of Active Surveillance for Very-Low-Risk Prostate Cancer in Sweden. *JAMA Oncol.* **2017**, *3*, 1393–1398. [CrossRef]
5. Hurwitz, L.; Agalliu, I.; Albanes, D.; Barry, K.; Berndt, S.; Cai, Q.; Chen, C.; Cheng, I.; Genkinger, J.; Giles, G.; et al. Recommended Definitions of Aggressive Prostate Cancer for Etiologic Epidemiologic Research. *J. Natl. Cancer Inst.* **2021**, *113*, 727–734. [CrossRef] [PubMed]
6. Epstein, J.; Egevad, L.; Amin, M.; Delahunt, B.; Srigley, J.; Humphrey, P. The 2014 International Society of Urological Pathology (ISUP) Consensus Conference on Gleason Grading of Prostatic Carcinoma: Definition of Grading Patterns and Proposal for New Grading System. *Am. J. Surg. Pathol.* **2016**, *40*, 244–252. [CrossRef]
7. Iczkowski, K.; van Leenders, G.; van der Kwast, T. The 2019 International Society of Urological Pathology (ISUP) Consensus Conference on Grading of Prostatic Carcinoma. *Am. J. Surg. Pathol* **2021**, *45*, 1007. [CrossRef] [PubMed]
8. Scholzen, T.; Endl, E.; Wohlenberg, C.; van der Sar, S.; Cowell, I.; Gerdes, J.; Singh, P. The Ki-67 protein interacts with members of the heterochromatin protein 1 (HP1) family: A potential role in the regulation of higher-order chromatin structure. *J. Pathol.* **2002**, *196*, 135–144. [CrossRef]
9. Zhang, A.; Chiam, K.; Haupt, Y.; Fox, S.; Birch, S.; Tilley, W.; Butler, L.; Knudsen, K.; Comstock, C.; Rasiah, K.; et al. An analysis of a multiple biomarker panel to better predict prostate cancer metastasis after radical prostatectomy. *Int. J. Cancer* **2019**, *144*, 1151–1159. [CrossRef]
10. Goltz, D.; Montani, M.; Braun, M.; Perner, S.; Wernert, N.; Jung, K.; Dietel, M.; Stephan, C.; Kristiansen, G. Prognostic relevance of proliferation markers (Ki-67, PHH3) within the cross-relation of ERG translocation and androgen receptor expression in prostate cancer. *Pathology* **2015**, *47*, 629–636. [CrossRef]
11. Hammarsten, P.; Josefsson, A.; Thysell, E.; Lundholm, M.; Hägglöf, C.; Iglesias-Gato, D.; Flores-Morales, A.; Stattin, P.; Egevad, L.; Granfors, T.; et al. Immunoreactivity for prostate specific antigen and Ki67 differentiates subgroups of prostate cancer related outcome. *Mod. Pathol.* **2019**, *32*, 1310–1319. [CrossRef]
12. Zellweger, T.; Günther, S.; Zlobec, I.; Savic, S.; Sauter, G.; Moch, H.; Mattarelli, G.; Eichenberger, T.; Curschellas, E.; Rüfenacht, H.; et al. Tumour growth fraction measured by immunohistochemical staining of Ki67 is an independent prognostic factor in preoperative prostate biopsies with small-volume or low-grade prostate cancer. *Int. J. Cancer* **2009**, *124*, 2116–2123. [CrossRef] [PubMed]
13. Epstein, J.; Amin, M.; Fine, S.; Algaba, F.; Aron, M.; Baydar, D.; Beltran, A.; Brimo, F.; Cheville, J.; Colecchia, M.; et al. The 2019 Genitourinary Pathology Society (GUPS) White Paper on Contemporary Grading of Prostate Cancer. *Arch. Pathol. Lab. Med.* **2021**, *145*, 461–493. [CrossRef] [PubMed]
14. Green, W.; Ball, G.; Hulman, G.; Johnson, C.; Van Schalwyk, G.; Ratan, H.; Soria, D.; Garibaldi, J.; Parkinson, R.; Hulman, J.; et al. KI67 and DLX2 predict increased risk of metastasis formation in prostate cancer-a targeted molecular approach. *Br. J. Cancer* **2016**, *115*, 236–242. [CrossRef]
15. Berney, D.; Gopalan, A.; Kudahetti, S.; Fisher, G.; Ambroisine, L.; Foster, C.; Reuter, V.; Eastham, J.; Moller, H.; Kattan, M.; et al. Ki-67 and outcome in clinically localised prostate cancer: Analysis of conservatively treated prostate cancer patients from the Trans-Atlantic Prostate Group study. *Br. J. Cancer* **2009**, *100*, 888–893. [CrossRef] [PubMed]
16. Fisher, G.; Yang, Z.; Kudahetti, S.; Møller, H.; Scardino, P.; Cuzick, J.; Berney, D. Prognostic value of Ki-67 for prostate cancer death in a conservatively managed cohort. *Br. J. Cancer* **2013**, *108*, 271–277. [CrossRef]
17. Tretiakova, M.; Wei, W.; Boyer, H.; Newcomb, L.; Hawley, S.; Auman, H.; Vakar-Lopez, F.; McKenney, J.; Fazli, L.; Simko, J.; et al. Prognostic value of Ki67 in localized prostate carcinoma: A multi-institutional study of >1000 prostatectomies. *Prostate Cancer Prostatic Dis.* **2016**, *19*, 264–270. [CrossRef]
18. Tollefson, M.; Karnes, R.; Kwon, E.; Lohse, C.; Rangel, L.; Mynderse, L.; Cheville, J.; Sebo, T. Prostate cancer Ki-67 (MIB-1) expression, perineural invasion, and gleason score as biopsy-based predictors of prostate cancer mortality: The Mayo model. *Mayo Clin. Proc.* **2014**, *89*, 308–318. [CrossRef]
19. Carroll, P.; Mohler, J. NCCN Guidelines Updates: Prostate Cancer and Prostate Cancer Early Detection. *J. Natl. Compr. Can. Netw.* **2018**, *16*, 620–623. [CrossRef] [PubMed]
20. Brembilla, G.; Dell'Oglio, P.; Stabile, A.; Damascelli, A.; Brunetti, L.; Ravelli, S.; Cristel, G.; Schiani, E.; Venturini, E.; Grippaldi, D.; et al. Interreader variability in prostate MRI reporting using Prostate Imaging Reporting and Data System version 2.1. *Eur. Radiol.* **2020**, *30*, 3383–3392. [CrossRef]
21. Fan, M.; Yuan, W.; Zhao, W.; Xu, M.; Wang, S.; Gao, X.; Li, L. Joint Prediction of Breast Cancer Histological Grade and Ki-67 Expression Level Based on DCE-MRI and DWI Radiomics. *IEEE J. Biomed. Health Inform.* **2020**, *24*, 1632–1642. [CrossRef]

Fanizzi, A.; Pomarico, D.; Paradiso, A.; Bove, S.; Diotaiuti, S.; Didonna, V.; Giotta, F.; La Forgia, D.; Latorre, A.; Pastena, M.; et al. Predicting of Sentinel Lymph Node Status in Breast Cancer Patients with Clinically Negative Nodes: A Validation Study. *Cancers* **2021**, *13*, 352. [CrossRef]

Saha, A.; Harowicz, M.; Grimm, L.; Kim, C.; Ghate, S.; Walsh, R.; Mazurowski, M. A machine learning approach to radiogenomics of breast cancer: A study of 922 subjects and 529 DCE-MRI features. *Br. J. Cancer* **2018**, *119*, 508–516. [CrossRef]

Gates, E.; Lin, J.; Weinberg, J.; Hamilton, J.; Prabhu, S.; Hazle, J.; Fuller, G.; Baladandayuthapani, V.; Fuentes, D.; Schellingerhout, D. Guiding the first biopsy in glioma patients using estimated Ki-67 maps derived from MRI: Conventional versus advanced imaging. *Neuro Oncol.* **2019**, *21*, 527–536. [CrossRef]

Pasquini, L.; Napolitano, A.; Lucignani, M.; Tagliente, E.; Dellepiane, F.; Rossi-Espagnet, M.; Ritrovato, M.; Vidiri, A.; Villani, V.; Ranazzi, G.; et al. AI and High-Grade Glioma for Diagnosis and Outcome Prediction: Do All Machine Learning Models Perform Equally Well? *Front. Oncol.* **2021**, *11*, 601425. [CrossRef]

Zaccaria, G.; Ferrero, S.; Hoster, E.; Passera, R.; Evangelista, A.; Genuardi, E.; Drandi, D.; Ghislieri, M.; Barbero, D.; Del Giudice, I.; et al. A Clinical Prognostic Model Based on Machine Learning from the Fondazione Italiana Linfomi (FIL) MCL0208 Phase III Trial. *Cancers* **2021**, *14*, 188. [CrossRef] [PubMed]

Bulloni, M.; Sandrini, G.; Stacchiotti, I.; Barberis, M.; Calabrese, F.; Carvalho, L.; Fontanini, G.; Alì, G.; Fortarezza, F.; Hofman, P.; et al. Automated Analysis of Proliferating Cells Spatial Organisation Predicts Prognosis in Lung Neuroendocrine Neoplasms. *Cancers* **2021**, *13*, 4875. [CrossRef]

Fehr, D.; Veeraraghavan, H.; Wibmer, A.; Gondo, T.; Matsumoto, K.; Vargas, H.; Sala, E.; Hricak, H.; Deasy, J. Automatic classification of prostate cancer Gleason scores from multiparametric magnetic resonance images. *Proc. Natl. Acad. Sci. USA* **2015**, *112*, E6265–E6273. [CrossRef] [PubMed]

Fan, X.; Xie, N.; Chen, J.; Li, T.; Cao, R.; Yu, H.; He, M.; Wang, Z.; Wang, Y.; Liu, H.; et al. Multiparametric MRI and Machine Learning Based Radiomic Models for Preoperative Prediction of Multiple Biological Characteristics in Prostate Cancer. *Front. Oncol.* **2022**, *12*, 839621. [CrossRef] [PubMed]

Zhou, L.; Peng, H.; Ji, Q.; Li, B.; Pan, L.; Chen, F.; Jiao, Z.; Wang, Y.; Huang, M.; Liu, G.; et al. Radiomic signatures based on multiparametric MR images for predicting Ki-67 index expression in medulloblastoma. *Ann. Transl. Med.* **2021**, *9*, 1665. [CrossRef]

Michaely, H.; Aringhieri, G.; Cioni, D.; Neri, E.J.D. Current Value of Biparametric Prostate MRI with Machine-Learning or Deep-Learning in the Detection, Grading, and Characterization of Prostate Cancer: A Systematic Review. *Diagnostics* **2022**, *12*, 799. [CrossRef] [PubMed]

Chen, T.; Zhang, Z.; Tan, S.; Zhang, Y.; Wei, C.; Wang, S.; Zhao, W.; Qian, X.; Zhou, Z.; Shen, J.; et al. MRI Based Radiomics Compared with the PI-RADS V2.1 in the Prediction of Clinically Significant Prostate Cancer: Biparametric vs Multiparametric MRI. *Front. Oncol.* **2021**, *11*, 792456. [CrossRef]

Xie, J.; Li, B.; Min, X.; Zhang, P.; Fan, C.; Li, Q.; Wang, L. Prediction of Pathological Upgrading at Radical Prostatectomy in Prostate Cancer Eligible for Active Surveillance: A Texture Features and Machine Learning-Based Analysis of Apparent Diffusion Coefficient Maps. *Front. Oncol.* **2020**, *10*, 604266. [CrossRef] [PubMed]

Chaddad, A.; Kucharczyk, M.; Niazi, T. Multimodal Radiomic Features for the Predicting Gleason Score of Prostate Cancer. *Cancers* **2018**, *10*, 249. [CrossRef] [PubMed]

Rodrigues, A.; Santinha, J.; Galvão, B.; Matos, C.; Couto, F.; Papanikolaou, N. Prediction of Prostate Cancer Disease Aggressiveness Using Bi-Parametric Mri Radiomics. *Cancers* **2021**, *13*, 6065. [CrossRef]

Zhang, G.; Han, Y.; Wei, J.; Qi, Y.; Gu, D.; Lei, J.; Yan, W.; Xiao, Y.; Xue, H.; Feng, F.; et al. Radiomics Based on MRI as a Biomarker to Guide Therapy by Predicting Upgrading of Prostate Cancer From Biopsy to Radical Prostatectomy. *J. Magn. Reson. Imaging* **2020**, *52*, 1239–1248. [CrossRef]

Meng, X.; Xia, W.; Xie, P.; Zhang, R.; Li, W.; Wang, M.; Xiong, F.; Liu, Y.; Fan, X.; Xie, Y.; et al. Preoperative radiomic signature based on multiparametric magnetic resonance imaging for noninvasive evaluation of biological characteristics in rectal cancer. *Eur. Radiol.* **2019**, *29*, 3200–3209. [CrossRef]

Lambin, P.; Leijenaar, R.; Deist, T.; Peerlings, J.; de Jong, E.; van Timmeren, J.; Sanduleanu, S.; Larue, R.; Even, A.; Jochems, A.; et al. Radiomics: The bridge between medical imaging and personalized medicine. *Nat. Rev. Clin. Oncol.* **2017**, *14*, 749–762. [CrossRef]

Stanzione, A.; Gambardella, M.; Cuocolo, R.; Ponsiglione, A.; Romeo, V.; Imbriaco, M. Prostate MRI radiomics: A systematic review and radiomic quality score assessment. *Eur. J. Radiol.* **2020**, *129*, 109095. [CrossRef]

Spadarella, G.; Stanzione, A.; Akinci D'Antonoli, T.; Andreychenko, A.; Fanni, S.; Ugga, L.; Kotter, E.; Cuocolo, R. Systematic review of the radiomics quality score applications: An EuSoMII Radiomics Auditing Group Initiative. *Eur. Radiol.* **2023**, *33*, 1884–1894. [CrossRef]

Disclaimer/Publisher's Note: The statements, opinions and data contained in all publications are solely those of the individual author(s) and contributor(s) and not of MDPI and/or the editor(s). MDPI and/or the editor(s) disclaim responsibility for any injury to people or property resulting from any ideas, methods, instructions or products referred to in the content.

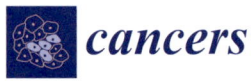

Article

Reasons for Discordance between ^{68}Ga-PSMA-PET and Magnetic Resonance Imaging in Men with Metastatic Prostate Cancer

Jade Wang [1,†], Elisabeth O'Dwyer [2,†], Juana Martinez Zuloaga [2], Kritika Subramanian [2], Jim C. Hu [3], Yuliya S. Jhanwar [2], Himanshu Nagar [4], Arindam RoyChoudhury [5], John Babich [6], Sandra Huicochea Castellanos [2], Joseph R. Osborne [2] and Daniel J. A. Margolis [2,*]

- [1] Department of Internal Medicine, New York-Presbyterian Hospital, New York, NY 10065, USA
- [2] Department of Radiology, Weill Cornell Medical College, New York, NY 10065, USA
- [3] Department of Urology, Weill Cornell Medical College, New York, NY 10065, USA
- [4] Department of Radiation Oncology, Weill Cornell Medical College, New York, NY 10065, USA; hnagar@med.cornell.edu
- [5] Department of Population Health Sciences, Weill Cornell Medical College, New York, NY 10065, USA
- [6] Ratio Therapeutics, Inc., Boston, MA 02210, USA
- * Correspondence: djm9016@med.cornell.edu
- † These authors contributed equally to this work.

Simple Summary: MRI uses magnetic pulses to create images of the body. PET scans use radioactive chemicals to determine what kinds of processes are going on in the body. PSMA is a chemical that is abundant on prostate cancer cells, so a PET scan using a radioactive chemical that attaches to PSMA shows where prostate cancer is, but this test has drawbacks: it is not widely available, it is expensive, and it exposes patients to radiation. However, a recent study found that PSMA PET was more accurate than MRI for finding areas where prostate cancer spreads. This study looks at the "false negative" cases—the specific cases where the MRI did not find prostate cancer when PSMA PET did—and how reading MRI can be improved.

Abstract: Background: PSMA PET has emerged as a "gold standard" imaging modality for assessing prostate cancer metastases. However, it is not universally available, and this limits its impact. In contrast, whole-body MRI is much more widely available but misses more lesions. This study aims to improve the interpretation of whole-body MRI by comparing false negative scans retrospectively to PSMA PET. Methods: This study was a retrospective sub-analysis of a prospectively collected database of patients who participated in a clinical trial of PSMA PET/MRI comparing PSMA PET and whole-body MRI from 2018–2021. Subjects whose separately read PSMA PET and MRI diagnostic reports showed discrepancies ("false negative" MRI cases) were selected for sub-analysis. The cases were reviewed by the same attending radiologist who originally read the scans. The radiologist noted specific features on MRI indicating metastatic disease that were initially missed. Results: Of 263 cases, 38 (14%) met the inclusion criteria and were reviewed. Six classes of mpMRI false negatives were identified: anatomically normal (18, 47%), atypical MRI appearance (6, 16%), mischaracterization (1, 3%), undercall (6, 16%), obscured (4, 11%), and no abnormality on MRI (3, 8%). Considering that the atypical and undercalled cases could have been adjusted in retrospect, and that 4 additional cases had positive lesions to the same extent and 11 further cases had disease confined to the pelvis, only 11 (4%) of the original 263 would have had disease outside of a conventional radiation treatment plan. Conclusion: Notably, almost 50% of the cases, including most lymph node metastases, were anatomically normal using standard criteria. This suggests that current anatomic criteria for evaluating prostate cancer lymph node metastases are not ideal, and there is a need for improved criteria. In addition, 32% of cases involved some element of human interpretive error, and, therefore, improving reader training may lead to more accurate results.

Keywords: prostate; cancer; MRI; PET; PSMA; whole-body

1. Introduction

Prostate cancer is the most common cancer in men and the second leading cause of male cancer mortality in the United States [1]. The lifetime risk of developing prostate cancer for a man living in the United States is estimated at 1 in 8. While prostate cancer often has a relatively indolent course, metastatic disease is not uncommon and carries a high mortality burden. The 5-year survival rate for patients with only local or regionally advanced prostate cancer is close to 100%, while the 5-year survival rate for patients with metastatic disease is only 30% [2].

Thus, it is clinically important to assess the presence and extent of metastasis in patients with prostate cancer. This has a major impact on treatment planning: patients with early-stage disease are eligible for surgical excision and localized radiotherapy, while patients with metastatic disease are generally limited to chemotherapy or androgen-deprivation therapy [3,4].

The assessment of prostate cancer metastasis has traditionally been performed by radionuclide bone scan and CT. However, these imaging methods cannot always accurately detect non-localized disease, resulting in disease recurrence even in patients initially treated with curative intent [5,6]. Meanwhile, magnetic resonance imaging (MRI) has been gaining increased recognition as a useful method of evaluating lymph nodes and distant metastases in patients with various cancers, including prostate cancer [7,8]. Yet, MRI, despite its advances, also still misses clinically relevant metastatic disease.

In recent years, a new imaging method has emerged for primary staging and assessment of metastatic prostate cancer. ^{68}Ga-PSMA-HBED-CC positron emission tomography (PET) imaging uses gallium-radiolabeled prostate-specific membrane antigen (PSMA), a peptide largely specific to prostatic tissue, including prostate cancer [9]. Although the spatial resolution of PET is lower than MRI, with lesions smaller than 6 mm not reliably detected, this is offset by its superior contrast-to-background. The major limitation of PSMA PET is that it requires the administration of novel radiotracers such as ^{68}Ga-PSMA-11. As a result, it is not widely available outside of large, resource-rich medical centers equipped with adequate infrastructure, and this limits its utility. Especially given that there is an order of magnitude more MRI units compared with PET units in the United States, with many states having only two or fewer centers providing this service and with many countries in the "global south" lacking PET altogether, one cannot count on PSMA PET availability despite the FDA having approved more than one formulation [10–12]. In contrast, while MRI is much more widely available, it misses a higher percentage of lesions compared to PSMA PET [13].

There is therefore a valuable opportunity to use PSMA PET as a standard of reference to improve the interpretation of MRI. This project aims to investigate whether the ability of MRI scans to detect metastatic prostate cancer can be enhanced using retrospective information provided by concomitant PSMA PET scans. To our knowledge, such an approach has not yet been taken. Improving the interpretation of MRI will allow more timely and effective diagnosis of metastatic prostate cancer in settings that lack PSMA PET imaging, and it will greatly benefit patients by allowing them to receive earlier treatment.

2. Materials and Methods

This study was a sub-analysis of an IRB-approved, HIPAA-compliant prospectively collected database of 263 patients who provided written informed consent for and participated in a clinical trial of ^{68}Ga-PSMA-HBED-CC PET/MRI comparing separately read PSMA PET and whole-body MRI and multiparametric MRI (mpMRI) of the prostate/prostatic bed from 2018 and 2021 at a single institution. Patients underwent concomitant PSMA PET/MRI for one of two general indications: (1) treatment planning or (2) biochemical recurrence based on serum prostate specific antigen (PSA) levels (defined either as PSA $\geq$ 0.2 ng/mL in radical prostatectomy patients or as 2 ng/mL greater than the nadir PSA in post-radiation therapy patients). Demographics are listed in Table 1. A formal description of the PSMA PET scanning technique has been previously reported, and 30 of the subjects analyzed herein overlap with this prior study, which focused only on subjects with biochemical recurrence [14].

Table 1. Demographics.

Subjects	263 Total	38 Met Criteria
Indications	(analyzed subjects only)	
	BCR, conventional imaging equivocal/suggestive for metastasis	2 (5.2%)
	BCR, conventional imaging negative for metastasis	20 (52.6%)
	High-risk primary cancer for surgical planning	3 (7.9%)
	Radiation/focal therapy planning for primary cancer	4 (10.5%)
	Biopsy planning for primary lesion	1 (2.6%)
	Other indication (not specified)	8 (21.0%)
Age	Average 69 years	range 46–88
Serum PSA	range 0.21–143 ng/mL	
Ethnicity reported	62%	
Hispanic/Latino	3%	
Race reported	50%	
White	91%	
Black/African American	6%	
Asian/Pacific Islander	3%	

In each case, the PSMA PET was read without first reviewing the MRI and vice versa, and the results were recorded. Subjects whose PSMA PET and MRI diagnostic reports showed discrepancies were selected for sub-analysis. Inclusion criteria included all patients whose PSMA PET was positive for metastases in the lymph node(s), bone, and/or other tissues while the corresponding MRI was negative.

Cases were excluded if (1) data were missing for one or both scans; (2) data could not be interpreted for one or both scans; (3) the MRI was found upon review to have correctly identified the lesion in question; or (4) the PSMA PET was a false positive based on biopsy results (with no subjects in this last category). See Figure 1.

Relevant cases were reviewed by the same attending radiologist who originally read the scans. The attending radiologist reviewed both the PSMA PET and MRI images and noted any common or stereotypical features on MRI (e.g., lesion size, location, or morphology) indicating metastatic disease that was initially missed. Six classes of false negative MRI were considered (Table 2).

Table 2. False negative classes.

False Negative Class (Number of Cases, %)	Description
Anatomically normal	This type of false negative occurred exclusively with lymph node metastases. The affected lymph node showed PSMA PET uptake but was anatomically normal in size (<10 mm in short axis for oval/reniform nodes or <8 mm in diameter for spherical nodes) and physiologic in shape on mpMRI.
Atypical MRI appearance	mpMRI appearance was abnormal but not suspicious and was not prospectively described.
Mischaracterization	The lesion was suspicious on mpMRI but was not initially reported.
Undercall	mpMRI appearance was abnormal but was described as "equivocal" or "low suspicion".
Obscured	Relevant area was difficult was to visualize on MRI because of technical or patient factors (e.g., hip replacement).
Negative	There was no focal structure on MRI to correlate with PSMA PET uptake.

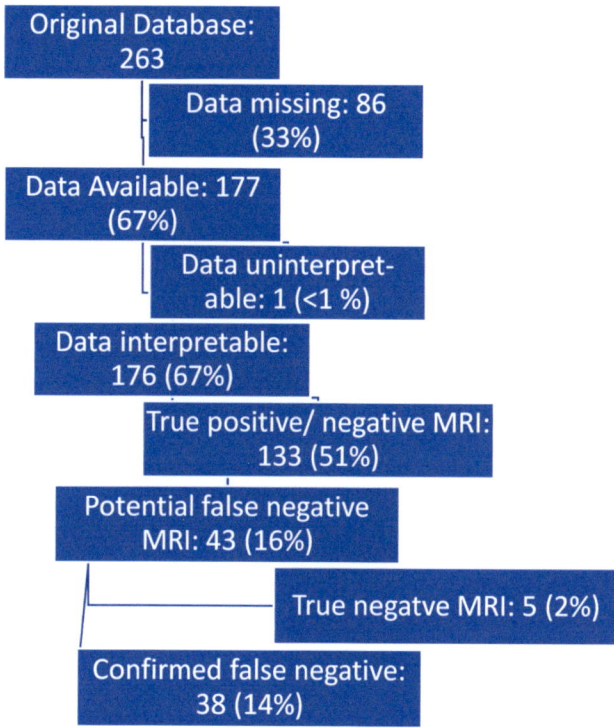

Figure 1. Flow diagram.

3. Results

Of the 263 subjects in the database, we identified 38 (14%) "MRI false negative" subjects that both met inclusion criteria and were not excluded by exclusion criteria. The average age at time of scan was 69 years (range 46–88). The maximum PSA at time of scan was recorded for 33 of 38 patients and ranged from 0.21–143 ng/mL.

The indications for imaging were the following (number of patients, %): conventional imaging equivocal or suggestive of prostate cancer metastatic disease (2, 5.2%); elevated PSA with no conventional imaging suggestive of metastatic or recurrent disease (20, 52.6%); planned for surgical extirpation (high-risk primary disease) (3, 7.9%); planned serial follow-up (i.e., focal therapy) with or without radiation therapy (4, 10.5%); planned for targeted biopsy of primary lesion (1, 2.6%); and other (8, 21.0%).

After the PSMA PET/MRI and mpMRI images were reviewed for each case, the 38 MRI false negative cases were found to fall into six broad classes. The common features associated with each class are outlined below in Table 3 and Figure 2.

Table 3. Breakdown of the six classes of MRI false negative.

False Negative Class (Number of Cases, %)
Anatomically normal (18, 47%)
Atypical MRI appearance (6, 16%)
Mischaracterization (1, 3%)
Undercall (6, 16%)
Obscured (4, 11%)
Negative (3, 8%)

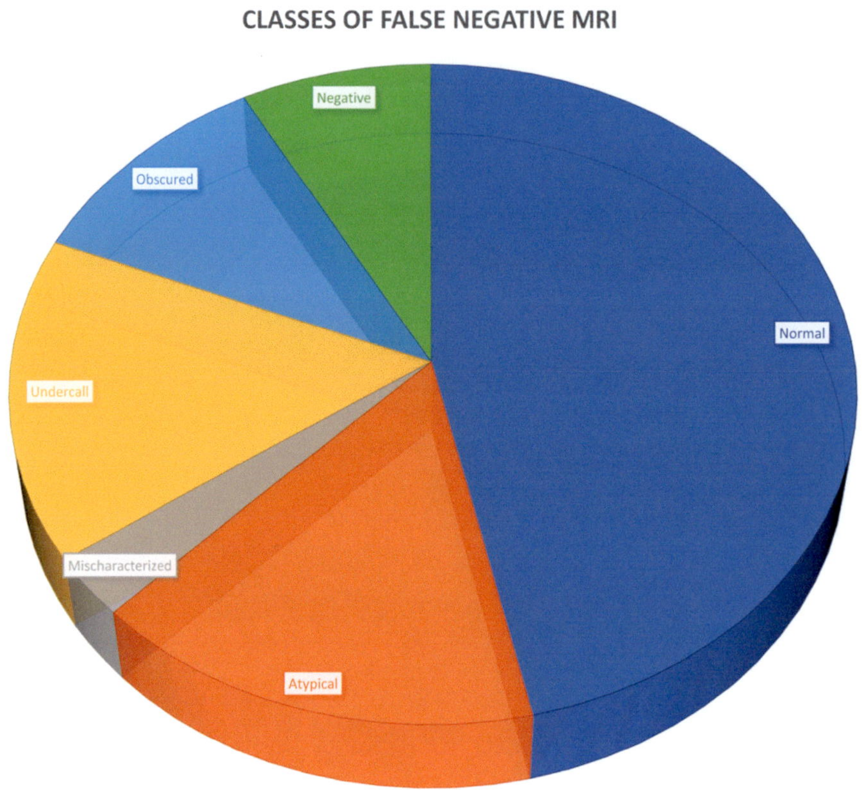

CLASSES OF FALSE NEGATIVE MRI

Figure 2. Six classes of MRI false negatives.

Upon further review, of those cases that were "false negative" on MRI, other sites of disease were found such that the degree of extent (local, regional, or distant) would not change in 4 cases (11%), such that management would not be altered. Additionally, 12 cases (32%) were either atypical or "undercalled", such that a change in reporting could have resulted in these cases being correctly classified. Regardless, the remaining 22 cases (58%) may have had disease not otherwise reported. However, of these cases, half (11, or 29% of 38) would have disease that would not have been included in a traditional pelvic lymph node and prostate bed radiation field. Compared to the entire dataset of 263 subjects, this results in 4% with undiagnosed extrapelvic disease.

3.1. Example 1—Anatomically Normal Lymph Node Metastasis

As seen in Figure 3, the largest class, comprising half of the cases, was anatomically normal. In other words, the size and morphology of the metastatic focus did not suggest an abnormality on MRI. This description applied to many false negative cases involving lymph node metastases. In this case, the initial mpMRI was negative for the lymph node metastases by size criteria, while the PSMA PET showed a PSMA-avid, subcentimeter, left-sided lesion (Figure 3C). Detailed review of the mpMRI confirmed that the lymph node in question measured well under 1.0 cm in short axis, with a similar "cold" contralateral lymph node with essentially the same characteristics (Figure 3A,B). There were no other features in the mpMRI that were suspicious for metastatic disease.

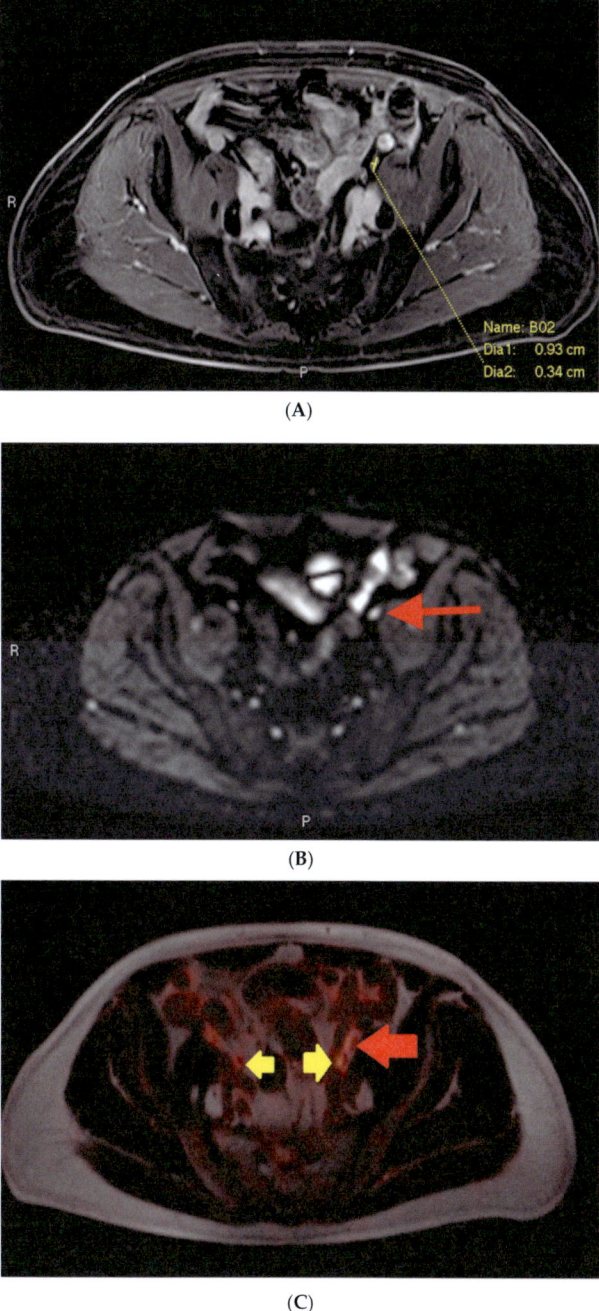

Figure 3. Post-contrast fat-saturated gradient T1-weighted image (**A**), diffusion-weighted imaging with b = 900 s/mm^2 (DWI) (**B**), and fused PET/single-shot T2-weighted imaging (**C**) through the pelvis. In Figure 3A, the lesion is marked with measurement calipers. In Figure 3B,C, the lesion is denoted with a red arrow. Yellow arrows indicate the ureters, which show physiologic PSMA PET uptake.

3.2. Example 2—Mischaracterization of Lymph Node Metastasis

Among the cases included in this analysis, there was only one example of a characterization issue, defined as an instance where a lymph node was suspicious on MRI on the basis of size but was not prospectively included in the report (Figure 4). This case involved a lymph node metastasis. The PSMA PET showed a PSMA-avid node in the left supraclavicular region (Figure 4C). The lymph node measured > 1.0 cm in short axis (Figure 4A). However, it also exhibited a benign morphology with an oval shape and a fatty hilum.

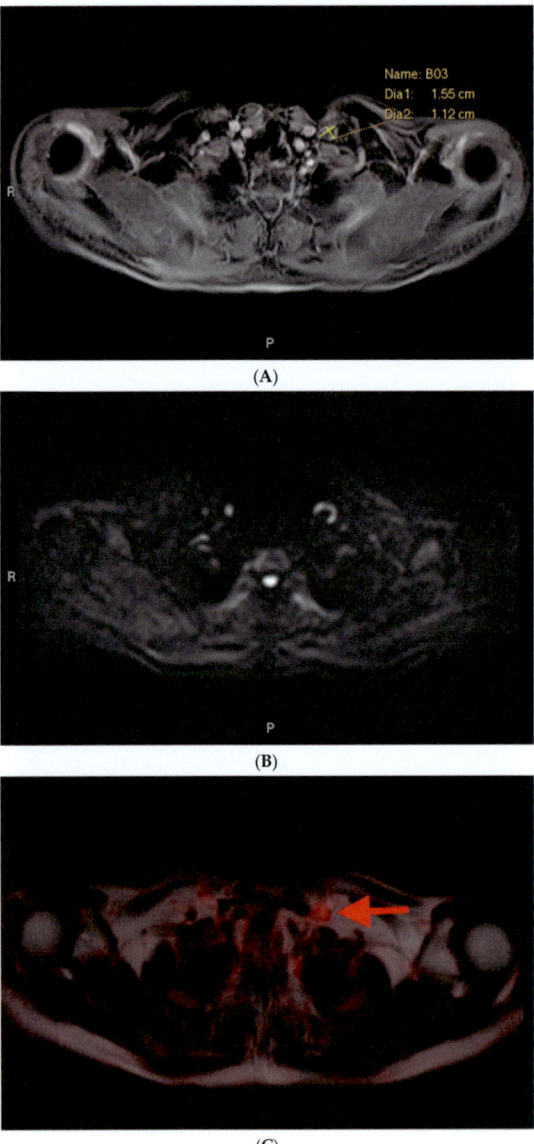

Figure 4. Post-contrast fat-saturated gradient T1 (**A**), DWI (**B**), and fused PET (**C**) images. In Figure 4A, the lesion is retrospectively measured (calipers). In Figure 4C, the lesion is denoted with a red arrow.

In terms of "atypical" and "undercalled" findings, with six of each, there were four "atypical" bone lesions: two rib lesions, one with signal loss but no T2 lengthening or restricted diffusion, and another with high signal on fat-suppressed T1/T2 but low signal on native T1/T2 and possible diffusion-restriction vs. T2 shine-through; one case of sternal subtle T1/T2 lengthening and possibly diffusion restriction also attributed to T2 shine-through; and one case of ischial T2-lengthening with an equivocal defect on T1 but no diffusion restriction. The other two "atypical" cases included asymmetric enhancement without restricted diffusion or a discrete mass in the seminal vesicles after radiation therapy, and thoracic lymph nodes that were slightly distorted from susceptibility artifact. The "undercalled" cases included five cases of lymph nodes that did not meet the size criteria but were either considered equivocal on the basis of round shape or short axis > 5 mm in the pelvic "landing zone" distribution, and one case where not all of the osseous lesions were identified. Obscured lesions included three cases of lymph nodes obscured by susceptibility artifact, either from lungs or metal, and one case where extensive degenerative bony change obscured an underlying focus that was PSMA-avid.

4. Discussion

This study aimed to classify major causes of MRI "misses" of metastatic prostate cancer when compared to PSMA PET, which was used as the standard of reference. In our analysis, the primary reason (47% of cases) why MRI missed metastatic lesions that were radiotracer-avid on PSMA PET/MRI was simply due to the lesions' normal appearance by existing anatomic size criteria. Although MRI has been shown to be comparable in sensitivity and specificity to some forms of traditional PET/CT, such as FDG-PET/CT and F18-choline PET/CT, and it is one of the most common methods of evaluating prostate cancer metastases, MRI interpretation still relies heavily on size as the main criteria for the evaluation of lymph nodes [15,16].

Our results suggest that the current standards for evaluating potentially metastatic prostate cancer lesions, particularly for metastatic lymph nodes, are not ideal. Current practice generally considers oval lymph nodes ≥ 1.0 cm in short axis or round nodes ≥ 0.8 cm in diameter as indicators of metastasis. However, these guidelines are optimized for increased specificity, not sensitivity [17]. As a result, MRI fairly frequently misses small metastases in "normal"-sized lymph nodes [13,18]. In contrast, PSMA PET, because it relies on PSMA expression and not solely on size criteria, shows superior performance in situations where metastatic lesions are more likely to be small. For example, PSMA PET has been demonstrated to have higher sensitivity than MRI in patients with low PSA values [19], as well as in patients with biochemical recurrence following radical prostatectomy [14]. Guberina et al. also found that PSMA PET/MRI was superior in detecting locally recurrent disease when compared to PSMA PET/CT [20].

Given the fact that MRI more easily misses smaller lesions using anatomic criteria alone, there is a need for multiparametric criteria to identify lesions that are functionally or biologically abnormal, instead of using purely size-based methods. One such alternative criteria has been proposed by Conlin et al. [21] Their group suggests using a four-compartment signal model of whole-body diffusion-weighted imaging, which appears to have promising potential to evaluate prostate cancer bone metastases

Additionally, 32% of the false negative cases analyzed were either characterization issues, atypical, or undercalled. In these cases, the lesions in question were initially seen on MRI but not given enough weight, often because they appeared in unexpected contexts. The one mischaracterized lesion, while significant by the size criteria, had a physiologic shape. Moreover, the supraclavicular region is an unusual location for solitary prostate cancer metastasis. These unusual features may have resulted in the initial interpretation of the lymph node as non-metastatic. Since there is some element of human interpretive error involved, improving reader training in terms of gauging suspicion may lead to more accurate results. The potential exists for clinical suspicion to inform the degree to which lesions are deemed suspicious on MRI.

The single case of "mischaracterization", where the single-reader failed to identify a lymph node in an atypical location but where the lymph note was clearly suspicious based on the size criteria, falls within normal radiology performance given the 263 prospectively enrolled subjects. The veracity of this finding could be reinforced by having a dual-reader or repeat single-reader analysis for inter-rater versus intra-rater assessment, respectively, but this was not part of the experimental design.

Ultimately, it is crucial to improve MRI interpretation because PSMA PET, though undoubtedly more powerful and superior to traditional methods, is currently limited by availability to high-resource regions [10–12]. PSMA imaging requires the use of radiotracers, which must be produced through a relatively laborious manufacturing process and which have relatively short half-lives [22–25]. Improving the interpretation of mpMRI has significant potential to positively impact the diagnosis and treatment of metastatic prostate cancer for many patients in developing and sparsely populated regions.

Future avenues of investigation include a deeper review of pulse sequence-specific features (e.g., diffusion restriction) to determine whether subtle pulse-specific abnormalities that indicate metastatic disease are present on the MRI. If present, such features may reveal new abnormalities in "normal" cases to help with diagnosis. Additionally, such features could be a valuable resource to improve reader training for atypical and potentially undercalled cases.

This study was limited by a fairly small sample size; out of 263 PSMA PET/MRI scans, only 38 cases (14%) had a false negative MRI result compared to PSMA. In addition, the cases consisted of patients with diverse clinical circumstances—some planning for initial therapy, others who had already received surgical and/or radiation therapy. This somewhat heterogenous sample size may also complicate retrospective MRI interpretation and could introduce bias in terms of analysis from a skewed population. Additionally, some of these cases (e.g., planning for focal therapy) might not normally entail whole-body MRI were it not for their participation in the prospective clinical trial. Whole-body MRI remains a relatively uncommon procedure, and while it holds the potential to be more widespread than PET scanning, issues including costs, time requirements, and expertise limit its value. Lastly, there is a possibility that some cases were "PSMA false positive" as pathologic confirmation was only available for a minority of cases.

5. Conclusions

In conclusion, it is rare that MRI will miss metastatic disease caught by PSMA PET, and rarer still that, if one does not consider atypical and equivocal cases falsely negative, only 4% of this cohort would have disease missed by conventional treatment planning. Regardless, improving multiparametric characterization of small lymph nodes holds the greatest promise to compensate for this, the most common class of false negative MRI.

Author Contributions: The authors claim sole responsibility as authors of this work. Data were analyzed by J.W., E.O., A.R. and D.J.A.M.; conceptualization, D.J.A.M.; methodology, D.J.A.M. and A.R.; validation, A.R.; formal analysis, J.W., D.J.A.M. and A.R.; investigation, all authors; resources, J.B. and J.R.O.; data curation, D.J.A.M.; writing—original draft preparation, J.W.; writing—review and editing, J.W., E.O. and D.J.A.M.; visualization, D.J.A.M.; supervision, D.J.A.M.; project administration, D.J.A.M.; funding acquisition, J.B. and J.R.O. All authors have read and agreed to the published version of the manuscript.

Funding: This research received no external funding.

Institutional Review Board Statement: The study was conducted in accordance with the Declaration of Helsinki and approved by the Institutional Review Board of Weill Cornell Medical College (protocol code 1706018301 approved 22 February 2019).

Informed Consent Statement: Informed consent was obtained from all subjects involved in the study.

Data Availability Statement: Data are not available for external review per institutional subject protection requirements.

Conflicts of Interest: John Babich is Founder, President and Chief Scientific Officer, Ratio Therapeutics, Inc. Daniel J. A. Margolis has received an ad hoc consulting consideration from Guerbet and Promaxo. None of these companies was involved in the funding or analysis of the data herein. The Corresponding Author assumes ultimate responsibility for the content.

References

1. Siegel, R.L.; Miller, K.D.; Fuchs, H.E.; Jemal, A. Cancer Statistics, 2021. *CA Cancer J. Clin.* **2021**, *71*, 7–33. [CrossRef] [PubMed]
2. American Society of Clinical Oncology Prostate Cancer Statistics. Available online: https://www.cancer.net/cancer-types/prostate-cancer/statistics (accessed on 25 September 2021).
3. Zerbib, M.; Zelefsky, M.J.; Higano, C.S.; Carroll, P.R. Conventional treatments of localized prostate cancer. *Urology* **2008**, *72*, S25–S35. [CrossRef]
4. Berry, W.R. The evolving role of chemotherapy in androgen-independent (hormone-refractory) prostate cancer. *Urology* **2005**, *65*, 2–7. [CrossRef]
5. Zumsteg, Z.S.; Spratt, D.E.; Romesser, P.B.; Pei, X.; Zhang, Z.; Polkinghorn, W.; McBride, S.; Kollmeier, M.; Yamada, Y.; Zelefsky, M.J. The natural history and predictors of outcome following biochemical relapse in the dose escalation era for prostate cancer patients undergoing definitive external beam radiotherapy. *Eur. Urol.* **2015**, *67*, 1009–1016. [CrossRef] [PubMed]
6. Eggener, S.E.; Scardino, P.T.; Walsh, P.C.; Han, M.; Partin, A.W.; Trock, B.J.; Feng, Z.; Wood, D.P.; Eastham, J.A.; Yossepowitch, O.; et al. Predicting 15-year prostate cancer specific mortality after radical prostatectomy. *J. Urol.* **2011**, *185*, 869–875. [CrossRef] [PubMed]
7. Machado Medeiros, T.; Altmayer, S.; Watte, G.; Zanon, M.; Basso Dias, A.; Henz Concatto, N.; Hoefel Paes, J.; Mattiello, R.; de Souza Santos, F.; Mohammed, T.-L.; et al. ^{18}F-FDG PET/CT and whole-body MRI diagnostic performance in M staging for non-small cell lung cancer: A systematic review and meta-analysis. *Eur. Radiol.* **2020**, *30*, 3641–3649. [CrossRef]
8. Zhan, Y.; Zhang, G.; Li, M.; Zhou, X. Whole-Body MRI vs. PET/CT for the Detection of Bone Metastases in Patients with Prostate Cancer: A Systematic Review and Meta-Analysis. *Front. Oncol.* **2021**, *11*, 633833. [CrossRef]
9. Maurer, T.; Eiber, M.; Schwaiger, M.; Gschwend, J.E. Current use of PSMA-PET in prostate cancer management. *Nat. Rev. Urol.* **2016**, *13*, 226–235. [CrossRef]
10. World Health Organisation Medical Devices. Available online: https://www.who.int/data/gho/data/themes/topics/topic-details/GHO/medical-devices (accessed on 20 May 2024).
11. Gallach, M.; Mikhail Lette, M.; Abdel-Wahab, M.; Giammarile, F.; Pellet, O.; Paez, D. Addressing Global Inequities in Positron Emission Tomography-Computed Tomography (PET-CT) for Cancer Management: A Statistical Model to Guide Strategic Planning. *Med. Sci. Monit.* **2020**, *26*, e926544. [CrossRef]
12. Subramanian, K.; Martinez, J.; Huicochea Castellanos, S.; Ivanidze, J.; Nagar, H.; Nicholson, S.; Youn, T.; Nauseef, J.T.; Tagawa, S.; Osborne, J.R. Complex implementation factors demonstrated when evaluating cost-effectiveness and monitoring racial disparities associated with [^{18}F]DCFPyL PET/CT in prostate cancer men. *Sci. Rep.* **2023**, *13*, 8321. [CrossRef]
13. Davis, G.L. Sensitivity of frozen section examination of pelvic lymph nodes for metastatic prostate carcinoma. *Cancer* **1995**, *76*, 661–668. [CrossRef] [PubMed]
14. Martinez, J.; Subramanian, K.; Margolis, D.; O'Dwyer, E.; Osborne, J.; Jhanwar, Y.; Nagar, H.; Williams, N.; RoyChoudhury, A.; Madera, G.; et al. ^{68}Ga-PSMA-HBED-CC PET/MRI is superior to multiparametric magnetic resonance imaging in men with biochemical recurrent prostate cancer: A prospective single-institutional study. *Transl. Oncol.* **2022**, *15*, 101242. [CrossRef] [PubMed]
15. Basso Dias, A.; Zanon, M.; Altmayer, S.; Sartori Pacini, G.; Henz Concatto, N.; Watte, G.; Garcez, A.; Mohammed, T.-L.; Verma, N.; Medeiros, T.; et al. Fluorine 18-FDG PET/CT and Diffusion-weighted MRI for Malignant versus Benign Pulmonary Lesions: A Meta-Analysis. *Radiology* **2019**, *290*, 525–534. [CrossRef] [PubMed]
16. Johnston, E.W.; Latifoltojar, A.; Sidhu, H.S.; Ramachandran, N.; Sokolska, M.; Bainbridge, A.; Moore, C.; Ahmed, H.U.; Punwani, S. Multiparametric whole-body 3.0-T MRI in newly diagnosed intermediate- and high-risk prostate cancer: Diagnostic accuracy and interobserver agreement for nodal and metastatic staging. *Eur. Radiol.* **2019**, *29*, 3159–3169. [CrossRef] [PubMed]
17. Zarzour, J.G.; Galgano, S.; McConathy, J.; Thomas, J.V.; Rais-Bahrami, S. Lymph node imaging in initial staging of prostate cancer: An overview and update. *World J. Radiol.* **2017**, *9*, 389–399. [CrossRef] [PubMed]
18. Jager, G.J.; Barentsz, J.O.; Oosterhof, G.O.; Witjes, J.A.; Ruijs, S.J. Pelvic adenopathy in prostatic and urinary bladder carcinoma: MR imaging with a three-dimensional TI-weighted magnetization-prepared-rapid gradient-echo sequence. *AJR Am. J. Roentgenol.* **1996**, *167*, 1503–1507. [CrossRef] [PubMed]
19. Kranzbühler, B.; Müller, J.; Becker, A.S.; Garcia Schüler, H.I.; Muehlematter, U.; Fankhauser, C.D.; Kedzia, S.; Guckenberger, M.; Kaufmann, P.A.; Eberli, D.; et al. Detection Rate and Localization of Prostate Cancer Recurrence Using ^{68}Ga-PSMA-11 PET/MRI in Patients with Low PSA Values ≤ 0.5 ng/mL. *J. Nucl. Med.* **2020**, *61*, 194–201. [CrossRef] [PubMed]
20. Guberina, N.; Hetkamp, P.; Ruebben, H.; Fendler, W.; Grueneisen, J.; Suntharalingam, S.; Kirchner, J.; Puellen, L.; Harke, N.; Radtke, J.P.; et al. Whole-Body Integrated [^{68}Ga]PSMA-11-PET/MR Imaging in Patients with Recurrent Prostate Cancer: Comparison with Whole-Body PET/CT as the Standard of Reference. *Mol. Imaging Biol.* **2020**, *22*, 788–796. [CrossRef] [PubMed]

21. Conlin, C.C.; Feng, C.H.; Digma, L.A.; Rodriguez-Soto, A.E.; Kuperman, J.M.; Holland, D.; Rakow-Penner, R.; Karow, D.S.; White, N.S.; Seibert, T.M.; et al. A Multicompartmental Diffusion Model for Improved Assessment of Whole-bodyDiffusion-weighted Imaging Data and Evaluation of Prostate Cancer Bone Metastases. *Radiol. Imaging Cancer* **2023**, *5*, e210115. [CrossRef]
22. Hofman, M.S.; Lawrentschuk, N.; Francis, R.J.; Tang, C.; Vela, I.; Thomas, P.; Rutherford, N.; Martin, J.M.; Frydenberg, M.; Shakher, R.; et al. proPSMA Study Group Collaborators Prostate-specific membrane antigen PET-CT in patients with high-risk prostate cancer before curative-intent surgery or radiotherapy (proPSMA): A prospective, randomised, multicentre study. *Lancet* **2020**, *395*, 1208–1216. [CrossRef]
23. Van Kalmthout, L.W.M.; van Melick, H.H.E.; Lavalaye, J.; Meijer, R.P.; Kooistra, A.; de Klerk, J.M.H.; Braat, A.J.A.T.; Kaldeway, H.P.; de Bruin, P.C.; de Keizer, B.; et al. Prospective Validation of Gallium-68 Prostate Specific Membrane Antigen-Positron Emission Tomography/Computerized Tomography for Primary Staging of Prostate Cancer. *J. Urol.* **2020**, *203*, 537–545. [CrossRef] [PubMed]
24. Yaxley, J.W.; Raveenthiran, S.; Nouhaud, F.-X.; Samartunga, H.; Yaxley, A.J.; Coughlin, G.; Delahunt, B.; Egevad, L.; McEwan, L.; Wong, D. Outcomes of Primary Lymph Node Staging of Intermediate and High Risk Prostate Cancer with 68Ga-PSMA Positron Emission Tomography/Computerized Tomography Compared to Histological Correlation of Pelvic Lymph Node Pathology. *Urol.* **2019**, *201*, 815–820. [CrossRef] [PubMed]
25. Martiniova, L.; Palatis, L.D.; Etchebehere, E.; Ravizzini, G. Gallium-68 in Medical Imaging. *Curr. Radiopharm.* **2016**, *9*, 187–2. [CrossRef] [PubMed]

Disclaimer/Publisher's Note: The statements, opinions and data contained in all publications are solely those of the individual author(s) and contributor(s) and not of MDPI and/or the editor(s). MDPI and/or the editor(s) disclaim responsibility for any injury to people or property resulting from any ideas, methods, instructions or products referred to in the content.

MDPI AG
Grosspeteranlage 5
4052 Basel
Switzerland
Tel.: +41 61 683 77 34

Cancers Editorial Office
E-mail: cancers@mdpi.com
www.mdpi.com/journal/cancers

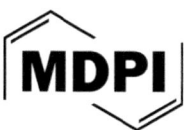

Disclaimer/Publisher's Note: The title and front matter of this reprint are at the discretion of the Guest Editors. The publisher is not responsible for their content or any associated concerns. The statements, opinions and data contained in all individual articles are solely those of the individual Editors and contributors and not of MDPI. MDPI disclaims responsibility for any injury to people or property resulting from any ideas, methods, instructions or products referred to in the content.

Printed by Libri Plureos GmbH in Hamburg, Germany